"This Terrible Struggle for Life"

"This Terrible Struggle for Life"

The Civil War Letters of a Union Regimental Surgeon

THOMAS S. HAWLEY, M.D.
Edited by DENNIS W. BELCHER

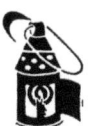

McFarland & Company, Inc., Publishers
Jefferson, North Carolina, and London

All letters unless otherwise noted used by permission of the Missouri History Museum, St. Louis.

The letters dated February 20, 1863, January 23, 1864, March 14, 1864, and December 22, 1865, are used by permission from the David M. Rubenstein Rare Book and Manuscript Library, Duke University, Durham, North Carolina.

The letters dated June 17, 1862, January 29, 1864, and February 3, 1865, are used by permission from Kathryn Breuer.

LIBRARY OF CONGRESS CATALOGUING-IN-PUBLICATION DATA

Hawley, Thomas S., 1837–1918.
"This terrible struggle for life" : the Civil War letters of a Union regimental surgeon / Thomas S. Hawley, M.D. ; edited by Dennis W. Belcher.
      p.   cm.
Includes bibliographical references and index.

ISBN 978-0-7864-6658-0
softcover : acid free paper ∞

1. Hawley, Thomas S., 1837–1918—Correspondence. 2. Surgeons—United States—Correspondence. 3. United States—History—Civil War, 1861–1865—Medical care. 4. Missouri—History—Civil War, 1861–1865—Personal narratives. 5. United States—History—Civil War, 1861–1865—Personal narratives. 6. Southwest, Old—History—Civil War, 1861–1865—Campaigns. 7. United States—History—Civil War, 1861–1865—Campaigns. 8. Missouri—History—Civil War, 1861–1865—Regimental histories. 9. United States—History—Civil War, 1861–1865—Regimental histories. I. Title.
E621.H37 2012
973.7'75—dc23   2012035681

BRITISH LIBRARY CATALOGUING DATA ARE AVAILABLE

© 2012 Dennis W. Belcher. All rights reserved

No part of this book may be reproduced or transmitted in any form or by any means, electronic or mechanical, including photocopying or recording, or by any information storage and retrieval system, without permission in writing from the publisher.

Front cover images: *from left* Thomas S. Hawley, 1873; letter written by Hawley on October 8, 1865 (both Missouri History Museum. St. Louis); circa 1860-1870 surgical kit by Tiemann (courtesy Jack W. Melton, Jr., photographer); background © 2012 Shutterstock

Manufactured in the United States of America

McFarland & Company, Inc., Publishers
  Box 611, Jefferson, North Carolina 28640
    www.mcfarlandpub.com

To Margaret

Acknowledgments

For 150 years the Thomas Hawley Civil War letters have been preserved and for the decisions made by various individuals over the years to care for these letters, I am very grateful. I offer my sincere appreciation to Molly Kodner and the Missouri History Museum Library and Research Center in St. Louis for their diligent efforts in preserving these letters and for their willingness to share them with the public. In addition, I am very grateful to Kathryn Breuer for the inclusion of three letters used in this collection. In addition, Ms. Breuer donated one additional Civil War letter and other materials to the Missouri Historical Society, including, four photographs. The descendants of Thomas Hawley have been of great assistance in completing this book. I want to offer my sincere thanks to Kathryn Breuer, Katherine McDuffee, Joan Garvin, and Georgina Joy Monahan for their unselfish contributions to this book. Thomas Hawley would be proud to have such fine relatives.

Due to the cursive style of writing, it was an effort to transcribe the letters, and I am very grateful to William Stolz, assistant director of reference at the Western Historical Manuscript Collection at the University of Missouri, for his invaluable assistance in transcribing the letters. He provided invaluable assistance in interpreting the difficult sections of the Hawley letters. I also express my appreciation to Mitch Fraas, reference librarian at Duke University, for his assistance with providing the information of the Hawley Collection at Duke.

I also want to acknowledge and express my gratitude to George Skoch, who is a recognized expert in Civil War era maps. George's expertise in map production is amazing, and he does an outstanding job. I cannot thank him enough for his efforts in the production of this work.

Table of Contents

Acknowledgments
vi
Preface
1
Introduction
5

One. 1861: Belleville, St. Louis, Rolla and Cape Girardeau
11

Two. 1862: Cape Girardeau, Corinth, Columbus and Holly Springs
52

Three. 1863: LaGrange, Vicksburg and Memphis
75

Four. 1864: LaGrange, Tupelo, Oxford, Missouri and Nashville
166

Five. 1865: Spanish Fort, Occupation of Alabama and Postwar Life
221

Chapter Notes
245
Bibliography
248
Index
251

Preface

The letters contained in this manuscript are from three sources. A total of ninety-seven Civil War letters have been preserved by the Missouri History Museum. The Hawley Collection of letters at the Missouri Historical Society includes additional letters not included in this book — 23 letters ranging from September 1856 to April 1861 and another 41 letters after March 1866. Another four wartime letters written by Thomas Hawley (January 20, 1863, January 23, 1864, March 14, 1864, December 22, 1865) are located at the Hawley Collection at Duke University. In addition, three letters are held by a descendent of Doctor Thomas Hawley, Ms. Kathryn Breuer. This work was designed to reflect the history of a tumultuous period in United States history from the eyes of a physician who participated in the western theater of the Civil War.

In August 1865, Doctor Thomas Swearingen Hawley prophetically wrote his thoughts about the two hundred letters he had composed in the war: "I suppose if all these ever collected, written during my five years of absence, rather think I would hardly follow all of them. Some breathing cheerfulness, hope and warm with love. Others full of strong desire and firm determination. Many almost with repetitions of former letters, some dull and are barely readable. Yet they have all been under peculiar circumstances. We are all creatures of circumstances. So of course these notes, by the way, must partake somewhat of the surroundings.

"If I have ever said anything wrong or calculated to wound any one's feelings, I chance pardon. If I have been amiss in duty, it was not through want of desire to do it, but because the body was weak or weary. I have always tried to comply with my promises and perform my duties near as possible. Often weak, weary and sick at heart. These 4 years of terrible war have been trying ones to me. Yet thank the Lord, his grace has always been sufficient for me. His shield has ever been over me in the hours of danger. How much I am indebted to the prayers of the righteous ones at home I can never tell."[1]

There is probably no better description of the author of the letters contained in this book than Hawley's own words. These letters chronicle the life and events over four and half years of service to his country. When Thomas Hawley joined the Union Army in the summer of 1861, he was a newly graduated physician and he struggled to find his place in a Union regiment. He was an ardent supporter of the Union cause and he was an excellent physician. During the war, he encountered poor officers and excellent officers and men who tried to take advantage of him and the best of friends. He served in the First Missouri Rifle Battalion in remote Rolla, Missouri, before that regiment became the 11th Missouri Infantry. He served as hospital steward and transferred to 111th Illinois Infantry for a short time before he transferred to hospital duty at Holly Springs, Mississippi, where he was captured during the raid commanded by Major General Earl Van Dorn in December 1863. Next, he commanded his own hospital near Memphis, and he was later part of the surgical support team during the Vicksburg campaign. He returned to the 11th Missouri Infantry in the summer of 1863 and was instrumental in medically salvaging the regiment which had suffered so greatly in the campaign. He finally was promoted to the rank of major and became the regimental surgeon of the 11th Missouri Veteran Volunteer Infantry. He campaigned with the regiment during the Battle of Tupelo, the Oxford, Mississippi Expedition, including the skirmishes at Abbeyville and Hurricane Creek. Next he marched with the regiment to DuValls Bluff, Arkansas, and joined in the pursuit of Major General Sterling Price during his famous Missouri raid in the summer and fall of 1864. He provided medical support to the regiment after they stormed into the Confederate line at the Battle of Nashville. The Confederate line was broken and the Union won the battle but the regiment of 325 men lost 90 men accomplishing this task. Hawley was on the field with these men and lost many friends that day. He concluded his war efforts by campaigning with the regiment in the siege of Spanish Fort in March and April 1865. Finally, his term of service carried him to central Alabama where the Union Army occupied and established order in the state after the war.

The transcription of the letters of Doctor Thomas Hawley was somewhat challenging due to the age of the letters and the cursive style of writing common to original Civil War records. The handwriting of physicians is poor in many cases but for the most part the letters by Thomas Hawley were written well considering many of these were composed in adverse situations. It should be noted a few peculiarities of the Hawley letters, including, the use of the word *you ens* which means "you" or "you all." It should also be noted the use of the abbreviations "inst." or instant and "ult." or ultimo. The inst. abbreviation refers to the current month. For example, a letter written on November 15 states, "I received your letter of the 5th inst.," indicates the author received a letter dated on November 5 of the current month. Likewise, the use of ult. or ultimo refers to a letter written the previous month. Otherwise, many of Thomas Hawley's letters can easily be read today as they could when they were written. One of the challenges in working with these letters was the habit of writing without punctuation or paragraphs. Often, a single page of the letter was written as a single sentence, and there was a need to include commas, paragraphs, question marks and periods. Punctuation was added to make the reading easier and efforts were made to ensure the intent of the Thomas Hawley text was not altered. There are certain cases where words are missing or clarification is needed and the added words are designated within brackets "[ ]."

Despite the events in the western theater of the Civil War, the real story of Thomas S. Hawley is his love and affection for his family — his mother, minister father, younger brother, and three younger sisters. Thomas Hawley was a good, ethical, moral individual involved in a bloody and dangerous war. He was called to perform operations that cause nightmares to imagine, but he never changed in his belief in God and the value of family. He never lost faith he was doing the right thing by participating in the war, despite the cost to himself and his family. This collection of letters not only details his four and a half year career in the army through firsthand accounts of the various campaigns and his various duties, he also chronicled his interactions with captured Confederate soldiers, interactions with pro–Southern and pro–Northern civilians in areas occupied by the Union army, his experiences with freed slaves and numerous other daily events in the great American Civil War. Thomas Hawley was a common man and his letters allow readers to view the war from his eyes. Finally, these letters offer a rare look at the Civil War from the eyes of a physician who supported a fighting regiment.

Introduction

Like the other Border States, Missouri struggled with its allegiance to the Confederacy or the Union as national divisions tore the country apart in 1860 and 1861. Although many issues precipitated the Civil War, none was more hotly contested than slavery, and Missouri was born under the cloud of slavery. The Missouri Compromise of 1820 allowed Missouri to enter the Union as a slaveholding state and prohibited slavery in any state north of the latitude of 36 degrees and 30 minutes. The Missouri Compromise avoided confronting the legal and moral consequences of slavery, although extremists on either side of the slavery issue were not happy with the outcome. Anti-slavery proponents were not pleased about the numerous men, women and children of color who were still slaves in the south. Pro-slavery supporters felt the compromise limited their constitutional right to own slaves.

The Missouri Compromise of 1820 held the country together for thirty years but in 1850 the slavery issue again exploded and another compromise was forged between anti-slavery and pro-slavery advocates. The 1850 compromise was reached in an attempt to keep the Union from splitting because of this issue. After the U.S.–Mexican War, the United States again gained new territory and the issue of whether slavery was going to be allowed in this new territory, had to be determined. The Compromise of 1850 and the Fugitive Slave Act temporarily pieced together an agreement which allowed California to enter the Union as a free state, abolished slavery in the District of Columbia, and appeased pro-slavery supporters with the Fugitive Slave Act.

By 1853 another crisis loomed as Kansas and Nebraska were opened for settlement, and in 1854, the Kansas-Nebraska Act was passed, which allowed each territory to decide through self-determination whether to allow slavery within its borders. This act directly impacted the state of Missouri because Kansas shared the western border of Missouri. Nebraska was considered a non-slave territory but many Missourians tried to influence the decisions about slavery in Kansas. Violence erupted and "Bleeding Kansas" fought for self-determination. It wasn't until 1861 that Kansas was made a non-slave holding state, but not before many more people were polarized on the issue of slavery.

Missouri in 1861

Abraham Lincoln was not the popular choice for president by the citizens of Missouri in the 1860 election. In fact, Lincoln only carried St. Louis and Gasconade County in the election. Lincoln finished in a weak fourth position in the election in Missouri, and because Lincoln lost so decidedly, many in the state questioned the direction the country was heading. Missouri was a slaveholding state but was increasingly becoming a state not tied to the values of many of the states of the Deep South. Missouri was a divided state on the issue of secession, and blood had already been shed with citizens of state being involved in Kansas for several years regarding the slavery issues in that state. Missouri's fourteenth governor, Claiborne Fox Jackson, had been elected from the Democratic Party in 1860, and he wanted Missouri to align with slave holding southern states. Jackson made clear his intentions when he placed the "current crisis squarely as the feet of Northern abolitionists who threatened millions of dollars of Southern slave property."[1] He felt the Southern states were not being represented by the increasingly industrialized North and he felt the Union had already been abandoned.

Governor Claiborne Jackson, Lieutenant Governor Thomas Reynolds, and others began "shaping political affairs so as to take the State out of the Union."[2] Most of the legislature opposed session, particularly representatives from St. Louis. The opposition from St. Louis could not be overstated because of its large population and strong commercial value. St. Louis also housed the United Stated military arsenal which contained a large number of muskets, powder, and other military supplies. St. Louis's mayor, Oliver Filley, and congressman, Frank Blair, were "Free-Soilers" and Blair was a personal friend of newly elected President Abraham Lincoln. Governor Jackson knew that if St. Louis was to be drawn to support secession, actions would have to be taken to accomplish this task. Not only was St. Louis pro–Union, most of the state was also. Despite the number of slaves held in the state, not all areas in Missouri aligned with the Union cause. Missouri, though not a large plantation state, did have many residents who had previously lived in Kentucky, Virginia and North Carolina. There was even an area of the state called "Little Dixie" because of the large number of people who had moved westward from other slave holding states. When Fort Sumter was shelled, the citizens of Missouri, while leaning toward preservation of the Union and compromise, were forced to decide where their allegiance would lie. After Fort Sumter, Abraham Lincoln called for 75,000 three-month volunteers, and Missouri was asked to furnish 4,000 of these men, but Governor Jackson flatly refused to provide them.

Both pro–Union and pro–Southern paramilitary organizations had been assembled prior to the Fort Sumter incident, particularly in the St. Louis area, where pro–Southern Minute Men and pro–Northern Home Guards were being trained in response to the deteriorating state and national situation. Governor Jackson's refusal to furnish the 4,000 recruits requested by Lincoln offered an opportunity for the pro–Union Home Guards to be mustered into service. The commander of the Union military forces in St. Louis was Captain Nathaniel Lyon, a hard line, pro–Union military officer whose experience in Kansas during the time when Missourians attempted to force Kansas to become a slave-holding state hardened his resolve against the South.

As Lyon mustered the Home Guards into service, the importance of protecting and controlling the St. Louis arsenal was clear. Lyon sent the military supplies that were not essential for the operation of the arsenal to Illinois. Lyon was also given authority to enlist 10,000 men to protect St. Louis and other parts of Missouri. The best laid plans of Governor Jackson seemed to be slipping away, but he began a plan to muster the state militia to better protect the rest of the state and counter Lyon's increased number of pro–Union troops being recruited. In addition, Jackson was "confident that Missouri would furnish 100,000 to the Southern cause."[3]

Doctor Thomas Hawley

It was amid this turmoil in Missouri the twenty-four-year-old, Doctor Thomas Swearingen Hawley found himself. Thomas S. Hawley was born on February 20, 1837, in Dayton, Ohio. He was the son of a Methodist-Episcopal minister and medical doctor, Nelson Hawley, and his mother was Elizabeth Swearingen Hawley. The Rev. Nelson Hawley was an itinerant minister and had connections in Robinson, Salem, and Olney, Illinois. Thomas Hawley had three sisters: Eva Bell (born 1856), Helen Francis (born 1848), and Maria Denning (born 1842). A fourth sister, Theodocia Goodale, was born in 1844, but she died in 1846 when a tree fell on her. Thomas also had a younger brother, Amos Augustus, who was born in 1840.[4]

After graduating from the St. Louis Medical College in 1861, Doctor Thomas Hawley began a four and a half year military career as a medical professional with the Union Army beginning with the First Missouri Rifle Battalion, then the 11th Missouri Infantry, next the 111th Illinois Infantry, and

Letter written by Thomas Hawley on February 9, 1862 (Missouri History Museum, St. Louis, Missouri).

Letter written by Thomas Hawley on October 8, 1865 (Missouri History Museum, St. Louis, Missouri).

finally he returned to the 11th Missouri Infantry for remainder of the Civil War. He began his military service as a hospital steward. Then he advanced to become an assistant surgeon and finally became a regimental surgeon. Over this career in the Union Army he worked in regimental hospitals and also divisional hospitals caring for the wounded and sick soldiers.

Approximately one hundred letters from Thomas Hawley written to his family from May 1861 through January 1866, when the 11th Missouri Infantry was mustered out of service, have been preserved. The letters reflected the organizational efforts of regiments early in the war, including, camp life at Rolla and Camp Girardeau, Missouri. There are only a few letters preserved for 1862. The letters in 1863 present an excellent overview of the Vicksburg Campaign from a hospital surgeon's perspective. In 1864, Doctor Hawley's letters highlighted the Battle of Tupelo, the Oxford Expedition and finally, the Battle of Nashville. In 1865, the regiment was involved in the siege of Spanish Fort and later occupied Alabama after the war. Only seven letters have survived which were written in 1865. Doctor Hawley was part of the 11th Missouri Infantry for most of the war, and this regiment was designated as one of the top fighting regiments of the Civil War.

Thomas Hawley was a prodigious letter writer, and it unclear how many letters he wrote during the Civil War, but in one of his letters he indicated he had written over 200 letters.[5] Obviously some have been lost, and others are in too poor condition to read. He promised to write his family every Sunday and he was fairly regular in the effort. His nicknames for his sisters were: "Fannie" for sister Helen Francis, "Myra" for sister Maria, and "Evie" for sister Eva Belle.

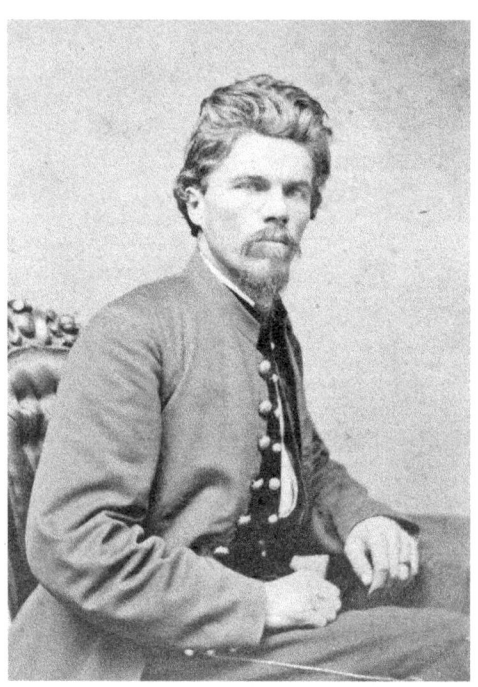

Thomas S. Hawley, M.D., ca. 1860s (courtesy Joan Garvin).

ONE

1861

Belleville, St. Louis, Rolla and Cape Girardeau

When Thomas Hawley made his decision to be part of the Union Army in 1861, he was a recent graduate from medical college and had not yet established a medical practice. He began his efforts to join the Union Army by trying to join the Eighth Missouri Infantry but he was unsuccessful. In 1861, many regiments were being formed and regiments had positions for four to five medical professionals. Therefore, medical positions were highly coveted and difficult to secure; and in mid–May 1861, Thomas was writing his family from Belleville, Illinois, regarding his efforts to find a position with a regiment.

St. Louis was the center of many factions in May 1861 and Union and pro–Southern factions both tried to influence Missouri's allegiance. Thomas Hawley went to Belleville, Illinois, a few miles east of St. Louis and met the soldiers organizing the 22nd Illinois Infantry whose colonel was Henry Doughtery and also the Seventh Illinois Infantry where Dr. James Hamilton served as surgeon. While attempting to enter military service, Thomas Hawley visited with his friends who were joining various regiments.

1861
Belleville [Illinois] Weds.
May 21

Dear Parents,

We arrived here safe Monday about night, went immediately to camp at fairgrounds, took lunch with the boys then Capt. Jackson let us out. Went to Priunns, saw the family, had a good time. I saw H. Roman Wed. morning. He is

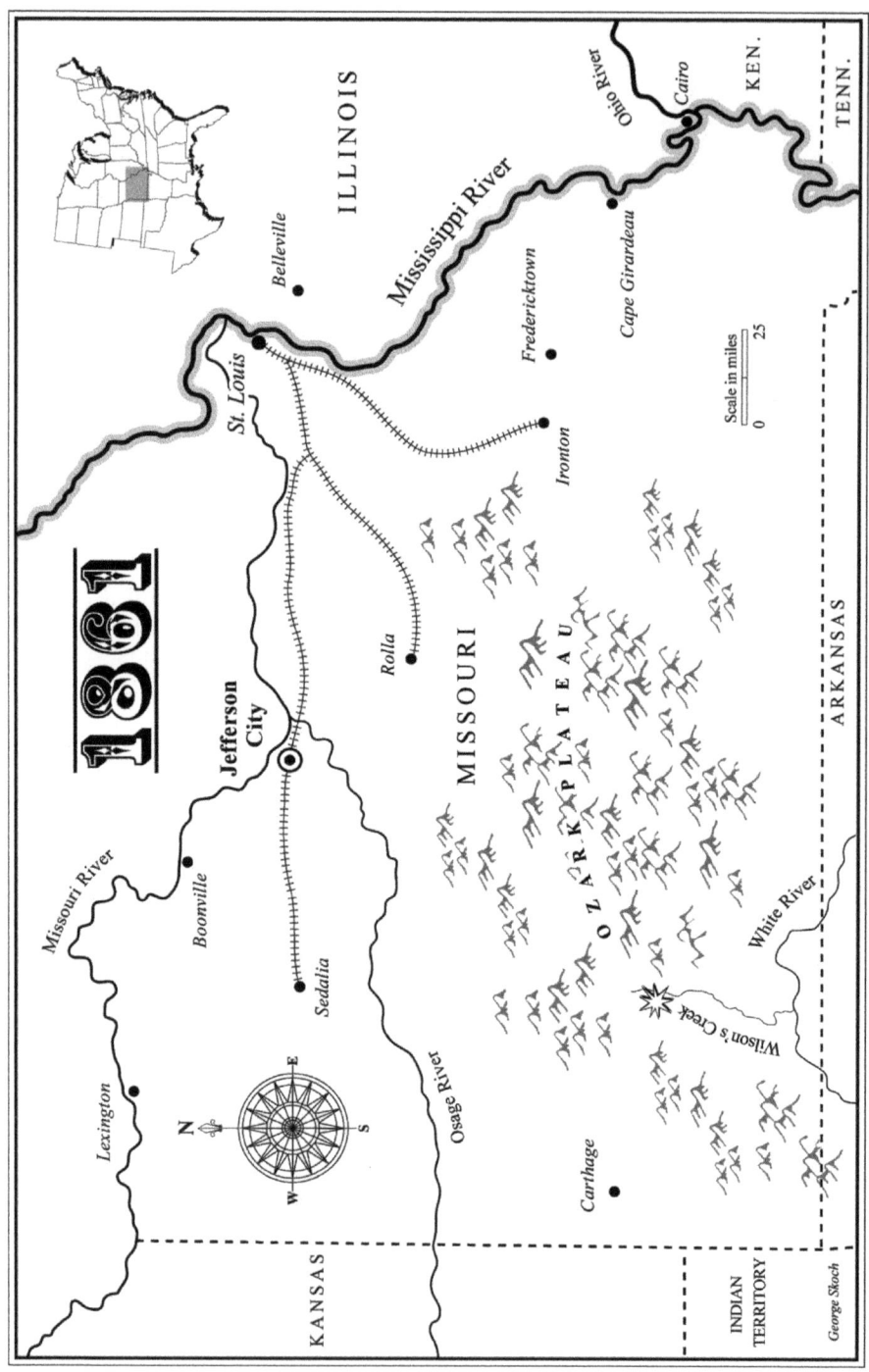

acting as physician pro tem and I hear has been offered the surgeon's place for good. I think he will probably accept. Dr. Hamilton is here from Bond Co., formerly from Crawford. I hear he said that he had applied for quartermaster, think he will come in. They and others are filled by the colonel.

Dr. Roman will assist me all he can and advises me to apply for the position of assistant surgeon. I guess they are not examined by any medical board until they are received into U. S. service. The election for field officers of this regiment came off on Monday. Col. Mr. Doherty [Henry Dougherty] from Clinton, major from Centralia but reported from Washington Co., that they might be accepted. His name is Probst. There is ten companys here. One from this place, Capt. Chancellor. The colonel will appoint the other officers as soon as he receives his commission which will be this week I guess.

Dr. Hamilton says he will do what he can for me. He is acquainted with the Colonel. Dr. Jefferys and Estis moved last week. He's taken her home.

All the friends are well. The little girl at the Widow Stooky's died on Sunday very suddenly. Attended a picnic on Friday. Took dinner at Mr. Ebermon's yesterday, will go out to Mr. B. N. West and Applegate's tonight perhaps.

I am well and doing well. Cannot say when I will go to St. Louis. Will write [to] you again in a few days. Let not your hearts be troubled for now I am old enough to begin the battles of life. I must not sever my pledges of love to you all. I will remain until the appointments are made, then write you the result. My undying love to all at home, the dearest spot on earth to me. Compliments to friends. Write soon as this is recvd. please.

You most affect. son and brother,

T. S. Hawley.

The Thomas Hawley letter of May 21 was written about ten days after the "Camp Jackson Massacre" in St. Louis where 28 people were killed and scores of others wounded when Captain Nathaniel Lyon, U. S. Infantry, captured a group of pro–Southern paramilitary militia. As Lyon marched these men through St. Louis a riot resulted. Although many were wounded or killed, the riot resulted in St. Louis firmly supporting the Union, and the incident further polarized the people of Missouri.

Belleville, Ill.
May 24, 1861
Dear Parents,

Just this moment recd. yours of the 23 inst. Very glad to hear from you.
Have been in camp most of the time since I wrote you, not visited much. Yesterday the appointment for surgeons was made. Dr. Roman Chief Surgeon,

Dr. Bond asst. from Randolph Co. They did not pass an examination. There was 7 or 8 applicants. Most of all of them sworn into service in this regiment. Dr. R. did all for me he could and that was a good deal. So also, Dr. Hamilton, but the staff officers were appointed from each company so that isolated against me some. I regret it some that I was not successful but feel far from being discouraged. Shall go to St. Louis soon. Thought of going west tomorrow afternoon but if you come, will wait until Monday or Tuesday. Dr. H. R.[Roman] advises me to get into the U. S. Service if I can as it will always be a recommendation. So will try in St. Louis, Mo. Will wait for you to come. They all want to see you all very much. Dined with Bro. Mitchell.

Yours,

T. S. Hawley
In love to all

By May 24, 1861, Thomas Hawley was aware he was not successful in gaining a position with the 22nd or Seventh Illinois infantries. He also found surgeons were not being appointed based on examinations, but by the colonels of the regiments. He found there were 7 or 8 physicians vying for the 3 or 4 medical positions within the regiment. Typically, regiments had medical positions for surgeon, the senior medical officer of the regiment, an assistant surgeon, and hospital steward. Some regiments also had a pharmacist and a second assistant surgeon. Undaunted, Thomas Hawley concluded to travel to St. Louis to find a position with another of the mustering regiments. His parents were traveling by train to the area and Thomas looked forward to their arrival before traveling to St. Louis.

By the end of May, Thomas Hawley continued his struggle to join a Union regiment. He met with Colonel Brown, presumably, Colonel Benjamin Gratz Brown. Colonel Benjamin Brown was the commander of the Fourth Missouri U. S. Regiment Reserves, and Brown was a very politically powerful person in Missouri. He was one of the founding members of the Missouri Republican Party and he worked diligently to keep Missouri from becoming a Confederate State. Brown was the grandson of Senator John Brown of Kentucky and he graduated from Transylvania University in Lexington, Kentucky, and Yale University.[1] Colonel Brown had already selected his regimental surgeon and was not planning to add other medical staff until the regiment was fully mustered but encouraged the young Doctor Hawley to continue his search for a position in another regiment.

Doctor Thomas Hawley diligently worked on a plan to join the Union Army including writing to Washington. He called upon his former professors for references and acquired information about other open medicals positions in the newly forming army. As he communicated his plan, he asked his father to speak on his behalf with Colonel Stephen Hicks of Salem, Illinois, who was forming a company of volunteers which would become part of the 40th Illinois Infantry.

St. Louis, Mo. Merchants Exc. May 31, 1861

Dear Parents Bro. & Sisters,

    I had quite a pleasant visit in B[elleville], came very near getting into that regiment which encourages me to continue, which I expect to do until success crowns my efforts. I have seen Drs. Pope and Linton from who I procured further testimonials and wishes for success. Mr. B. will do all he can for me. I walked yesterday several miles and was introduced to Col. Brown. He has appointed the first Surgeon. Said he had thought of waiting until the regiment was called into active service before he appointed the assistant surgeon. Said he would think of my application and that my references were good. I shall procure more, have called but did not find the other professors at home. Think I shall write to Washington soon if I procure no satisfaction here. Shall go to the Arsenal tomorrow, must get pass today. It rained all morning. Pa, I wish you would write Dr. Leass and find out where Dr. Gipson is. Also when you see Col. Hicks if he forms a regiment, I may have a chance there. We are all well, cannot say when I will return home. Will write you often and in the meantime, I do hope you will not feel too gloomy. There is no cause for fear. All is well. My unspeakable love to all and every one. Also compliments to inquiring friends. The family all send best wishes etc.

Good bye,

Yours, Tho. S. Hawley M. D.

No letters survive reporting

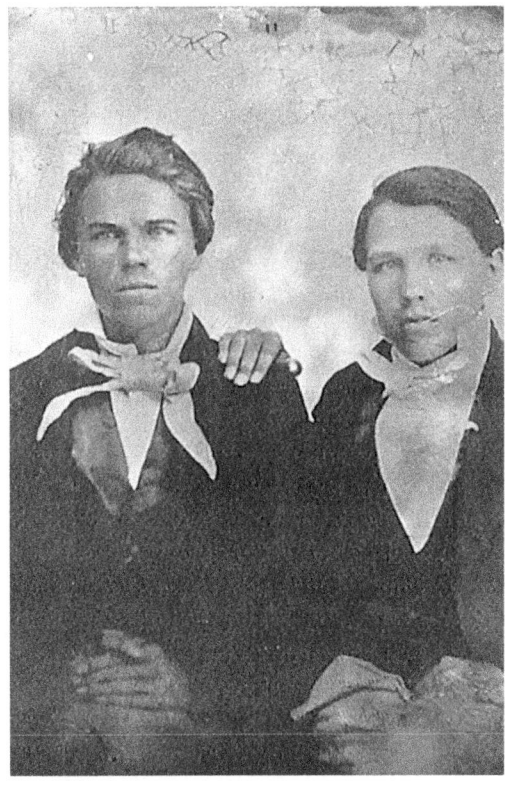

Thomas Hawley (left) and his brother, Amos Hawley in 1858 (courtesy Georgina Joy Monahan).

Thomas Hawley's activities in June and his next letter was written to his family on July 2, 1861, from St. Louis, Missouri. Hawley continued his search for a position in the military and explained that his friends occupied their spare time by playing baseball. The hospital which the medical staff was trying to convert into a functioning facility was so dreadful the soldiers chose to suffer with their medical problems rather than be treated under the deplorable conditions of the hospital. Despite the overall poor living conditions at the camp, the hospital was decidedly worse. In the letter of July 2, Doctor Hawley wrote he expected the United States Congress to increase the number of Union soldiers and this provided further hope he could find a position with a regiment of volunteers. In this letter he made his first reference to Doctor Thomas Smith, surgeon of the First Missouri Rifle Battalion, a three-month infantry regiment.

Amos Hawley, Thomas Hawley's younger brother, suffered from poor health and concern for his health was a constant worry for Thomas. In his July 2 letter, he encouraged his brother's activities but cautioned about his over exertion.

St. Louis, Mo. July 2, 1861

Dearest Friends,

I received your truly, doubly welcome and good letters on last Thursday and did not, as is my custom, answer on Sunday as I had hoped to have some news by this time. But none has been received up to this hour in this office near the third story window. Hall has gone to his ball club, Morning Star. Goes out half past five, plays an hour sometimes longer. None of the family up. Quite cool last night. Yesterday H. and I went to Caseyville [Illinois]. First one I saw to know was Chas. Hamilton as he and Hall were old play mates in R. They had a good time. He is assisting his father who is commissary so he could pass the sentinels any time. We first went to the hospital, an old brick and stone building, north of the town and over a mile from Camp. This Hosp. is two storys high on side hill, one story under ground, no floor to this. Two rooms below used as kitchen and officer's quarters. Two rooms above — no mattresses, no bedsteads, no straw — each man had his blanket (pen played out), another, and a fine carpet of dust and dirt, filth, tobacco juice & cuds. Thousands of flies and duch [Dutch] Surgeon and steward. No wonder only 10 or 15 report themselves, yet near 300 of our duty laying around camp. This, though bad, is preferable to the Hosp.

I spoke to col. [colonel], has appointed first surgeon and he said asst. Dr. Elliott thinks the present incumbent will not give satisfaction and be ousted, then Dr. E. and his friend have the promise. One has gone to Springfield. Dr. E. goes this week. So you see, no good for this child. There [is] no news from any other quarter. I saw several friends from B.—Mr. Peiper Throp, Wm. & Bennie West, seem all well. Your Bro. Houts seems well pleased and I guess all the men and officers are satisfied. I saw Dr. Smith Sunday, had not organized the regiment yet. I shall see some of the men soon and if they are willing, I can assist to raise men. Pa, for the offer of your vest, I am much obliged. Have one in Salem, bought for 75 cts, nice wearables, white vest new socked in the Mississippi but so clean and white, need nothing else but hat, will get military cap, oil cloth for 50 [cts]. So, soon as congress convenes, more men will be called out. Then I will have an additional chance and will soon go to Springfield. Am glad Amos is going to Bro. Js. Wist. I could go to[o] [for] a few days. My dear Bro. take good care of your health, do not overheat your blood. I hope you will enjoy the visit much.

H. F.[Helen Francis], I thank you forty times for that short, sweet letter. Please write often. Myra I thank for good intentions. [I] hope you will write soon. I saw your friend Chas. Black on cars coming from camp. Told him to call and see the folks in Salem. I wrote to our friend black or Black but forgot to give information as to directing letters. Tell him please when you write to Olney send my compliments to friends. Amos, please write to me. Eva Bell, I send you 40½ kisses. Wish I could see you soon. Love to all.

Your affect.,

Thos. S. Hawley, MD

PS. Ma, I send you Stars & Stripes. Pa, thank you very much for the remittance. Wm. B. offers me some if needed.

As Thomas Hawley described the deplorable conditions of the hospital which included thousands of flies and no beds for patients, the political situation within Missouri deteriorated drastically from May 31 until July 2, 1861. During this time, the pro–Southern Missouri governor, Claiborne Fox Jackson, successfully pushed through the Military Act on May 14, 1861, which was designed to disband the old Missouri Militia, and instead, replace it with a military force which would defend Missouri from an invasion by the Union Army. This newly created Missouri State Guard was commanded by Major General Sterling Price. Price was a native Virginian and was active in the Missouri legislature and had served in the U. S. House of Representatives. He was elected governor of Missouri serving from 1853 to 1857. He commanded the Second Regiment, Missouri Mounted Volunteer Cavalry, during the Mexican War.

A temporary truce was achieved between the factions in Missouri on May 20 by General Sterling Price and Major General William S. Harney who commanded the U. S. Army Military Department of the West. The Price-Harney Truce stated, "General Price, having by commission full authority over the militia of the State of Missouri, undertakes, with the sanction of the governor of the State, already declared, to direct the whole power of the State officers to maintain order within the State among the people thereof, and General Harney publicly declares that, this object being thus assured, he can have no occasion, as he has no wish, to make military movements, which might otherwise create excitements and jealousies which he most earnestly desires to avoid."[2] This temporary solution initially calmed the deepening division within the state, but the extremists on both sides were not happy with the compromise. Governor Jackson used this time to strengthen his efforts to guide Missouri toward the Confederacy and General Nathaniel Lyon continued to push for greater enlistments for the Union Army. Finally a meeting was held on June 11, 1861, between Nathaniel Lyon, Sterling Price and Governor Jackson and after four hours it became apparent that no agreement could be reached and Lyon was quoted as stating that rather than give up any part of Missouri to non–Union control, "I would see you, and you, and you, and every man, woman, and child in the state dead and buried."[3]

As the hopes for peace faded, Nathaniel Lyon was promoted to the rank of the brigadier general and assumed command of the Union Army of the West on July 2, 1861. The Missouri executive government in Jefferson City fled the capital on June 13 and on June 15 General Lyon arrived there with 2,000 Union troops. The pro–Southern troops of Jackson and Price moved to southwestern Missouri in July, and Union troops from Kansas, Iowa, and Illinois joined Nathaniel Lyon's Union troops in St. Louis and in other locations within the state.

For Thomas Hawley, July 1861 was an important month because he was successful in finding a medical position with a three-month regiment, the First Missouri Rifle Battalion, which was stationed in Rolla, Missouri. The summer of 1861 was one of unpleasant heat and humidity as described in Hawley's July 8 letter. Doctor Thomas Smith informed Thomas Hawley the First Missouri Rifles needed a hospital steward and Thomas Hawley's efforts of securing a position, at last, were successful. He was ordered to join the regiment on July 9 in Rolla, Missouri, and planned to travel from St. Louis on the Pacific Railroad (P. R. R.).

The reference to Brother Brooks in the letter written on July 8, 1861, was to the chaplain of the First Missouri Rifles, Joseph Brooks. Brooks was born in Ohio on November 1, 1821. Brooks received his education at Indiana Asbury University and became a minister of the Methodist Episcopal Church after his ordination in 1840. He developed quite a reputation as a staunch abolitionist when he lived in St. Louis prior to the war. He was the editor of the *Central Christian Advocate* while in St Louis.[4] Brooks was forty-one years old and was a man determined the Union would win the war.

July 8, 1861
St. Louis, Mo.

Dearest Friends on Earth to Me,

Parents, Bro. and three sweet little Sisters, how much I want to see and kiss you all from the least to the greatest.

Hot, hotter, hottest, but all well and not much sickness in this city. All quiet. No perceptible indications of a storm. Col. Wymans the 13th Ills. Regiment passed through this city, came and left on the P. R. R. Saturday for S. W. B.

Afternoon— Well, I received marching orders— a letter from Dr. Smith asking me to come to Rolla soon if I had not changed my mind. Dr. said he could get the position of Hosp. Steward for the time being and would most likely, as soon as the regiment is fully organized, get the appointment permanently. So I go yet with some regrets but having faith in that motto "Patient waiting, No loss." Dr. sent me a pass, will start tomorrow. They think the reg. will be organized this week. Bro. Brooks is going to Springfield for two companies.

Nine O'clock. Just returned from Bro. Brooks. He just [arrived] from Rolla. Says Dr. S. [Smith] wants to see me immediately, thinks they will be organized this week or next. Will start tomorrow, $8.20 get to Rolla [this] evening. More troops going. Military train. Will write you as soon as settled. [My] unbounded love to all, each & every one.

Yours ever,

T. S. Hawley

Dear Sister Myra,

Many thanks for your kind letter. Can't think of any way to compensate you but by promising to kiss your fat, rosey cheeks, 14½ times & bit once. Couldn't think of doing it though before I return to your town of Salem.

Glad to hear that you appreciated my fine singing at last. But that is the way with all our pleasures and blessings. Never know of what comfort they are to us until deprived of them. I never more than now knew or felt the value of a pure, sisterly love, when there was a likelihood of my being separated from the direct interchange of our sentiments but we can chit chat through the medium of pen and paper. Well, I cannot kiss you just now so will commission [some] body else's brother to fulfill that unpleasant duty. Golly, how I want one smack!! Had a good time out to Bro. Cantines, eh? Glad to hear it. Wish I could have been along. Blackberrys, cherrys & cream, I suppose? I spent a pleasant evening last week at Wm. McNeely's, special invite to call again soon. Spent the 4th at home, had bonfire, sky rockets, Roman candles, ten balloons there at night. Fannie, Alice wants to hear from you very much. Please write soon. Often. Wishes you were here. Does not go to school. I handed Dr. Elliott the communication *from Pa. I have been here so long it seems like home. They express regrets at my leaving. Have been very kind, could not have been more so. Will call to see if Brooks has returned from Rolla. Please write soon.*

Your affect. bro.,

T. S. Hawley

Send poetry by Mr. B. Very good.

Rolla, Missouri, was the western terminus of the Pacific Railroad and as the political situation in Missouri deteriorated in 1861, much of the elected civil government of Missouri was in exile. The Missouri State Guard under command of Major General Sterling Price maneuvered throughout Missouri looking for opportunities to thwart Union control of the state. As a way of quickly moving troops from St. Louis to the interior part of the state, Rolla became a site of thousands of Union troops and any further westward movement was accomplished by marching, wagons, or horseback. Rolla was a town of 600 inhabitants at the beginning of the war and the Union Army immediately took control of the town, including, using the courthouse as a hay storage barn. It was later converted into a hospital.

Thomas Hawley recorded an excellent description of the travel from St. Louis to Rolla on the Pacific Railroad in his July 13 letter. Doctor Hawley provided some, not so flattering, descriptions of the farmers and inhabitants from this part of Missouri.

Once Thomas Hawley arrived at Rolla his life was a flurry of activity. He was met by his new superior officer, Doctor Thomas Smith. Doctor Thomas Smith was the ranking medical officer of the First Missouri Rifles and later held the same position in the 11th Missouri Infantry. Doctor Smith was one of the oldest persons in the regiment. Thomas Smith was born on July 17, 1808, in Lancaster, Pennsylvania. Smith began his career as a school teacher and when he was 20 years old he married Martha McKay. When he was 28, his wife died and he moved to western Pennsylvania and began studying medicine under Doctor John Hassen. He next resided in Cincinnati, Ohio, and he graduated from medical school with honors and began to practice medicine in Cincinnati in 1848. By 1854, he had moved to Keokuk, Iowa. Later, he moved to St. Louis in hopes of improving the health of his second wife, and in 1861 he joined the First Missouri Rifle Battalion.[5]

Camp Rolla, Phelps Co., Mo. July the 13th 1861

Headquarters of Medical Officers at the Hospital

Well Dear Father, Mother, Bro. & Sisters,

Since I last wrote you I have had some experiences in camp life and have

One. 1861

been very busy dealing out medicines to the sick of which we have today 28 in the hospital and about the same in quarters. I left St. Louis as I told you in my last, had a pleasant ride of one hundred and 15 miles through hilly, stony country. A few miles from St. L. the country is fine & fertile but soon becomes stony. Several miles [of] high bluffs almost perpendicular for 200 feet and a few little rises on the other side, the Merimack, I believe. We went to Franklin 30 miles from St. L on the P. R. R., layed over one hour. This village of F. has 200 or 300 inhabitants of which half has left. The P. R. R. runs on and soon comes to Missouri River, thence to Jefferson City. From Franklin, the south W. B. [west bound] of P. R. R. running in a south wly [westerly] direction over a ruff almost barren country, terminates at this place. Has been built for one year by stockholders of St. Louis mostly and must have cost the men a vast amount. We passed through 2 tunnels, over many deep gorges and through deep cuts. But for the last 60 miles the road runs most of the time on the south side of a long ridge and often I could catch a glimpse through the scrubby oak of a fine panoramic view, hills covered with small trees with here and there a garden spot then the long shadows stretching out far to the east into the richer valleys for the hills are very stony, while the valleys resemble our prairie of Illinois (i.e.) in soil. The hills are rich in iron ore with some lead. This place is only a few miles from the Ozark Mts. The nearest point being an elbow in the chain pointing northward. Country new, not many farmers and they not enterprising. Men being of that class designated by a (Colored person) as "poor white trash." Of course from the "sacred soil," where flourish their boasted chivalry of the C. S. of A.

I arrived at this city and Tuesday evening was met by Dr. Smith on the platform when he conducted me to headquarters. After remaining there a few moments, we went or came to this place. Next morning was installed in office of Hosp. Steward and have not had many spare moments since. The sick having just moved to this house this week, we had all to fix up and had 20 or 30 patients every day but not much medicine. On Wednesday, received 4 boxes medicines. These had to be packed, checked, some opened, the rest repacked and by this time we had to prescribe for near 50 patients of which 25 remained in hospital. I did not leave the house for two days but medicines arranged, everything organized on yesterday and today all moves as smoothly as a manger bell.

Yesterday, Dr. S. concluded he must go to the city in the evening, said Col. Bayles had been asking for or about me. Then he wanted me to go over with him. So I ran over, the col. was unwell. We went in, spoke to him. He had several letters and dispatches, was giving orders. We had just received word that a soldier from this place had been stabbed by another soldier 5 or six miles from town. The Col. immediately commanded a sergeant to select 4 of his best and most trusty men with each on horse. Men armed and equipped to go with these messengers of which there was 3 and find the man. And told me to be in readi-

ness with instruments to accompany the others. Would do so with pleasure. This was near 7 o'clock or 8, fine night, moon shinning & cool. I came here, got case of instruments, camphor, brandy, cod, ammonia, bandages, etc., returned. On the way felt most gloriously good at the prospects of a little fun, would get a sword and rise of some Lieut. and perhaps meet "secesh," found the men armed already when the order was countermanded. I felt disappointed. After questioning the messengers, their reports conflicted. The col. thought it was a trap layed and it was too far to send a few men at night. We had no fears and urged the matter [or] the poor man must die. Today I hear a man was bayoneted in abdomen and brought to this place. He wounds looked bad, said he will die. I wish we could have gone.

Well, we are doing well. Plenty to do. I guess we will not stay long but soon go back to St. Louis to organize for 3 years. Then I hope to see your mail goes. Now must leave some blank paper just for want of time. My inexpressible love to all. Write soon to this place. I can get it. Yours in love,
T. S. Hawley

Immediately after joining the regiment, Thomas Hawley was immersed in caring for the sick and wounded, seeing about twenty to thirty patients a day. The medical supplies for the regiment were sparse and undoubtedly the sanitary conditions were limited at this stage in the war. Also, during the first days with the regiment, Hawley was introduced to the colonel of the First Missouri Rifles, David Bayles. David Bayles was a native of Ohio, and had military experience, having fought in the Mexican War. Prior to the beginning of the Civil War he worked as a "collector, water license" in St. Louis. Bayles recruited men for the First Missouri Rifles with his friend Captain Rufus Saxton. As the regiment was being organized Saxton intended to command the First Missouri Rifles and Bayles planned to serve as his subordinate, presumably, lieutenant colonel. At this time, Bayles was nominally referred to as colonel. Poor health plagued David Bayles and he suffered from dropsy which is often accompanied by swelling in various parts of the body.

In Thomas Hawley's July 13 letter, he referred to the increasingly dangerous situations in the countryside near Rolla, Missouri. Despite what turned out to be a real medical emergency, an attempt to send medical assistance to a soldier who was bayoneted was cancelled due to fears the message was false and a trap was prepared to capture Union soldiers. Unfortunately, according to Hawley's conclusion, the unfortunate soldier was brought to camp the next day and presumably died of his wounds.

In Hawley's next letter, on July 15, he recorded the large number of soldiers congregating at Rolla resulted in some interactions with old acquaintances, but Thomas Hawley was busy with the medical conditions of the soldiers at the post. The soldiers were experiencing some illnesses resulting in fevers and chills. The hospital was a confiscated house of a Southern sympathizer and the management and supervision of medical and cook staff was a new skill for the young doctor. He was challenged with a cook nicknamed "Hog" and also dealt somewhat intemperately with a lazy Frenchman. Doctor Hawley recorded the regiment was not yet organized and appeared to be lacking the necessary number of men to be mustered as a full regiment. Civil War regiments generally contained ten companies and each company could contain a maximum of 101 men. So a fully staffed infantry regiment ideally had 1000 soldiers and also a regimental staff which included, a colonel, a lieutenant colonel, a major, an adjutant, a chaplain, at least three medical officers, commissary sergeant, quartermaster, musicians and a sergeant major. The letter of July 15 made reference to General Butler's contraband and this term referred to the slaves that had escaped or in some other manner came into the hands of the Union Army. These individuals were fortunate to no longer be slaves, but often they struggled finding a decent occupation and living facilities.

During this time, the opposing forces were garnering their strength and began to identify their respective military objectives. The Southern sympathizing Missouri State Guard under the command of Colonel John S. Marmaduke met the advancing Federal forces under command of General Nathaniel Lyon near Boonville, Missouri, in early July 1861. A small skirmish resulted with the total casualties of less than a 100 men. The result of this battle was the removal of Sterling Price's State Guard from central Missouri to the southwestern part of the state and the battle shed the blood of Missourians further dividing the state and nation. Soon after the skirmish at Boonville, another skirmish occurred at Carthage, Missouri, on July 5, 1861, with slightly greater than 100 total casualties.

July 15

Monday. No train yesterday. I was so much engaged this morning could not get to [the] train in time. This will be a long letter and a long time coming, I guess you will think. Almost every day find some old acquaintances in connection with our Battalion as it is now. Dr. Smith will not return from St. Louis for two or 3 days. Today all passed off smoothly, prescribed for only 40 patients. Bow Griffin is here from St. Clair, the same boy, Mr. Parker from Lebanon, Father Risley's son, Wm. Hoyt's son of Lebanon.

Our Hospital is a new secesh house, frame. Front and back porch, six rooms and kitchen, one story with cellar full of water. No well. We must carry water 2 hundred yards. I now have two cooks and one nurse. My first cook, Hog by name & nature, I promoted to mess, has an old steam boat crank, for the *present does fine. For dinner today fine beef & bean soup, coffee, sugar, no milk. Buttered biscuit with army crackers and beef steak tonight. The Ills. 13*th *captured near 4 horses, some grocery stores, guns, knapsacks, old guns and other contrabands. They have also taken charge of a grocery in this place meaning that the proprietors were in the Southern Army. Today one of Gen. Butler's contrabands came to the Ills. 13*th*. They sent him off. My cooks took him into the kitchen. Gave him his breakfast. Some of the men wanted me to keep him in the Hosp. I could not, do not know where he is now. Heard no preaching, only a few words from our back porch yesterday. I keep the Hosp. stores, and cooksmith such things, for barely at noon, I was fixing up some medicine, an old Frenchman, not sick but lazy, brought in his plate with a nice beef steak for some vinegar. I very deliberately took down a bottle of Epsom salts in sol [solution] coalesced with spirit of lavender but horrid stuff and poured it on his beef steak. He has not called for more.*

Sickness chills — cure Quinine, will try to write again this week. We may stay here for some time perhaps for only a few weeks. Not yet organized. The regiment could not get some men near Salem for 3 years or war time or so [they] say. Please write soon— T. S. H. Rolla, Phelps Co., Mo.

Lots of love to to all, your most aff.,

T. S. Hawley, MD

On July 18, Doctor Thomas Hawley was still diligently ministering to the sick and ill soldiers. The first hint of conflict between Thomas Hawley and Thomas Smith was noted in this letter. Although Hawley quickly moved past his comment about Smith, it was evident the relationship between the two men was not all that Doctor Hawley had hoped. The most important comment regarding Doctor Smith in this letter was Thomas Hawley's statement, "I know he is not infallible." Smith either thought that he was always right or Hawley had observed something Smith did which he did not agree. Despite the friction between Hawley and Smith, one of the most humorous events in this letter by Thomas Hawley was Doctor Smith's extraction one of Hawley's healthy teeth. Thomas Hawley recorded Doctor Fuller was the third medical professional of the First Missouri Rifle Battalion.

The regiment was still not organized by July 18 and Hawley wrote that he did not think the organization would occur for some time due to a conflict of who would be named as officers. The First Missouri Rifles was a three-month regiment and the expiration of the term of service was rapidly approaching. The difficulty in organizing the full three-year regiments from the men of a three-month regiment was maintaining an adequate number of soldiers who were willing to re-enlist. Hawley recorded Company B was going to St. Louis and unhappiness with the officers was likely to result in the soldiers permanently leaving the regiment. On a positive note, Doctor Clark Hendee, acting captain, arrived in camp with a company of men ready to enlist.

Camp Rolla, Phelps Co., Mo. July 18, 1861
 In the Hospital many miles from home with hills, rivers, towns and villages intervening and separating me from my
 Parents and other Dear ones at home. You will not be surprised that I should sometimes become lonely. But up to this time every spare moment has been occupied how I have already informed you. Our no. [number] of sick has not much decreased but we have matters better arranged, consequently we have more spare time. Afternoon is quite pleasant but warm, yet the weather has been fine for this time of year.
 We treat from 50 to 65 patients every day and have on an average 25 in hospital. When I left you in haste I had no idea it would be this long before I should see you again, [or] I could not have left as I did. How much and how often I have wished to see and kiss and embrace you, one and all, you cannot tell. But as for the time this is desired, to hear from you as I did in St. Louis. Would be a great source of pleasure but it appears so, for even this pleasure is denied me. I assure you, to go to war for that alone would afford no attraction for me. My motives as you well know are far different. Home has too many attractions for me to think one moment of giving place to it in my affections. The battlefield or the military camp which latter place will stand no comparison to my home with its great gravitation drawing me ever towards it, no matter wheresoever it be. If Father, Mother, bro. and sisters are there, there is home. I have no old family clock, rocking chairs, where mother has rocked me & herself many years ago. No pleasant nook in the fine old garden where we children were want to hide away and gather currants, strawberries. No fine old spring in some sequestered glen. I have none of these to draw or deride my love for home, nor do I regret it as it is all my love centered on those dear flesh and blood relations and not in inanimate objects. In His good and righteous cause I think I have already passed through the most trying scene, leaving home and seeing the sudden and heartfelt gush of tears from those I so fondly love. Yet the prospect of soon seeing you again soon softened, and still does, the aches over my leaving you for some time. I need not assure you that I will use all fair means to see you and that might [be] soon. Yet, I may be doomed to disappointment.
 My health so far is tolerable. Good, yet it might be better. Dr. Smith is not exactly the man I thought him to be but an upright conscientious man I have not the least doubt. I have never known him to acknowledge himself in the wrong and he is more stern and commanding than I have been used to. Yet I know he is not infallible. Dr. Fuller, who is now acting as assistant surgeon, is a jolly, and

so far as I have seen, a fine clever fellow, understands medicine well, has had lots of practice, so he says, in or near Springfield, Ills. As to the other officers I cannot say much as I have not seen them much. The regiment is not, and I think will not be, organized for some time. There is some difficulty among the officers or would be such, too many aspirants for the good of all.

Mr. Bayles, acting I understand as col. for the time, is a fine man. Capt. Saxton of the regular army is to be our col. and his reputation as a soldier and a fine man is established beyond care. Of course the regular officers, especially medical staff, are not as yet appointed permanently. I think I am safe for the present position and perhaps for a better. Am getting along smoothly so far. I told you in my last of the col. requesting me to be in readiness for the evening's march to attend a wounded man. I had a severe attack the other day but stood firm & the enemy retreated only carrying away a tooth. I had a slight tooth ache. Not being well, so I concluded, as Dr. S. had some reputation as a tooth drawer, to have mine extracted. I showed him the offending one. He took his forceps, layed hold, held my head, pulled and hauled. I heard something crack. He could not come it, changed instruments and out it came. BUT LO! it proved to be a sound tooth. He said he had pulled many hundred but never a harder one. Had to use lots of force. I stood it like a soldier never paralleled. But soon felt faint, took some brandy. It made me sick for two days and will for more. I would not have lost the tooth for $50 but it's gone.

I saw two soldiers have a citizen in tow a few moments ago. He was caught hollering for Jeff Davis. Poor Feller. I guess he was drunk. Today we had news that a provision train was attacked between here and St. Louis, Mo., no harm done, I guess. One company, that is Comp B, say they are going to St. Louis Monday. Their time is out for 3 months and most of them want to see their friends before they join or enlist for 3 years and I think some of them and perhaps half, will not return. So they will have to recruit more and longer. Many of them say if they cannot have a change of officers, they will not enlist for 3 years. If you see a good opening for me in Ills., just send word immediately and I can come for I am under no special obligation to remain longer. If Col. Hicks wants assistance, I can come. I think I will soon see if I can go for recruits as we never have things organized. I give the patients medicine, attend to the household matters, generally have two good cooks and one nurse. I have not heard from home since I left St. Louis, Mo. but heard from Mr. B. twice. I shall continue to write long, and I fear uninteresting letters, to you. Dr. looks for Mr. Reed and wife here the first of next week. Mr. Brooks has gone to Keokuk, Iowa. I do not know what for. I saw the letter you wrote to Mr. Reed and think you was right as to the recruiting. Part of Dr. Hendee's com [company] from Clay & Richland Co. came here this week. He is in St. Louis, so I hear.

Please send me a paper, the <u>Western</u>, for instance. I have not seen it for a

long time or the <u>Salem Advocate</u>. Myra, give my most sincere love to your friends who inquire for me and now, do all write soon. Well, I hear the drum and fife for tattoo of the Ills. 13th regiment who are camped just back of our house. So I close but not until I have renewed my oft expressed sentiments of endearing attachments to you all of which I cannot find words strongly enough to express. Your affect. son,
T. S. Hawley

In the letter written on July 21, there was a sense of urgency regarding the organization of the regiment. The condition of the regiment was not good. Doctor Thomas Smith had departed for St. Louis leaving the medical duties of the regiment in the hands of Thomas Hawley and Doctor Fuller. The rumor was the regiment had marching orders while several of the companies were planning to leave the service due to the dissatisfaction with the officers.

Thomas Hawley described his meeting with an old acquaintance, Doctor Clark Hendee, a thirty-six-year-old, Vermont-native. Hendee was instrumental in organizing a company from Clay County, Illinois, and he personally paid to transport the men of the company to St. Louis for enlistment from his own money. Clark Bentley was elected 1st lieutenant of the newly forming company. Bentley was a 33 year-old painter living in Louisiana, Missouri, and he was born in New York. Hawley also recognized Mark Sappington although Sappington did not recognize him. Missouri native, minister and farmer, Mark Sappington was living in Clay County, Illinois, prior to his enlistment.[6]

Bushwhacking was common as small bands of soldiers tried to make an impact on the organizing armies in Missouri. The local Methodist minister, the Rev. Stanford Ing, led a Union patrol that captured 30 Southern sympathizers. The captured men were the center of attention in the camp. Hawley surprisingly found these men looked normal and he stated the captured captain was a rather fine looking man.

Camp Rolla, Mo. July 21, 1861
My Very Dear Parents, Bro. & Sisters,

Although I mailed you a long letter only two or 3 days ago, I will send you this tomorrow, Monday. We have no train here on Sunday consequently no news and today, no Sunday school, no preaching and nothing to distinguish it from another day of the week except that it rains and has rained all day. We have not been out of the house today (i. e.), Dr. Fuller and I. Dr. Smith left yesterday morning in post haste for St. Louis. We understand that this battalion had orders to march by next Wednesday and surely every man who knows anything of our condition would say nothing could be more deleterious to us in our present condition. Only 3 or 4 companies of three months volunteers & their time almost expired. Most, or at least many of the men, dissatisfied with their commanders and wanting to go home, if not to stay on furlough for 3 or 4 weeks.

You can see to march such men without suitable equipage 50 or 60 miles farther into this state would be, to say the least of it, highly injudicious. Not that there would be any danger from secesh. But recruits could not be easily sent there as here on the R R. Those whose time would soon run out would want to go home and their mileage would be so much the more and when once they had gone they would not be likely to return. I think we will not go until the Rifle Regiment is fully organized and the officers are making strenuous efforts to accomplish that purpose now. Parts of two companies came in last week, one, Dr. Hendee from Olney. The men, most of them are Clay & Richland Cos. I have not seen all the boys. Yesterday I saw Huzzy formerly of Olney and today Mr. Sappington formerly of the Southern Illinois Conference came into the office with Leut. Bentley. As soon as I saw Sap[pington] I knew him and stepped forward and cordially shook him by the hand. He barely spoke. I saw he did not know me so I kept cool, gave him medicine for his sick boys and told him to call again when any more was needed. I shall soon see him again and will make myself known. He has no officers as yet so I hear, looks ruff and hairy.

Last Thursday Companys D and K numbering about 175 men from the Ills. 13th under command of Lieut. Col. Georges started on a scouting party guided by Rev. Ing of the Mo. Con. [Missouri Methodist Conference]. (Here he is now on the porch—large, tall man, black felt hat, dark eyes. His head run through a hole in the large piece of oil cloth. He is getting up a company of cavalry, has now 45 or 50 men. There, he's gone now out into the rain). Well this party went 25 or 30 miles from here and captured 30 men and as many horses, among the former a captain and lieutenant who rode into their camp the second night they were out. The men made no noise. These men did not see them. They took charge of them but the captain, etc., claimed to be good loyal citizens. The boys kept them. Next day they were recognized and acknowledged and showed their papers being secesh. The boys were shot at 4 times and captured the men who shot. Two boys rode up to 8 mounted and armed men, captured them without a shot. About an hour ago they came in, marched by here and up to the camp. I mean the whole party. I went into camp and saw secesh marched into the cold wet tents called guard houses. I watched the expression of their continuances. Some chaffed and ground their teeth. Others walked up to the tent door, lifted the canvas looked in, hesitated one moment, stooped and stepped in intently as a dog driven into his kennel. A few appeared to be pleased with the change although I should think the prospect was anything but inviting. I saw one gray headed man but he appeared hale and hearty. The captain was rather a fine appearing man. Most of the men looked exceedingly ruff and seedy and the horses to match. I have not heard the particulars. Will write the rest in my next.

One of our captains stopped on the steps a short time ago and said he did not like the ways things were working with our battalion. Said he heard Col. Bayles was under arrest in St. Louis. Things are very uncertain. I wish I knew just what to do and what would be done. I received your welcome letter of the 17 inst. on the 20, it being the first time I had heard from you since I left St. Louis, have heard from there once or twice. Sorry you could not write longer letters. All write some please. I guess we will stay here. I get along well with the boys. Mr. Parks is from Lebanon. My patient's friend say the boys like me well. He writes some time for the <u>Democrat</u> signed P. from Rolla. Undivided love to all each one, has more than I can tell of.

Your affectionate son,

T. S. Hawley

The Phelps Co. Court House situated in Rolla on the brow of a hill running east. The house fronts north and is south of most of the town. This view as you see is from the northeast and does not do justice to the house which is built of brick with limestone corners. They have a strong burglar proof jail. The railroad

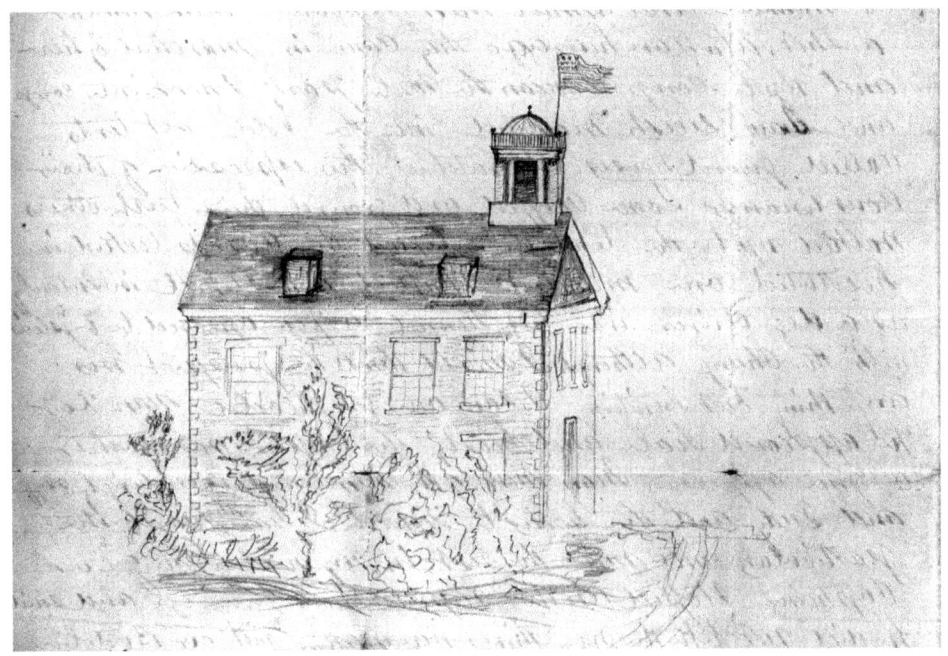

Drawing of the Phelps County Courthouse from Thomas Hawley's letter of July 21, 1861 (Missouri History Museum, St. Louis, Missouri).

runs north and west of the courthouse. Its general course being northeast and southwest and is graded some miles from here. Half a mile from town there is [a] cut 75 feet deep where I got Myra gold which I sent her in my last. Will try to find some more specimens.

The Sunday of July 28, 1861, found Thomas Hawley still tending to his medical duties in Rolla, Missouri, but the organization of the regiment was closer to being finalized. The First Missouri Rifles were due to depart Rolla on July 29 for St. Louis to be organized into a 3-year Union regiment. The threat of attack was ever present for the Union soldiers in Rolla and in Hawley's letter he related the rumor of attack was far worse than any actual threat. Hawley mentioned the result of a small skirmish between a group of 22 Missouri Home Guards (Union) and 65 Missouri State Guard (Southern) troops near Rolla. The skirmish showed the confusion and lack of experience of many of the soldiers at this stage of the Civil War. The Missouri Home Guard officer felt he was outnumbered and fled; however, most of the soldiers stayed at their post and successfully repulsed the attackers. Some of the wounded were returned to Rolla and Doctor Hawley described in detail the impact of musket or minié balls on human bones. He indicated one musket ball shattered a bone into 50 pieces. It was this type of wound that would be so devastating in the upcoming war and which caused so many amputations.

Sunday
Camp Rolla, Mo. July 28, 1861

Dearest Friends at home I recd. yours of the 24 inst. in due time, cannot give you a shadow of the pleasure it afforded me. I have received your letters as written for the last week. Dr. Smith left for St. Louis last Monday, has not been heard from since. Any information in regard to his whereabouts will be thankfully received by the undersigned. If not sent by 10 o'clock tomorrow, may keep cool for the undersigned and his worthy assistant (i. e.), Dr. A. B. Fuller, will start in hot pursuit and will stop at the U. S. Arsenal in St. Louis, Mo. for an indefinite period and will be happy to attend to all calls, professional or otherwise. In short, this Battalion is under marching orders to go to St. Louis tomorrow and today we have been packing part of the time. This morning heard the Chap[lain] of the Ills. 13th preach in camp, had his hat on and most of the sermon was read. Not many of the men present. Music by the band. I stood under a small tree with my arm upon it, cap on and paying close attention, psalm and sermon in connection. We have had some exciting times since I last wrote. 3 or 4 companys of the Ills. 13th have been out on a scouting expedition, have been sending flying reports of their successes and reverses at one time. Sent in a courier on a foaming steed reporting that their men were surrounded, then Madam Rumor with her ten thousand tongues started flying. Reports of 7 or 800 secesh near. At night all the town was in fear and soldiers were looking for a night attack. Some of the men slept on their arms. Most of the battalion has left, gone to St. Louis. I guess we go today, if cars enough.

Last Thursday a company of Home Guards, 22 in number were drilling near a log house some 15 or 20 miles from here and about 3 o'clock in the afternoon, they were attacked by 65 secesh mounted who came rushing down upon them. The capt. of the Home Guards ordered a retreat rather than stand against such odds. 7 of the men obeyed. The other 15 in number remained and fought like tigers, killing men and horses in numbers, losing one killed, 1st lieut. and two others wounded. Secesh concluded it wouldn't pay and seceded in disgust leaving their dead and wounded on the field. They were all brought here on Friday last. 3 left in the Ills. 13 and two brought here but all under the care of Dr. Plummer, 1st Surgeon of the Ills. 13th, but his assistant Dr. Law was out scouting. Dr. Fuller and I assisted in the operations of the two that came here. One a Union man body, soul and all, was shot just above the elbow, the ball passing clear through the arm breaking the bone in 50 pieces making a hole I could put my finger in easy. Dr. F. gave chloroform. I held the amputated limb. Dr. P. cut and a slow one it was, occupying at least an hour. He tied at least 5 more ligatures than was necessary and tied next to the bone where, if he had been an anatomist, could or would have known there was no artery. But after all, it was done up right well and the man is doing well. The other man that was brought here a secesh, a young, married man, black hair and with all, rather good looking fellow. Was shot through the leg just above the patella breaking the lower part of the femur into a dozen fragments and opening the capsular ligament. The ball passed out lower than where it entered from. 36 to 40 hours had passed from the shooting until the operation. The men had to be conveyed over 15 miles of very rough road. Well, we do not go until tomorrow. For time, I cannot finish this letter.

Write soon, your affect.,

T. S. Hawley

P.S. Write next to St. Louis as usual.

By August 2, 1861, Thomas Hawley and the First Missouri Rifle Battalion were back in St. Louis and Doctor Hawley related in his letter one of the most convincing anti-liquor lectures of the war. His letter described the result of drinking "bad" liquor on the part of a Doctor Burnes who had recently died. Doctor Hawley described in detail the autopsy which was performed on the body as 5 doctors and 4 attorneys observed the procedure. On an humorous note, as the effects of the bad alcohol were observed in the vital organs, the observers consumed two bottles of the brandy. Doctor Hawley thought he might lose his position in the army due to the observers becoming intoxicated during the autopsy.

At long last the First Missouri Rifle Battalion was beginning to be organized after the three-month enlistment period. The new regiment, mustered into service on August 5–6 in St. Louis, was called the 11th Regiment Missouri Volunteer Infantry and this regiment was a three-year regiment. Because many of the county quotas were filled in Illinois, men from Illinois enlisted in Missouri regiments which were not filled. The 11th Missouri Infantry when fully mustered was predominantly made up of these men from Illinois. Nine of the ten companies were Illinois companies and only Company K had a majority of the men from Missouri.

Thomas Hawley made a passing reference in the August 2 letter to another doctor who would become one of his closest friends in the regiment, Eli Bowyer. Bowyer was born in Warren County, Ohio on March 20, 1818. Bowyer taught school for two years prior to studying to become a physician. He graduated from the Ohio Medical College in Cincinnati in 1844 and moved to Mason, Ohio, to practice medicine. He moved to Indiana and finally, in 1860, settled in Olney, Illinois, as he tried to find a geographic location which was beneficial to his health.[7] Both Bowyer and Hawley would serve together throughout the war, become roommates and closest friends.

St. Louis Aug. 2, 1861
Dearest Friends,

As you see by the date of this, I am in St. Louis again after a short term of camp life which I have given you a history of except the two or 3 last days. I formed several pleasant acquaintances during my short stay in Rolla among which was Dr. Burnes, a graduate of some school in Canada. Was not over 30 years of age. No family, no relations, had removed from Arkansas to Rolla in April. Soon after coming to Rolla commenced drinking and had been under the influence of stimulants to a greater or lesser degree ever since until last Thursday night. Was attacked with premonitory symptoms of <u>mania a potu</u>. He continued to grow gradually worse. Was not wild and raving at any time. Dr. Fuller and I called in on Sunday. He was then one mass of living, dying, jerking, quivering flesh. Eyes glaring wildly, his pulse was feeble and irregular, limbs cold and clammy. The Dr. had prescribed for himself the first two days of his sickness. He then called in Dr. Thrallkill. He took large quantities of stimulants opiates. When we saw him we knew he must die but sent over a vial containing equal parts of tine, opiates and viratril. Nothing did any good. He died Monday morning. Some of his friends called Dr. Fuller and I over, said they wanted the body examined. We went and all said I must perform the work. The house or office *was full 4 or 5 MDs, 3 or 4 lawyers. We first examined the brain, congestion was evident everywhere by the livid (Aug. 4) appearance of the face, ears by the large amount of blood in the scalp and by the blood oozing out of skull. When the scalp was separated, we found the brain full of effusious serum and blood water in the ventricles, brain somewhat hardened. Weighed 49 oz. (Avoirdupois).*

The heart was next examined, found large clots of fibers in each opening of left ventricle. These clots look like organized muscle so firm and as large as my finger. These clots were, I think, whipped out of the blood during the irregular beating of the heart. The stomach was literally burnt up, could push my finger through the walls, gangrene having set in, contents like mucus. Liver much enlarged and congested. We examined no farther because the ravages of bad whisky was evident in every vital organ and this was the strongest temperance lecture that could have been heard or in this case seen. Yet it was unheeded for there was two bottles of brandy emptyed during the examination and two got quite tipsy. And I regret to say one of them could have [been] the existing cause of a present spell of sickness to that afternoon's drinking and I fear will lose a position in the army on the same account.

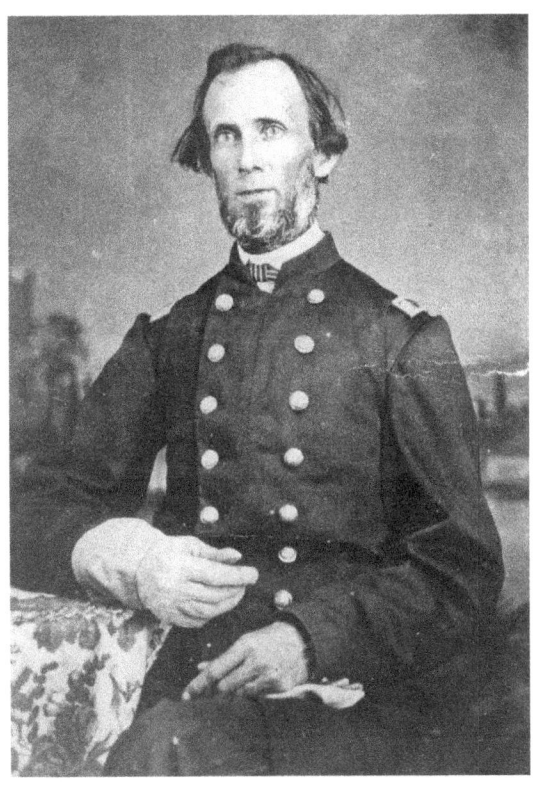

Assistant Surgeon Eli Bowyer (USAMHI).

I speak of Dr. Fuller, finer little fellow cannot be found. I have attended him during the last week. He is now almost well. Our quarters are now at the Marion Hospital but I come to Mr. B. every other night until our regimental Hospital is finished. I find several friends in the new companies, Elmore Ridgely from Olney, Jim Notestine, Henry Kaley, Saml. Conrad, Saml. Donald, Lewis Gray (no friend of mine) and some others. There are 740 men there now. 4 or 5 companies organized. All the officers green with one or two exceptions. I will probably hold my present position for some time yet for I think Dr. Bowyer of Olney will come in as asst. I will try and come home in a few weeks. So far all well. *Please write soon and give all the news. I have no time now to write more for I must be at the Marion by 9 o'clock to give medicine at 10. Bro. Brooks will preach for us.*

My unbounded love to all and 40 kisses.

Aff. son & bro.,

T. S. Hawley, M D

After the 11th Missouri Infantry was mustered into service it was immediately sent to Cape Girardeau, Missouri, which was considered the southernmost Union held territory in southeastern Missouri. The regiment was mustered into service on August 5 and 6 and on August 7 the regiment traveled by steamboat to Cape Girardeau where the soldiers were housed in old mills. The regiment immediately was put to work enhancing the defenses of the town and rumors abounded that Southern forces were planning a surprise attack on the city.

As soon as Doctor Hawley was mustered into service things began to happen very quickly. Shortly after arriving at Cape Girardeau, the first major battle of the Civil War in the west was fought at Wilson's Creek, Missouri, on August 10, 1861. This had a sobering effect on the soldiers in Cape Girardeau because the Southern forces in Missouri defeated the Union forces under Brigadier General Nathaniel Lyon, the outspoken supporter of Union sentiment in Missouri. Not only were the Union forces defeated, but Lyon was killed in the battle. The realization this new Civil War would be bloody and hard-fought was clear after August 10.

Doctor Hawley wrote his next letter to his parents and siblings on August 25 and he described how busy he was. Thomas Hawley was still serving as hospital steward, Doctor Eli Bowyer was serving as assistant surgeon and the regimental surgeon, Thomas Smith, rounded out the medical staff of the 11th Missouri Infantry. As was common in the early days of the war, diseases were wide spread as sanitary conditions were limited and as the throng of men was thrown together in close quarters contagious diseases spread easily. The regiment contained about 950 men and over 120 of these were medically treated on August 24. Two-thirds of those ill suffered from some form of intermittent fever, such as, typhoid fever or malaria.

Not only were medical conditions limited, the men were without uniforms, although they were expected shortly. There was a hint of some problems yet to be revealed as Hawley reported Doctor Thomas Smith and Colonel David Bayles were not present with the regiment. On a lighter note, the cost for washing Thomas Hawley's shirt was ten cents and he was appalled at such a price.

One. 1861

Camp Fremont, Cape Girardeau, Mo. August 25, 1861
Dear Parents, Bro. & Sisters,

I suppose when you get this, Pa will be in Robinson and you will indeed be lonesome. How is Amos? Why don't he write or you? Say now, that last letter was, or appeared to me, too short. But then Pa was leaving and Mr. Allyn's family was leaving or staying and Myra had to get the supper. I should like to step in and say your efficiency in the culinary department, but not so much for the eating as the social, filial and kissable feast. Your humble servant has [been] slightly indisposed for the past two days. Only becoming acclimated to this malarious and noxious district. Yesterday we had 120 patients, ⅔ of the diseases, or those affected, partaken of an intermittent character. This morning many complained of colds, pains & aches caused by exposure for many had no blankets, coats and are half naked. They have promises of uniforms tomorrow at the farthest. Dr. Smith, Rev. Banks & Col. Bayles are neither here nor have been for 2 weeks. Dr. S. never has one send a small lot of medicines. Capt. Livingston just now said he saw all our uniforms packed up & it would soon be here. He is just from Olney, said Tom Scoot was in feeble health. Also Henry Spring. They both served some in Cairo. What you say of Mr. B. & family I hope is fully appreciated and hope to in some respect repay if not now, in some future time. I regret to hear that you are and do suffer so much from the heat.

I wrote to Mr. B. to send some of my clothes. But I find that it won't pay. What! Ten cents for washing a linen shirt which I have paid twice. I see some made of flannel of a grey or purple color and in the same manner of a linen. They do ~~not~~ look well and do not require washing, ironing so much. If I should come home soon, you must not expect me to be in full officer dress, starched up, etc. But rather shabby yet, as I hope full face healthy and as I know full to overflowing with love for one and all. Can't say for which I have the most love in store. Our boys which I told you of as being shot are almost well and all sick doing well and getting better. Both remarkable cases to recover from.

Have heard no preaching today, was in hopes to but could not. How long does Pa remain in Crawford? I should like to hear from them, Link and Gran Pa. We have a most excellent cook now, and have good healthy meals. Yes Myra, if you could see some of his cooking, you would be surprised. His stove is a ditch dug in the ground 8 inches deep, 4 feet long and ten feet wide. This lined with stones and built up 5 or 6 inches, has an iron bar across. It does well. 2 large camp kettles, one frying pan, with this he prepares our luxurious, good, healthy food.

At present, no excitement. Myra, did you give my love to Emma?
500 camp kettles full of love. Love to all. All write soon.
Myra do, Amos do, Fannie do write to your

Affect. son & bro.,

T. S. Hawley

By the end of the first week in September 1861, the regimental elections were held and Thomas Hawley and the rest of the officers of the 11th Missouri Infantry were elected for the various positions. Among the regimental staff was David Bayles, elected as colonel, and Lieutenant Colonel William Panabaker. William Panabaker was another of physicians who made up the officer ranks of the 11th Missouri Infantry. By all accounts, William Panabaker was a colorful and skillful officer. Not only was he a physician, but he was also a Methodist minister. He had served in the army during the U. S.-Mexican War and had traveled to California during the gold rush.[8] He was instrumental in recruiting men to form Company A and when he was elected to the rank of lieutenant colonel, he was replaced as captain of Company A by Captain Cyrenus Elliott, also a physician. Major Benjamin Livingston was the final ranking officer of the regimental staff. Livingston was a 30 year-old attorney from Olney, Illinois. The immediate plans for the regiment were various garrison and scouting duties throughout the fall at Cape Girardeau.

The friendship between Thomas Hawley and Eli Bowyer was evident in the September 8 letter. Bowyer was older than Thomas Hawley and acted as mentor to the younger doctor. Bowyer's leadership within the medical staff was exhibited as he fended off efforts of a Doctor Browning who tried to gain a position within the regiment. After conversing with Doctor Browning, Eli Bowyer refused to speak with him again and Hawley referred to Browning as a "rascal."

Cape Girardeau, Mo. Sept 8th, 1861

Dearest Parents, It has been some time since I last heard from you. Then Ma wrote a good long letter. Maria & Fanny each a short one. I had a long one partly written, finished that and another. I have forgotten now what I wrote you. So if I should mention the same thing twice, do not be astonished. We have had an election in the regiment lately for field officers. Col. D. Bayles was unanimously chosen as such. Capt. Pennabaker [Panabaker], Lt. Col., Capt. Livingston as Major. Dr. Smith's office was confirmed with Dr. Bowyer's and mine. Most of men now have their uniforms & look well. Not many of the officers have theirs for they have to go to St. Louis and as yet have not had time. Col. Bayles is now commander of this post as Col. Marsh is gone and is now on his way to Cairo. Our troops have charge of the breast works and artillery. From this and a few other reasons, we conclude it possible that we may remain here for a few weeks longer. I have a certificate from Dr. Smith & Col. Bayles saying I served in the Rifle Battalion for 1 month as asst. surgeon and asking an order for the money which is now due. Indeed most of the men in the battalion have been paid off. When I get that I can, and will, prepare myself for the campaign. I sent the certificate to Mr. Baker. He will collect it for me if he can, then I hope to have time to go and get it. There is several troops in this place which are only passing through on their way to Cairo. Gen. Prentiss was here. So also Gen. Grant and more. They are all bound for Cairo & Kentucky where I think there will soon be fighting done.

I hope to hear from you soon. Perhaps there is a letter on the way now. I suppose Pa has returned from Crawford by this time. I received a letter from James Palmsteer saying Pa had been there. Did he collect enough to pay our taxes? I hope so but fear not quite. A number of our debtors has gone to the war so I hear. Sam Mann, Theo and Isaac has gone some other place. Ellis Johns is in Capt. Dollahan's Comp[any]. Bro. Brooks preached yesterday but I did not hear him, have not been very well for two or 3 days but feel better today. We are getting more help. Will have more time for reading and writing, not being so much confined, we will feel better ourselves. Dr. Smith has been unwell, is better now—

Dr. Bowyer is a very agreeable companion and cares for me like a brother, said at one time I should have my position if he lost his. There was a Dr. Browning here trying for one or the other and Dr. Bowyer and he had quite a talk. Dr. Bowyer does not speak to him now. He is most evidently a rascal. I have not heard from Mr. Baker for 8 or 10 days. I had supposed some of them would pay you a visit for this summer as they have usually done. I suppose, and hope, you will remain in Salem another year for another move at this time will not do. Will not pay and I think the people of S. cannot do better than keep you and you might do more by remaining. I should like to see you in Salem about Conference time but should love to spend hours or days unalloyed by the entrance of a stranger. We anticipate no danger from Rebels here now, have driven most of them to other "Sacred soil." Col. Cook's regiment came in today 8th. He being the senior commander, Col. Bayles will be superseded in command. I hardly know what to say about Amos going to Crawford on the farm. Is his general health good? If so and you can find a friend in whom you have confidence, I think it might do him good. I know his great anxiety to do something if he could only find some healthy and lucrative employment near home, I would be happy but how can he do that? I will take great pleasure in answering questions from each and every one. Write soon all of you while I remain as ever your most

Affect. son,

T. S. Hawley

Many changes occurred within the regiment and within Doctor Hawley's life by September 29 as the deteriorating relationship between Thomas Hawley and his superior officer, Doctor Thomas Smith, continued. The autocratic rule of Smith chaffed Hawley but luckily the calm hand of Doctor Eli Bowyer made the day-to-day existence acceptable. Doctor Hawley severely criticized

Smith for his slow efforts in securing proper care and stating the delay resulted in unneeded deaths.

The medical situation continued to be an arduous task for the doctors of the regiment and greater than 10 percent of soldiers were under medical treatments. The number of ill had begun to decrease slowly by the time of this letter, but typhoid fever and measles took a toll as the deaths of the soldiers testified. The soldiers were treated in a confiscated house which served as a hospital which made caring for the sick much better than previous locations.

Also of interest in the September 29 letter was the replacement of Colonel David Bayles by newly promoted Colonel Joseph Plummer. David Bayles, disappointed, was mustered out, honorably, from the army on September 30, 1861 after appealing unsuccessfully with Major General John C. Fremont, his superior officer. Newly appointed Colonel Joseph Plummer was an excellent soldier. He was born on November 15, 1861, in Barre, Massachusetts, and he was a school teacher after completing his education. In 1837, he obtained an appointment to the United States Military Academy at West Point, New York. He graduated, joined the United States Army and was commissioned as a second lieutenant in 1841. Plummer did not participate in the Mexican-American War due to illness. He served on the Texas frontier from 1848 to 1861. By the time Colonel Plummer joined the 11th Missouri Infantry he was carrying a remembrance from the Battle of Wilson's Creek, a wound that would contribute in part his death in 1862.[9]

Thomas Hawley wrote a paragraph in the September 29 letter about the condition of the war. He felt the ethical and moral values of the United States favored the Union troops and asked if the Confederates won, "Will civilization, morals, and religion be advanced?" Clearly, the Confederate victory at Lexington, Missouri, was on his mind as he blamed, not the common Union soldier for the loss, but the officers. The Battle of Lexington, or the Battle of the Hemp Bales, occurred from September 13 to 20, 1861. After the Confederate success at Wilson's Creek in August, General Sterling Price's forces marched on Lexington, Missouri, and forced the garrison of 3,500 Union soldiers to seek protection behind fortifications. On September 20, Price's men advanced on the Union troops behind mobile fortifications, hemp bales, until they were close enough for the final assault. Price forced the entire Union garrison of 3,500 men to surrender.

W. H. Mores House (contraband) Hospital
of Mo. 11th Regiment Camp Fremont, Cape Girardeau, Mo.
Sunday afternoon 3 pm Sept 29, 1861
My very dear Parents, Sisters & Bro.,
I have not heard from you since I left home, have written once to Pa, once

One. 1861

to Maria. Pa, perhaps you will think I have not been strictly faithful to my promise having only written to you once instead of twice a week. Well, I must say I could not. My duties have increased instead of diminished since I returned from Salem. Dr. Smith appears to think his duty is confined to issue orders and have them obeyed to the letter. Dr. B[owyer] left for home on last Friday night, will pass through Salem, I guess on Monday, and return on Wednesday or Thursday. [He] said would see you if [he] could. The more I see and know of him, the more I admire and esteem. But to think or contemplate the characteristics of his colleague, my feelings take the opposite course from the former.

As you see, the Hospital is changed from the old mill and two story small farm house to a private residence. The former proprietor of which is in the secesh ranks and now Uncle Sam concludes to take charge of house and furniture. So you see we live at home. Nice office, chairs, large looking glass, office in front parlor. Back—large bedstead, feather bed and hair mattress. This room I occupy with the quartermaster for the present, Dr. B. when he returns. The furniture is stacked up in this. Sliding door between it and office. Long hall back then dining room where the patients eat and runs off for the kitchen and store room and two or three out houses. 7 rooms upstairs for sick. The list is gradually decreasing just now. 4 have died since I returned—typhoid fever, one nearly well, then relapsed. The two first died on Thanksgiving day, the two last will be buried today. The whole regiment turns out in full uniform with unused arms and fire three volleys over the graves. The chaplain performs the funeral rites. We have one or two more cases of typhoid fever and I have fears for them under their present treatment. I cannot rejoice so much at our occupying of this house when I think by proper management of our Sen. Surgeon, we could have had it two months ago and perhaps saved the lives of two or three men. I hear nothing in regard to our being removed. For the last week our sick list has average "per diem" 170 men. Yesterday I was not out of the house but twice, then not far, and had not 20 minutes spare time. The day before we were running until 10 o'clock at night. Yet today when the col. called returns, he said, "You medical men must have a peach deal to do, from the sick report I see this morning." Dr. Smith said yes, he had nearly [a] hundred himself down, had it all to do now the assistant was gone.

I called to see the medical purveyor in this state at St. Louis. They don't examine medical men in this state until there is some objection found with them. You will see by the papers that we are under command of another col. or he will soon take command. I was introduced to him today and like his appearance much better than the present commander at least for good sound judgment. Col. Plummer former captain in the regular service and command[ed] with distinguished bravery at Wilson Creek. No preaching today, have not had time to go had there been any. But hope to have time to pay a visit down town tonight and if possible find out where those flowers came from. I have them yet on the mantle. We have evergreens in the yard, was called just now post haste to see a man in quarters, had serious cramps and pains in stomach.

I have written to Mr. B. once and answered a letter from James Palmsteers. I will try to write once more this week. I hope you can see Dr. Bowyer and chat with him.

I suppose the clergy of the S. Ill. Conf. will convene at Salem and deliberate on the best means and ways of promoting the moral and religious interest of Egypt. Right nobly have they performed their duty so far. The cloud of moral darkness has been gradually dispelled until now and now it is fast disappearing below the horizon and I hope never to rise again. But what! If this monster rebellion should come off victorious in the present conflict? Will civilization, morals and religion be advanced? No. For its government and their institutions are entirely adverse to the advancement of all good characteristics. It cannot. It will not. It shall not conquer. Yet we so far of the north have met with adversities on every hand. And I fear all by the mismanagement or neglect of our officers. Instead of sorrow from our defeat at Lexington, I was MAD. Price's advance on this place was known 3 weeks before his attack. They might have sent troops from Washington. There has been a number of boats passing today.

The medical purveyor from Cairo was in today and passed around the ward, said he would have things fixed up today or tomorrow. Please write soon. Give my love [to] all enquiring friends at Conference. My ever abiding, unchanging and always giving but nonetheless love to all. Divide to suit the receiver and until I return.

I remain as ever your affect. son,

T. S. Hawley

This half sheet contraband.

By October 2, the division between Thomas Hawley and Thomas Smith continued to widen as Hawley wrote he could not like his superior officer and was even considering refusing to work under his command. Hawley went farther and described Smith's medical methods as being archaic. Hawley reported the desperation of one of the patients who feared he would die and pleaded with his physician to save him. The medical staff struggled to control typhoid fever, the major illness in the regiment. Finally, Hawley also wrote of his happiness with Colonel Joseph Plummer's command of the regiment.

Headquarters U. S. Hospital Department
Camp Fremont, Cape Girardeau, Mo. Oct 2nd 1861
Dear Parents, Sisters and Bro.,

This week I write to you twice and trying in part to redeem my promise to write often. No news from home and yet I wait for each slow and uncertain mail to bring me news from "The dear ones at home." Now you are nearing one of the annual periods which is of great interest to those in the Itinerancy. Shall we be required to remove from these near and dear friends to be placed among entire strangers? Each one will scrutinize our various movements. Or will the changes be for the better? Strangers receiving us with a bro.'s kindness caring for our wants. I hope it may be so in your case. If it should be necessary for you to change which considering the present times, I think will hardly be done.

After passing through the wards, arranging and searching, giving directions to nurses I again stop to chat a while with home. I did think a call down town would be my pleasure tonight but after all dutys are performed it is after seven o'clock. All are well pleased with the change of commanders. Col. Plummer is a thorough military man of the regular army and our former col. had not the knowledge, experience or judgment that the present one has.

Thank you [a] thousand times for that nice long letter written on the 28. It just came to hand by Dr. Smith and I wish he had not got hold on it. I cannot like him & my mind is almost made not to serve with or under him. If it was not for Dr. Bowyer who I find so different, I could decide in one moment. The men all like me and some come to me first and so far I have found the officers pleasant and agreeable. Dr. B. is home on furlough, will be back this week I hope.

I read your good letter with great pleasure, it being the first news I had from home since I left. I regret that I did not write from St. Louis. I most sincerely wish you a fine, glorious, happy time during Conference. May the Lord be with that noble body of self sacrificing men and guide their deliberations. I did regret somewhat to hear that Charley & Saroney had passed into other hands. I know Ma will miss them more than any other one. Pa will soon find some other horse that will do as well as two. The fair, I do not doubt, you will or did enjoy. Wish I could have been there with you.

The same letter I speak of, I mean the last that I received from you, came to hand just in time to cheer my dreary spirits. I had the blues. I could not do a thing to please him [Dr. Smith]. I had to do this and must do that. Then I was performing the dutys of the office's steward and assistant, had not been out of the Hospital more than two minutes at a time. He prides himself on his military authority. To work this way I cannot stand but my health is improving slowly. I received a letter from L.[Lincoln] G. Swearingen this evening. He belongs to the 5th Cavalry regiment, Col. Updegraff commanding, Camp Butler, Illinois. He said he hated to leave but could not stand it any longer. Well, we will hope for the best and bear and forbear like a good soldier. We have several cases of enteric or typhoid fever and Dr. S. does not treat them properly, not according to modern practices as I perhaps told you before. We have lost 4 and will, I fear, soon lose more. I just passed round the wards. One poor fellow plead[ed] with me to stay longer with him. Said he did not want to die & could not. My unbounded love to all with two cans of kisses each. Please write often, all and each one.

T. S. Hawley

You affect. son

Between October 4 and November 24 significant events occurred in the Civil War in Missouri which impacted Thomas Hawley's life. Two battles occurred and one involved the 11th Missouri Infantry which Hawley referred to as the "gallant Mo 11th" in deference to the regiment's actions in the Battle of Fredericktown, Missouri, on October 21. In this battle, Colonel Joseph Plummer commanded the Union forces against the Southern sympathizing forces of the Missouri State Guard commanded by Brigadier General M. Jeff Thompson. Although Thompson was greatly outnumbered, he tried to lure the Union forces into an ambush. The Union forces avoided the trap and were successful in the battle. The 11th Missouri Infantry participated in the battle and received the recognition for its actions.[10] It is not known if Hawley marched with the regiment to Fredericktown and participated in the battle. The regiment lost one man killed-in-action and only a few others were wounded, but two wounds were severe. On November 24 Hawley mentioned in his letter the possibility the Union forces could take Memphis in the fall of 1861.

The other battle which occurred since Hawley's last letter was the Battle of Belmont in which Brigadier General Ulysses Grant attacked the Confederate forces of Brigadier General Gideon Pillow. On November 7, 1861, Grant attacked and overran the Confederate camp at Belmont but the Southern forces regrouped, and counterattacked Grant's force. Grant withdrew his Union troops back onto riverboats and returned to Cairo, Illinois. The casualties totaled greater than 1,400 for both the Union and Southern forces.

The fourth medical professional of the 11th Missouri Infantry was mentioned for the first time in Hawley's letter of November 24, Doctor Zeba French. Zeba French was a 23-year-old doctor who resided in Sumner, Illinois, prior to the war and he was recruited to be the apothecary for the regiment which was very helpful for Thomas Hawley. Hawley, who served variously as hospital steward, surgeon and apothecary, was grateful for the reduction in his workload in whatever manner it occurred. French was not yet a member of the medical staff of the regiment but this was the first mention he might be added. Hawley commented in the November 24 letter he felt Doctor Smith would not want to add the new apothecary because Hawley was already performing that duty. The regiment continued garrison duty into November at Cape Girardeau.

One. 1861

Cape Girardeau, Mo. Nov. 24, 1861
Sunday Afternoon

Dear Parents,

Just received your kind letter. Glad to hear all well. Was not much disappointed to hear the medical board had adjourned. I have not had much time to read but hope to have more and Dr. B. and I will read regularly and in accordance with the memorandum sent by you for which, and many other favors, I am much obliged.

There is some talk of our leaving this place. Of one thing I am quite sure that there is a expedition being fitted out for the great western floating army in connection with superior land forces. Consequently as the gallant Mo 11th has been tested, we may be called upon to participate in this movement instead of remaining inactive during the winter months. 200 seamen have gone to Cairo. A large number of rifled cannon and these also with ammunition and gun boats. All these taken in connection with other equally important movements, if the administration permits to the coming conflict. Gen. Halleck told Col. Plummer he should winter in Memphis which for winter is more pleasing than these cold hills, barren country. Yet I say that I love this city of marble and think it would be a very pleasant home. The scenery as I have before told you is fine while the commercial advantages are unbounded. Besides there is some fine and excellent folks and so far as I am acquainted, am pleased with the citizens. But there is some whose feelings, sympathies are entirely with the south, with such I have nothing to do.

I made a requisition for clothes last week. 2 pr uniform dark blue pants, 2 pr woolen drawers, 2 soldiers shirts, 2 pr socks, 1 overcoat, army blue, 1 black seal skin blanket. I purchased 1 officer's cap, 1 pr heavy kid gloves lined with lambskin. So you can see I [am] pretty well furnished with wearables this time. Oh yes, I also got one soldier's jacket and blouse which I can wear under in going out or in the office. I have a supply now of all the necessarys that I think of. May purchase a overcoat or, I mean, dark blue cloth coat. Cannot say when the paymaster will come up this way.

Nothing has occurred worth mentioning since I last wrote you, in or about this place. Dr. B. and I went to Catholic Church today. House crowded—half soldiers. Quite a fancy house, organ and all completed. You can see the front of the house in the letter I sent you which is correct.

Just now came down from Ward No. 1 having applied a blister to Pat Flin's breast. Dr. B. said Dr. pull that man's tooth and I will give you something. I pulled it in a short motion then he showed me two letters, one from you the 20th inst. Another from R. Stuz of Mt. Carmel inquiring if there was such a thing as an apothecary in the army, saying he had nothing to do. Business was stagnant and he wanted something to do. I shall answer him immediately that there is such a place in each regiment. All other regiments, of which I have an acquaintance, has one man serving in that capacity as druggist except the Mo. 11th Regt. and I have that and the duty of Hospital Steward besides. But Dr. B. and I have a man engaged to act as nurse, a young Mr. French from Lawrence County, Ills. whom when he returns we propose to install as druggist. I cannot say but I think Dr. S. will say I am the chap. But he cannot make me do more than my legitimate duties and he can find no clause in the army regulations which says the Hospital Steward must attend to pouring up medicine. So we will have a man in his place. I mean as druggist. I shall do all I can for Rudolph but have not much hopes. He says nothing about the family nor the friends in Mt. Carmel.

Dear Sister. I am much obliged for your kindness in procuring those things for me and especially that counterfeit of yourself. But where in the world can I or will get them and if we move to Columbus, Ky., I have almost a mind to take the telegraph and run up some night by Salem and St. Louis. Why don't some of Mr. B. family wright, I mean write to me. I have not heard directly from them for a long time. Folks, when will, or can, you send me your pictures? Almost daily some of the Mo. 11th pass Salem. Many have gone on furloughs and will return in the next two weeks. For the last ten days it has been quite cold. Most of our men recd. thin overcoats and jackets last week with the addition of one blanket, they are now, I think, comfortable. Ma, I love you. Amos, Fannie, all please write right soon. For those kind letters already sent, I thank you. I love the ones who sent me those newspapers I recd. All at one time, please scatter them a little. I am glad Dr. Eliott made an easy trip. Yours in love all over and up to the ears with many kind wishes, etc. I remain

Yours affectly.,

T. S. Hawley, MD

One of the most endearing facets of Thomas Hawley's letters was his love and appreciation of his family. In all his letters, he unfailingly offers his affections to his family members and often reflected on familial scenes and experiences. He constantly inquired of the activities and health of the family members. Hawley's letters also demonstrate his religious upbringing and being the son of a Methodist-Episcopal minister he strove to attend religious services whenever he could.

In Hawley's letter at the end of November, he presented a very interesting and enlightening description of the escape of Charley, an ex-slave. Charley spent two months on the run from his master in Arkansas and revealed the Confederates were training slaves in anticipation of the upcoming conflict. Charley was also a very interesting person, and being the slave of a member of the U.S. Congress he was a well-traveled individual having visited Buffalo, Chicago and Indianapolis. Though it is difficult conclusively to describe the position the soldiers of the regiment took regarding slavery, several regimental records showed a strong abolitionist leaning. Doctor Hawley wrote in his letter that despite the order of General Henry Halleck requiring escaped slaves to be removed from Union control, Charley was hired by the regiment and allowed to remain.

Thomas Hawley also wrote in his letter he would like to receive a promotion. The role of Hospital Steward was satisfactory for him, but he desired to become an assistant surgeon in a regiment. He continued happily in his current role and he was busy caring for the ill of the regiment. About 20 soldiers of the regiment had died since the regiment was mustered, and the primary causes were typhoid fever and measles. Thomas Hawley also mentioned the massing of infantry and the Union Navy as preparations were made to open the Mississippi River to Union control. He promised the Union armada would "speak in tongues of thunder."

Sunday Morning
Hospital Office Mo. 11 Regt.
Cape Girardeau, Mo. Nov 30, 1861
Dearest Friends,

I hope this epistle may find you well, happy and cheerful. And when you are seated around the family fire side, think of the absent one not regretfully, but as one of the family circle gone forth to lend a helping hand in this hour of our country's peril and you heroes & heroines who remain at home but granting permission to one whom I know you all love, to absent himself from you for months and perhaps years. Think not that you will receive no reward for this sacrifice. And in reflecting on my position remember (for the present at least) I have a pleasant comfortable home, plenty to eat and plenty to wear and better than all that, have good health. So far I feel satisfied with my position and as to my office am well pleased with it and think when we become better organized, will like it better. But at the same time I shall continue to look for and strive for higher positions. I feel a natural and honest ambition for promotion but shall do nothing dishonest to gain a higher office. I well know the best policy to pursue is to fill well the one which I now occupy and gain the friendly intercourse and confidence of those whom I meet. So far as I know and hear this point has been gained, although not especially sought. I had some hopes of my being enabled to stand an examination but now look for advancement some other way. Yet if the opportunity should come up for examination, I shall embrace it speedily. But not so quick as I would you.

The young man last spoken of in the other letter as coming to act as apothecary, Mr. French from Lawrence County, has returned. We have spoken to Dr. S., but he is not disposed to favor us anymore than can be helped.

The sick list has continued the same for some weeks. We have lost nearly twenty since first coming here. No more cases of the measles. I see they are raging in some other camps. Not so many cases of typhoid fever but more of the inflammation character, many coughing from bad colds. The officers have repeatedly spoken of preparing for winter quarters but as yet nothing definite has been done. First, they will talk about building barracks then of repairing some old mill and consequently nothing is done. It is hard to tell whether this is from pure neglect or only to deceive the men as to the character of their future aspirations. For if they go into permanent winter quarters no forward movements will be made. So, secesh can rest secure for a few months but I cannot think this is the design of the Federal Army, at least of the western department.

Several gunboats have gone down this week. Thousands of men are coming from all avenues of the great west and valley of the "father of waters" to open a free communication with the gulf. I think there can be no doubt that the greatest fresh water armada ever fitted out will soon descend the broad bosom of the mighty Mississippi and speak in tongues of thunder to the fire eaters. This armada will float directly through the heart of Rebelliondom carrying death and destruction in its wake to all who dare oppose.

While in these quarters we shall try to enjoy them to their fullest extent. But shall not make to ourselves any fair promises for fear of a sudden disappointment.

We had quite a snow storm yesterday, or rather Friday night. But yesterday the genial rays of sun induced most of it to take wings & fly away. They never have much sleighing in this climate but plenty of mud and disagreeable weather. Col. Plummer has gone on some mission to the city of Washington. May be gone 3 or 4 weeks and some think much longer but others think will return our col. The non-commissioned staff to which I belong got up a paper setting forth our good opinion of Col. Plummer wishing him success in his mission, a pleasant visit, hoping he would return to us safe and sound and our colonel.

Friday evening a big stalwart Negro stepped up to Dr. B. and asked, "Is this your Drs. surgery?" He had been sent to the hospital by the head capt. Then Dr. interrogated him. He left Arkansas two months ago. His master commenced drilling him with 750 others. Charley concluded to skedaddle. Left one night, traveled 30 miles, layed low during the day. Found some good friends who would tell him the way and gave something to eat. He came up to New Madrid. When he saw the very men whom he had drilled with, he spoke to them from a cornfield. Tried to persuade some to come with him. Could not. He passed Memphis, saw them working on gunboats & building breastworks as "high as this house." Secesh told him they would make a wind up of it this time. Charley said they were drilling a great many Negroes but the blacks would not fight if they could help it. Charley came by Greenville, saw Jeff Thompson. Came in our camp. He went from Covington, Ky. 4 years ago, was taken by a slave dealer to New Orleans, sold for $1350 to his last master Mr. Ross. Dr. B[owyer] knew his first owner in Ky., was living near a relation of his. When his straight story was told, Dr. B. told him, he was now a free man upon which intelligence he was full to overflowing with joy. We concluded to keep him. He attends chores about the office and kitchen, also attending the Dr.'s horse. We find him very ready. He went with his first master to Chicago, Buffalo, Indianapolis and attended two sessions of Congress, his master being a member. Charely is six feet, straight as a gun barrel, pleasant countenance, bushy head, showey ivorys, kind and obliging, ever ready to do. We will stand by him. Maj. Gen. Halleck to the contrary, not withstanding, and only the other day after an order was read on dress parade to send all contraband Negroes outside of the pickets, but he was before that a free man and engaged here for a compensation.

No letter last week. The orderly acting as postmaster just stepped in, pulled out two letters. I said I'll bet some for me. Generally get mine on Friday, Saturday or Sunday. But Lo! They were for Dr. Smith, none for your humble servant, told the orderly I would give a quarter for a letter. Never mind. I know some are coming. How can I get those things from St. Louis? No news from Mr. B.'s family. Thanks for those papers. But you need not send the <u>Democrat</u> nor <u>Republican</u> as I can get them much earlier here. Some boys in hospital generally buy them the day after. Much love to all whom it may concern. A word to the wise is sufficient.

Your affctly.,

T. S. Hawley

The 11th Missouri Infantry and Thomas Hawley remained in Cape Girardeau through the end of 1861. The medical staff was successful in getting the illnesses under control as much as possible, but illness and deaths as a result of disease continued throughout the war. Measles and typhoid fever appeared to finally be controlled. Doctor Thomas Smith and Thomas Hawley continued to be on bad terms and Eli Bowyer counseled Hawley to stay with the regiment. Fortunately, Doctor Zeba French had officially joined the medical staff as apothecary by December 9 despite the reluctance of Smith to accept him.

While 11th Missouri Infantry made Cape Girardeau their winter quarters, there was time for fun and love. Lieutenant John Cowperthwait found time for a wedding. Lieutenant Cowperthwait was a native Missourian and he was a 26 year-old, engineer living in St. Louis prior to entering service with the 11th Missouri Infantry. Among the members of the regiment Hawley mentioned in his December 9 letter were Lieutenant Mark Sappington, a 31-year-old minister from Clay County, Illinois; Lieutenant James Wilson, a farmer from Springfield, Illinois; and Private John Holt, a 44-year-old minister from Fairview, Illinois.[11] The influence of Hawley's upbringing was evident as he described how he was almost forced to take part in dancing. He appeared to have enjoyed his time at Cowperthwait's wedding and apologetically confessed to his family he had danced.

Camp Fremont   Dec. 9, 1861

Dear Ma & Pa, Dear Bro. and Sisters, especially the smallest. What great pleasure one sweet kiss would give your absent son and bro. But for the present such sweets are denied me so I can only enjoy them in imagination and this is so strong sometimes it almost amounts to a reality. But such counterfeit reality, only one can enjoy unless both think at once. I received yours of the 3rd inst. on last Friday night. You speak of one written on the day before that I have not received. Having so short time to prepare, got leave of absence to meet the board in Cairo beside the uncertainty of a berth and the fear of losing this. All these things I consulted with Dr. B. who knows my situation better than anyone else and has my interest at heart. We both came to the conclusion that I had better remain. But if the time would have been longer, think it most probable I would have gone. For the past few days I have had more leisure than usual, or at least, have not been so closely confined to the office. Do not have to put up medicine now as we have an apothecary, Mr. French a fine young man. Heard Mr. Brooks once yesterday. Said the other day he would send for my things at his house. Mr. B. has been unwell is now better. The sick list is decreasing. None but what I think will get well, in hospital at this time. One of the prisoners of war died last Saturday. We have had two buildings as hospitals for the past few months but will soon condense them into one. I hoped soon to be furnished here [with] ready money for purchasing butter, chickens, eggs, etc., necessities for the sick; (milk, etc.) and cannot be provided by the army quartermaster.

Lieut. Cowperthwait of Co. D was married the other day. Some of the officers gave him a reception party at his boarding house. Lieut. Wilson of Co. B and I sent notes and escorted each a lady to the house. Found the regimental band, then a sitt was formed to dance. One was wanted, therefore, I must dance. My pardners danced. I consented without thinking much about it. Lieut. Sappington of Co. D was the chief manager, as I understand, of the party. He was there but did not dance. We had a very pleasant time although I did not enjoy the dancing much but the music was fine of which we had plenty after the dancing. I enjoy society but cannot say I like or enjoy dancing, think that will be the last if I know before-hand that there will be dancing. Yet I cannot say that I regret that little hop much under the circumstances. It was at a private house in a private parlor among a few private friends. Lieut. Sapping[ton] formerly of S. Ills. Conference you well know. Mr. Holt was here, private in Co. E, Capt. Hollister commanding. If I could get off without losing my place here I would go. But guess the chance of a berth in Mo. is as good as one in Ills. For according to the Gov.['s] letter, candidates are numerous. I wish your letter had come to hand sooner. No papers for 3 to 6 days, water too low for boats to pass, four or 5 up on bars now. Please write soon and send lots of love.

Love I send you and love I give unto you. Yours aft.,

T. S. Hawley

As might be expected from Hawley's last letter of 1861 which was written three days before Christmas, his thoughts were of home and of past Christmases. The regiment recently went through an official review. Thomas Hawley also wrote of a young lady and her mother he met and his interactions with them.

Thomas Hawley also wrote the 11th Missouri Infantry was mustered into service incorrectly and there was some concern it wasn't officially a regiment. Certain records indicated the regiment only mustered 954 men and Company K did not have a required minimum of soldiers. Because the number of soldiers in Company K was below the minimum, it was disqualified as a company and the regiment officially only had nine companies instead of the required ten companies. Although, this was quickly solved by transferring some soldiers from the other nine companies to Company K, it was cause for a little excitement in the 11th Missouri Infantry. In addition to this error, Hawley also wrote he was not sworn into service yet, and this error was also quickly corrected.

[Camp Fremont Dec. 22, 1861]

Back room, arm on center table two hundred miles from you. I take up my pen and consult my muse this icy Sabbath the 22nd day of December 1861 at Cape Girardeau, Mo.

With Christmas coming and almost here I think of you and speak of you. Yes and dream of you. Thinking of the happy time we all had together one year ago. I again wish you each one and all a Merry, oh Merry Christmas. Think of the pleasant time we enjoyed with our Christmas tree and far better, each other's society, then put two or three such together and you have an idea of the Merry Christmas I wish you. Do not let my absence mar your pleasure during the Holy days. I cannot be with you. Oh, how much I wish I could if it was only to spend a few short days. But I shall try to enjoy myself and no doubt will. It is my duty, yet that shall not lessen my desire to be with you. Dear Little Evie Bell, my heart yearns for her so much and Fannie with her round, rosey face surrounded and bounded by ringlets which I love so much. But I cannot specify, for to tell half the love I have for each would require a steamboat load of letters which I have not time to write just now for our apothecary is sick and I still have all the work to do. I have not heard from you since the letter informing me that the board would meet in Cairo to examine medical applicants for surgeons. Since then there has been a grand review at this place, Gen. Rensellear, Sturgis & Sweeney, which passed off in fine order last Wednesday, a fine bright warm summer day. The Mo. 11th, Ills. 13th, Sappers & Miners, Heavy artillery comp., Cavalry comp. 2. In all 3,000 men, I suppose. I did not appear with the men or non-commissioned staff but among the spectators and finely. Lieut. Orr and your humble servant, marched with 3 young ladies to their respective homes. One of them almost took me prisoner, at least captured some booty. Young and fair, dark, hazel eyes, black hair which fell over the shoulders in beautiful ringlets. The countenance, when not animated by conversation rather sober but when speaking the eyes sparkle, the rosey lips and whole countenance eloquent and lively, yes & lovely. I called the other evening, had a pleasant chat, formed the acquaintance of the mother, found them very loyal. Said she would gladly lose all her slaves if the south would all lose theirs and she hoped they would. The mother is a widow and has lost thousands of dollars by debtors running off. During the evening pound cakes and canned peaches was brought in by a slave woman. We had some music. So the evening passed off pleasantly, I assure you. But the worst of all is this ideal of beauty is soon going to St. Louis to school with her uncle which I very much regret. Now Myra don't say that I'm gone for. It is all in fun & is not the same one I used to speak of. There was a grand ball on the <u>Memphis</u> last week. I did not go.

  The paymaster has paid off this regiment and your most obedient servant received for two months wages $47 U. S. scrip. I now have over $50 and hardly know what to do with it. But think I must send Mr. Baker some for the $20 I borrowed but will not send until I have a safe way. I would be most happy to pay you some and if you need any, I will send. I have received pay up to Oct. 31, have drawn according to their present charges $25 dollars-worth of clothing and will have to buy some more. I shall not draw any more I think for they charge us exorbitant prices which is taken out of the men's wages. They are entitled to draw $3.50 worth of clothing per month. If they exceed that amount it is subtracted from the pay you get. It has been decided that this regiment, so called, is not one in reality. Not having 10 companies with the required amount of men. Co[mpany] K has only 40–50 men therefore they have been mustered in illegally. Some of the officers have not been sworn in and cannot now get their pay. But I think it will soon be all right especially if Col. Plummer returns. We have been baffled around from pillar to post long enough. I have not been sworn in according to Gen. Halleck's orders, neither do I as yet think it necessary but I have as I suppose been mustered in and drew my pay and consider myself virtually obligated to perform the duties of my position which I can say I have done and more than I was duty bound to perform. Yet I do not regret having performed these duties.

Again I miss you my dear parents, bro. & sisters. A Merry, Merry Christmas and hope to hear from you soon and doubt not that I will ere you receive this. The news from the sea coast is encouraging and we do not think of a war with England until this rebellion is put down and when we take Columbus and they come up from the coast and capture New Orleans, the navigation of the Mississippi will be open. Then we will have the rebellion squelched. The news from this state is good. If the administration or Congress would organize some position policy in regard to slavery, its emancipation and colonization of the blacks in Central America or some equally genial clime to the constitution of the Negro, all would soon come right. And we again be at peace and harmony at home as well as abroad and the champion nation of the world. I have perfect confidence in the ways and means of providence for I think He has this war in His hands and is on our side. No church today. Raining nearly all the time. Hospital remains full, some cases of pneumonia. Myra, I will send you a piece of music if I can get it. Harry has those things that Miss Mc. brought down to him. He will send the first chance. Much love to Ma, Pa, Myra, Amos, Fannie and last but not least Evie Bell, is sent by your most affectionate son & bro.,

T. S. Hawley

Thomas Hawley's final letter of 1861 was written on December 22, 1861. This was a fateful year for the young physician and for the country. Hawley recorded his efforts to gain a medical position with a Union regiment and he was successful through the series of events which resulted in traveling to various locations—Belleville, Rolla, St. Louis, and Cape Girardeau. He was a Hospital Steward in the one the most effective fighting regiments in the Union Army in the Civil War, and he was surrounded by good friends and acquaintances. Even though his relationship with Doctor Thomas Smith was not good, he had a good friend and mentor in the level-headed and greatly respected Doctor Eli Bowyer.

Throughout the year the country struggled with the terrible state of affairs and clearly the breach that had occurred was not repairable before good men and women would pay the ultimate sacrifice for their country. The resolution to the war would not occur for four years. A young doctor in the 11th Missouri Infantry was only one cog and part of the large machine determined to ensure the United States would not be permanently pulled apart.

Two

1862

Cape Girardeau, Corinth, Columbus and Holly Springs

The new year found Doctor Thomas Hawley and the 11th Missouri Infantry in Cape Girardeau, Missouri, where the activities of the regiment were concentrated on making the city impregnable to attack from the Confederate Army or Navy. The regiment served as part of the brigade commanded by Colonel Joseph Plummer and by all indications, Plummer was well respected and efficient. There was also great pride in the regiment as Captain William Stewart, Company K, recorded in a letter he sent to his parents, "Our regiment (the Eleventh United States Volunteer of Missouri) has quite a name for courage and fighting ability — and they will no doubt be assigned important work to do."[1] As was often in the case of many newly formed regiments in the Civil War, sanitation and hygiene were important aspects of camp life because the spread of disease was often quick and disastrous. During the first four months of service the regiment recorded twenty-six soldiers died of diseases, including measles, chronic diarrhea, typhoid fever, pneumonia and other various maladies. Two additional men were killed-in-action.

In Hawley's letter of February 9, 1862, he cited the recent Union victory at the Battle of Fort Henry along the Cumberland River on the Kentucky-Tennessee border. On February 6, Brigadier General Ulysses Grant in conjunction with Flag Officer Andrew H. Foote coordinated an attack against an earthen fort commanded by Confederate Brigadier General Lloyd Tilghman. Most of the Confederate garrison escaped and moved to Fort Donelson about ten miles away. Grant and Foote attacked Fort Donelson on February 14 and 15 and were successful in capturing the fort. These were significant victories. Once Fort Donelson was captured by Grant, the Southern forces were unable

Two. 1862

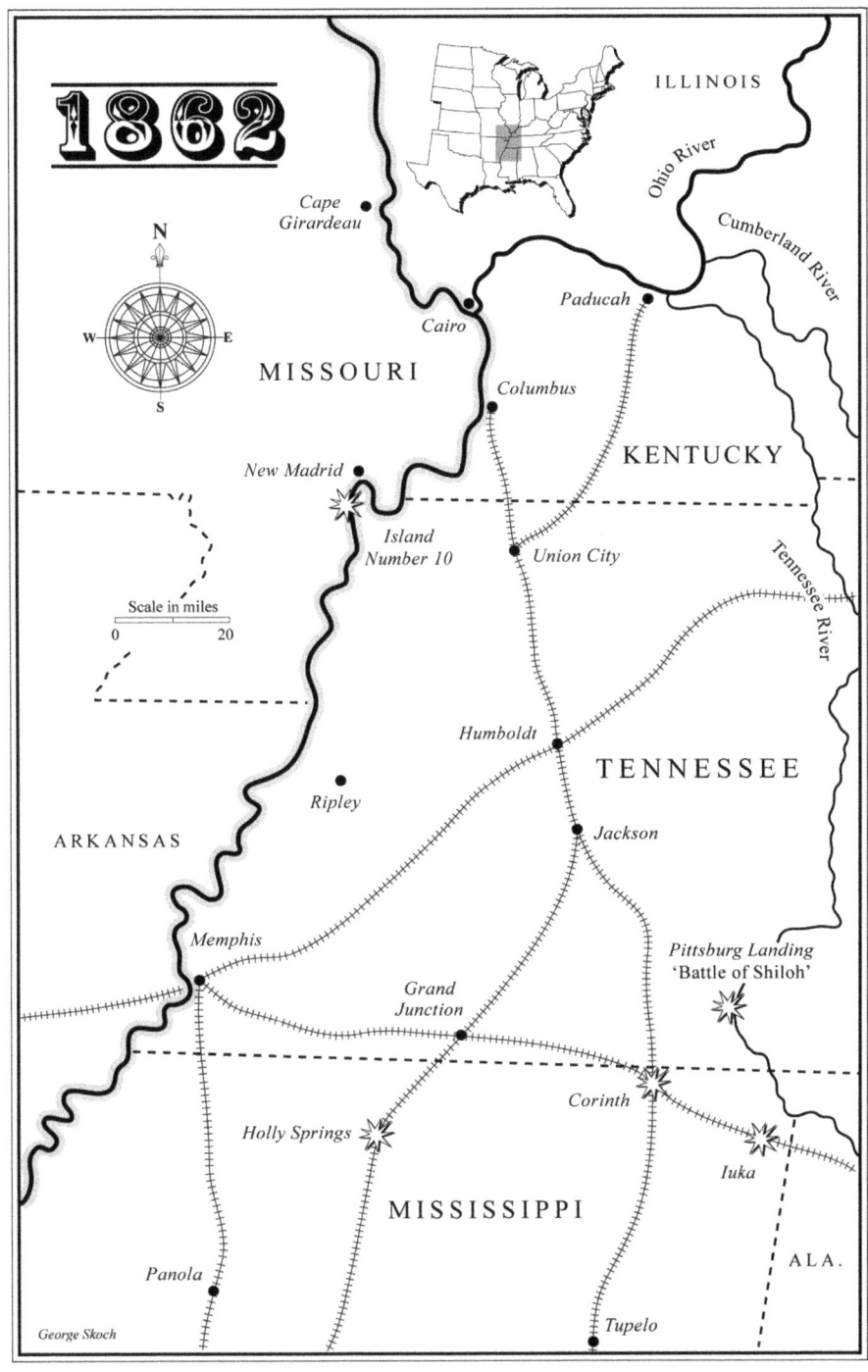

to maintain their strategic position in southern Kentucky and middle Tennessee. The valuable river systems, including, the Tennessee and Cumberland Rivers, and the railroad lines in this area were available for use by Union troops.

For Thomas Hawley, he had labored for the past six months under his difficult superior officer, Doctor Thomas Smith. Doctor Smith was 25 years older than Hawley and Hawley's impression of his superior was he was autocratic, inflexible and had not kept up with modern medical methods. Smith's leadership caused Thomas Hawley to seek a post with another regiment and only Assistant Surgeon Doctor Eli Bowyer's support kept him with the regiment. However, Thomas Hawley was pleased and surprised when in February 1862 Smith left his post with the regiment. Doctor Thomas Smith, who officially resigned on April 4, 1862, stated his reason for leaving the regiment was due to the extreme "labors of the past two months having so impaired my health, as to render it necessary that I should have some relaxation from active duty for a time..."[2]

Hawley's February 9 letter included a discussion regarding contraband slaves, which were runaway or captured slaves; and at this point in the war, these slaves were still the legal property of their owners although they were separated physically. It wasn't until March 1862 when the United States government forbade the return of these persons to their previous owners. The handling of the slaves was a very sensitive issue in February 1862 and Hawley recorded the 11th Missouri's Lieutenant Colonel William Panabaker had sent a contraband slave to his home in Lawrence County, Illinois with disastrous consequences. As described by Hawley, the reception to this arrival by some Illinois residents resulted in the man escaping to Canada to secure his freedom.

Hospital, Mo. 11th Regiment, Camp Fremont
Cape Girardeau, Mo. February 9th 1862
Dear Ma, Pa, Sisters and Bro.,

I did not hear from you last week as I usually do. But doubt not a letter was sent but it must have come to a halt some place above. Boats are passing in quick succession for the last 3 days filled with troops which smacks of business not far in the future. The 17th Ills., bag and baggage, left this place yesterday for Fort Henry as they say—

Glorious news wasn't it, the capture of Ft. Henry in Tennessee. Once more that fine emblem of liberty floats defiantly on the soil of Tennessee. As Maj. Gen. Halleck says, "and there it will float forever," and so slowly but surely we fulfill the steps as indicated in that able document—the president's message. England has quieted down and is satisfied. The rebel generals and papers see the fatal coil and almost feel its fearful noose. All are despondent. The boys say six boats passed this place today all ladened with troops for "Dixie land."

My throat has been sore for some days but does not amount to anything dangerous.

No special news in this department. I have found Col. Plummer's lady very pleasant and sociable. He is beloved by all. Yesterday [he] gave orders for inspection to come off 10 o'clock Saturday instead of 10 o'clock Sunday and preaching twice each Sunday instead of once, at 10 A.M. & 3 P.M. We had been preaching at 3 P.M. and only once.

I have answered all your letters except perhaps one of Myra's and one of Pa's or rather a question of his. It does my heart good to hear that your spiritual blessings are great and notwithstanding the wild rages of war with all its exciting and demoralizing influences. Stars are being added to your crown almost daily and will not

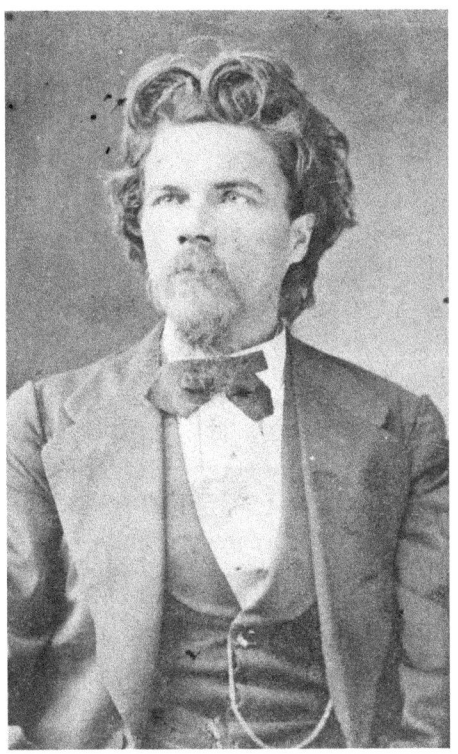

Thomas S. Hawley, 1873 (Missouri History Museum, St. Louis, Missouri).

those of the family, who with you have born the "heat and burden of the day," have a large share of the divine blessings. I hope and pray and trust they may. Oh, what eternal blessings await those who have come up through great tribulations- the family faithful. I have a hope that it will be my happy lot to greet you all inside the pearly gates of the New Jerusalem. I pray we may in the Eternal City, as here, form an undivided family. My heart leaps with joy to hear Br[other] Amos is on the only sure path to happiness. That he studys his bible much is a sure indication of his following its precepts. Dr. B[owyer] and I, as you have already heard, try to read our bible at least once a day. And attend Church as often as we can. Our position is very fortunate. We seldom hear any profane swearing and need not allow it about the hospital, at least by the hospital attendants over whom we have control. I distribute books and pamphlets through the wards when I can get them. It does the men good. They have not confidence enough in the Chaplain to read his tracts or books. When I go through the wards I joke with those who are convalescent and see to the wants of the sick and needy.

Dr. B. says he will do all he can for my promotion. He went to see Col. Murdock who has over 300 cavalry but found out there was two or three applicants of the col.'s acquaintance. The men are mostly from this part of the state, are rough but good hearted fellows. Many have been driven from their homes. Have lost all they had. I spoke of them in my letter last month. I hope and think I will be promoted yet. When is the examining board of Ills.? When do they convene again? Where is Dr. Greene and Dr. Elliott? There is a string of questions for you.

A little contraband about 7 or 8 years old came to the hospital a few days ago and says he wants to stay, that his master Jno. Bedford is in the south and that they scold him at home and he didn't want to go back. Says that he belongs to me. Can black boots, chop wood, carry wood chips and water, is a bright little fellow. I hardly know what to do with him. If those secesh and pro-slavery stay-at-home cowards in Ills. would not make so much fuss, I would send him to you, then he could be civilized and educated and perhaps become a missionary and in turn could save you many steps. Col. Panabaker sent a darky home and the vile traitors there raised a great storm and formed a committee to paint on the raiment of color and politely invite[d] him to skedaddle and he left for Canada.

The col. has always been a democrat but when they go to war they soon become abolitionized, at least some do and I hope all may do the same. Then we may look for a speedy termination of this gigantic Civil War.

We may soon leave this place. All to us is unknown. Dr. Smith is now past surgeon and that will increase our labors. We have a house full, still have not lost any for some weeks. I hope Evie Bell is now well and so also all the rest. Some cases of measles and mumps now in hospital. Some say smallpox in Jonesboro. Don't think it's true. Some mud just now. Dr. French, Lieut. Orr and I called at the Catholic college, found the students pleasant fellows, gay and happy, formed the acquaintance of one who knew Mr. B. and family in town. He was well posted.

I have not had an opportunity to send Mr. B. that $20. Almost afraid to trust the mail but will soon if he don't get it some other way.

I often wish some of you could come to see me. Much unalloyed love, I send each.

Write soon.

Affctly. Your son & bro.,

T. S. Hawley MD
Hospital Steward
11th Regt. Mol. Vol.

The 11th Missouri Infantry left Cape Girardeau in late February and traveled to Commerce, Missouri, to join in the Army of the Mississippi's offensive on New Madrid, Missouri, and Island Number 10. The Confederate Army had selected Columbus, Kentucky, to be the primary military obstacle on Mississippi River south of the Union-held Cape Girardeau, Missouri. Once Fort Donelson and Fort Henry fell into Union hands, the Union Army was in a position to surround and capture the Confederate stronghold at Columbus. The Confederate Army abandoned Columbus before this could happen. The next significant Southern fortified position on the Mississippi River was Island Number 10 which was a large island in the middle of the Mississippi River and just up-river from New Madrid, Missouri. Major General John Pope led his Army of the Mississippi to this location with the intent of removing the Confederate resistance at New Madrid and Island Number 10.

Doctor Thomas Hawley and the 11th Missouri Infantry arrived at New Madrid in early March 1862 and participated in the siege. The 11th Missouri as part of the Fifth Division was detached about five miles south of New Madrid to Point Pleasant, Missouri, on March 6, 1862. Brigadier General Joseph Plummer's Fifth Division was given the duty of preventing any Confederate naval or ground forces from relieving the siege from the south. The siege continued until April 8 when the Southern forces surrendered.

During the month of March into early April, the regiment slept in the outdoors and at the end of the siege the soldiers of the 11th Missouri were suffering the affects of exposure to the elements. By April 8, Doctor Hawley and Doctor Eli Bowyer were dealing with numerous medical problems with double digit reports of men sick from each company. Most of the diseases were a result of the living in the cool, damp conditions the soldiers experienced during the siege and only one man in the regiment suffered an accidental wound which resulted in the loss of some of his toes. During the first three months of 1862, another eighteen soldiers of the regiment died due to disease.[3] In May, the newly appointed regimental surgeon of the 11th Missouri Infantry was Doctor Melancthon Fish. The thirty-four-year old Fish was born in Delaware County, New York. As with many of the physicians in the regiment, he began his career as a school teacher and he lived in various locations including Texas. He also was employed as a tutor at the Wesleyan Seminary in Michigan in 1847 and 1848. The versatile Doctor Fish served for six years in China as vice-consul.[4] Fish was a talented, highly energetic and excellent physician. The relationship between Fish and Hawley was good and there were no unfavorable remarks from Thomas Hawley in his letters like ones made in regard to Doctor Thomas Smith.

Thomas Hawley traveled with his regiment down the Mississippi River after the capture of Island Number 10 to a spot along the river called Mosquito Point, Arkansas. By all indications the location was aptly named because of the numerous, large and abundant creatures. The regiment next traveled up the Mississippi River and along the Cumberland River and participated in the siege of Corinth in April and May 1862. The Battle of Shiloh was fought on April 6 and 7, 1862, and the Union Army seized the strategic initiative against the Confederate forces in northern Mississippi. Three Union armies, the Army of the Mississippi, the Army of the Ohio, and the Army of the Tennessee, converged on the entrenched Confederate forces at Corinth, Mississippi. Doctor Hawley's 11th Missouri Infantry lost three men killed and another twenty-two wounded during the actions around Corinth. In late May 28, the Confederate forces abandoned Corinth and the Union Army pursued them until June 12 when they returned northward to the Corinth area.

Camp Near Corinth, Miss.
June 27, 1862
Dear Sister [Myra],

Your earnest plea to write soon has been heard. I proceed to comply immediately and am again at your feet, i. e., in imagination asking not if you are engaged or how soon can I visit you but rather to hold a pleasant tête à tête with your own sweet self. I love you, oh so much. Did you ever hear those three words before, if so did they sound sweetly to your ears? You say stop quizzing and go on with the pretty talk. Well, you did right in stopping the correspondence but wrong in continuing it so far without throwing out 64 pd. hints, that in accordance with your feelings all epistolary communication would cease immediately. Yet I suppose it was some fun. Well about Bob, does he still continue his messages? It is a treat to read one of his [letters]. They are full of fun oddities, jokes, queer sayings, etc. I suppose he is destined to live the life of single blessedness, notwithstanding his gallantry and handsome face. Well, nearly all of our friends in Olney have seceded and yet there is plenty of time for us to wait for our hero and heroines. But then I tell you confidentially I came near finding mine in that same old town a [illegible] month ago. One rainy day after school hours I took a pleasure trip into the country (a queer time you say). Bro. was driving and by his side sat a buxom lassie with rosey cheeks & fair hair. But by my side was another far different of medium height and graceful form dressed tastefully but not richly beautiful, wavy hair which if let alone and not confined, fell over the fair brow and neck in silken ringlets not dark as the raven's wing but a fair dark brown. Her countenance at first sight rather sad or thoughtful. But when lit up by the theme of conversation all was lovely and highly interesting, then the depths of those pure dark hazel orbs. To see was but to love.

You, Myra, have seen her but not often, yet know her well. I'll tell you some time her name, but not now. Knows nothing of my sentiments, indeed, I hardly know them myself, but feel queer. Now tell me of your hero or must you wait until he returns from the battlefield all covered with glory? This is a terrible place, such horrid oaths and vulgar epithets and but a few are exempt. A brave few are.

The weather is warm, rather hot. We are getting along well. My health is good, So is Jos. & Robt., Frenchies, Freds and Dick, but my most cherished friend, Dr. Bowyer, is quite unwell and has been for two weeks, is still confined but improving slowly, has mild typhoid fever. I hope he soon will be able to go home and see his wife & children. The health of the regiment is improving under whose treatment? Last Sunday 101, now 75 sick in quarters, sent them to Genl. Hospital. Finley Notestine, 2nd Sergeant in Co. E, sends his compliments, is well and looks well. Came near having sun stroke on one of our long marches from Boonville, but I soon cured him up. Capt. Hollister by whom I sent home 50 dollars left last Tuesday for Olney and his merry, many spring so I hear.

Old Bonypart, strange to say since I cannot draw rations for him, is improving, looks much better. All remains quiet at our old camp. Please give my l__e and compliments to the Miss Scotts, Miss E. Merritt, Mattie Prinn, the Miss Eberman, Angie Stookey and all your correspondence & friends generally. But don't say anything about my heroine for I tell you it all. So give my compliments to Mollie Hersha, etc. How is Fannie, I know she must be improving greatly. And little Evie Belle, those sweet messages she sent to me, I shall never forget. So sensible for her, or one of her years. Kiss her often for me and give my best wishes and purest love to all, Ma, Pa, Fannie, E. Bell, Dear Brother and retain a Sister's portion in your own keeping. But write soon and answer all the questions for your affectionate Bro.

T. S. Hawley

On July 20, 1862, the 11th Missouri Infantry was camped at Clear Creek near Corinth, Mississippi. Although the surgeons were not involved in the direct combat with their enemies, they still marched and rode along with the regiment as it traveled from one location to another. During the battles the regimental surgeons were located close to the fighting to provide medical assistance to any of the soldiers who were wounded. Almost a year after the regiment formed, the medical professionals were accustomed to constantly attending to the needs of the soldiers. The regiment camped near Corinth on July 20, 1862, which provided an opportunity for the soldiers to rest and recover. There were approximately 525 soldiers present for duty with 11th Missouri at this time and only five men were sick enough to be placed in the hospital although another 60 suffered from a variety of ailments.[5] Throughout the war, Hawley would be closely attached to his family and he took the opportunity to tease his sister in a letter about her affinity for shoes by suggesting she might even want to marry a shoemaker.

Camp 11th Regt. Mo. Vols. July 20 [1862]
Darling Sister Myra,

How often the thought of home with all its attractions come before the soldier's mental vision, daily, hourly, even in the thickest of the strife or in the still and starry night. Almost every moment of these periods, he is wandering up and down the pleasant shade of the old door yard and all around are loved ones. But soon he finds that he is yet a soldier enduring the hardships and fatigues, fighting to maintain the institutions of our country, of freedom and liberty. Oft such am I, though you may say I do not fight. Yet I think the same is to labor in the cause — protect, help and care for the sick & wounded, not shrinking from the path of duty if it is one of danger.

Well, how soon do you think of housekeeping or presiding as mistress of a hotel. It appears you have been engaged. I — to — Hadn't you better engage a shoemaker. You know Pa used to advise that you should marry one of that profession? Have you got a good pair of shoes now? If not, you perhaps better have your measures taken. Well now, Fannie was naughty to tell on her poor little housekeeper. Have you the audacity to ask [for] another letter in confidence after exposing all the sacred secrets of the first. Nary time, my dear. I will defer them until I shall have the felicity of unfolding them to my lady as the morning sun unfolds by kissing the sweet rosey leaves and dries up all the pearly dew drops. But you may tell me whom you thought it was and if your guess was right, why — well —

Health better at this camp. We now have three large fine hospital tents nearly as large as your parlor, 14 × 16, eleven feet high in middle and four at sides. Only 5 sick in hospital and near sixty in quarters. Dr. Bowyer has just returned and is well. Had a fine time in Olney, saw Dr. N. Hawley only a few moments. F. Notestine, health is good as usual, saw Leander Johnson a few days ago, is well, has picture of a nice lady & child. Well, please write often and give my compliments to all inquiring friends.

Your affct. bro.,
T. S. Hawley

The August 1862 undated letter written to Fanny Hawley holds few historical items, but the letter revealed the affection and support Thomas provided for his family despite his absence. Helen Francis (Fanny) Hawley was born in 1848 and was about 14 years old at the time this letter was sent. The letter served as an encouragement for Fanny to think of more mature things and to work hard on her studies.

[August 1862]
Camp Gaylord 11th Regt. Mo. Vols.

Darling Sister Fanny,

> *My dear little miss*
> *Oh, I'd like to give you a kiss*
> *One, two, three or four*
> *If you'll cry, I'd kiss more*
>
> *Then your ginnie castle*
> *And I'd have a wrestle*
> *I should pull his ears*
> *And he would shed tears*

The rest of this beautiful piece of manuscript tumbled over the shelf in the back of my brain and I regret to say has never been found. Evidently a great loss.

A man is generally pardoned for bad writing but a young lady never, especially when in correspondence with young gents. But brothers will always excuse, yet would be too happy to see school misses improving. And now, my dear little sister, do please strive hard to improve in all your studys. Press each golden moment into service and make it furnish for you some jeweled thought. By little effort you can soon exceed all your mates. Remember you are almost a young lady in years. Please try hard to be older in mind, thought, ideas, etc. At your time of life, time is precious. I am confident you possess rare genius for composing. Please write to me often. Each one will not advise so much as this. I hope sometime you may be able to graduate. I shall help you.

Run and romp and play, when you do play, but when you study, study hard.

I wish you had a little pony to ride upon. The exercise is so fine and delightful. It's a poor plan to build castles in the air only to throw them down again. Children do that with blocks. Do you play with blocks? Well now, my dear sister, write often when others write to me and tell me all your thoughts, desires, wishes. Please do. Your most

Affectionate bro.,

T. S. Hawley

The fully medically qualified Doctor Thomas Hawley had served as a hospital steward in the 11th Missouri Infantry for over a year by the time his August 10 letter was penned. It was apparent from his letters he had a genuine affection for Doctor Eli Bowyer who held the rank of assistant surgeon of the regiment and his letters revealed Hawley had many friends within the regiment. However, he wanted a higher rank and position of authority and the appointment to a post of assistant surgeon. None of the letters written at this point in war recorded his relationship with the new regimental surgeon, Doctor Melancthon Fish. Prior to the letter on August 10, 1862, Doctor Eli Bowyer made a formal request on behalf of Thomas Hawley to Colonel Joseph Mower, commander of the 11th Missouri Infantry, to be granted leave to meet with the Board of Examiners as a step to his promotion to the rank of assistant surgeon.[6] The August 10 letter was the request for a formal examination for that purpose.

Camp Gaylord
11th Regt. Mo. Vols.
August 10th 1862
Dr. Nogen President of the Board of Examiners of Mo.
Dear Sir,

I desire a leave of absence and an order for examination and appeal to you as an old friend of my preptor Jas. A. Roman of Belleville, Ills. He gave me a letter of introduction to you. I called a few times but spent more time studying than visiting. I graduated at the St. Louis Medical [College], have references as to my qualifications for military service. Have been in this regt. since August 6th 1861, enlisted as hospital steward, served 5 months as asst. surgeon. Most of it had entire charge. All of which I have certificates for. If you can possibly comply with this request, a great favor will be conferred.

Most respectfully yours,
T. S. Hawley M.D.

Many changes occurred from August to the Hawley's next letter in November 1862. He left his post in the 11th Missouri Infantry and was promised an appointment as assistant surgeon in the 111th Illinois Infantry. During the three months between the letters, Doctor Hawley spent some of the time with his family in Illinois before joining his new regiment. The 111th Illinois Infantry was mustered into service on September 18, 1862 at Salem, Illinois, and the regiment was organized under the command of Colonel James S. Martin. The regiment originally consisted of 11 companies from Marion, Clay, Washington, Wayne and Clinton counties in Illinois. After being mustered into service the regiment remained in Salem until October 31 when it moved to Cairo, Illinois, and then to Columbus, Kentucky, where it remained until March 1863. The regiment moved from Cairo in the side-wheeled steamer, the *Maria Denning*, to Columbus, Kentucky, about 30 miles south of Cairo on the Mississippi River. Brigadier General Jefferson C. Davis commanded the Union troops at Columbus and the regiment worked on the construction of fortifications and railroads while serving on garrison duty.

Hawley left the 11th Missouri Infantry just before that regiment fought two bloody battles at Iuka on September 19, 1862, and Corinth, Mississippi, on October 3 and 4, 1862. The regiment lost about 150 men during these battles but gained positive recognition for its ability to battle the Confederates.

Columbus, Ky. Nov 1st / 62
Dear Parents,
Once again our communications must be through the medium of pen, ink and paper. My second parting with those I hold most dear was harder ten-fold than the first. I cannot account for it except that I knew in reality and by sad experience what it was to be separated from you. The 111th left Salem Thursday about 8 o'clock and a sad parting to nearly all it was. Fountains of tears was shed but all bore it bravely. We left Tonti about 11 o'clock and arrived at Cairo at 12 am which last place we left 10 today and arrived here safe. Expect to leave for Jackson at 4 in the morning. We have a few sick on [our] hands. Mr. Simmonson is better. Nothing new that I know of. Some expect a fight soon. I do not. If we remain at Jackson long, I will try and see the 11 Mo. I sent you the papers from Salem that I had to Newton. It is near 8 o'clock at night. Our tent is pitched on the banks of the Mississippi in this famous town and in sight of that bloody field, Belmont. I bid adieu to the Salemites without shedding many tears. Saw Mr. Celiff at Tonti [Station]. Old cap, old coat, old man unless it was an optical allusion. Oh yes. We came down on the <u>Maria Denning</u>. She has been repaired to some extent. The 72nd Ills. is stationed at this place. One of the Board of Trade Chicago regt.
We got a nice dispensing wagon, traveling apothecary shop from the medical purveyor today. Saw 5 or 6 hundred rebel prisoners at Cairo today taken at Perryville. The weather remains pleasant. I shall try and keep you posted and someone please write often to your Doc. Give my love to all the friends diluted with compliments. But to each member of the [family], take it pure and unalloyed.
Yours in haste and full of affections for all,
T. S. Hawley

Although Thomas Hawley had left the 11th Missouri Infantry to join the 111th Illinois Infantry, his exact duties within the new regiment were somewhat unclear; but he was appointed second assistant surgeon for the 111th Illinois Infantry. He reported to Doctor James Phillips, regimental surgeon, of the new regiment and found his initial responsibilities were the medical care of the soldiers who were in the hospital and also those soldiers who worked on the railroad. Despite being with the 111th Illinois Infantry, Hawley did not lose touch with the men of the 11th Missouri who at that time, were involved in Grant's movement toward Vicksburg. Grant began his Central Mississippi Campaign in November 1862 with the intent of capturing the Confederate fortress at Vicksburg commanded by Lieutenant General John Pemberton. Grant sent his troops along two routes. The first route was taken by Major General William Sherman who moved downstream from Memphis to the Yazoo River just north of Vicksburg. Grant's other wing moved south along the railroads through north central Mississippi, and the 11th Missouri Infantry was part of the overland assault. It is important to note Hawley's strong connection to the 11th Missouri Infantry because he would rejoin this regiment in the spring of 1863. Meanwhile, the 111th Illinois Infantry remained garrisoned at Columbus, Kentucky.

Columbus, Ky.
Head Quarters Medical
Department 111th Ills. Vols. Nov. 15, 1862

Dear Parents and all others to whom this may come greeting, as I expect to be very busy tomorrow my usual day of writing. I came to this conclusion to improve this pleasant evening after the labors of the day in a short chat with the dear ones at home. I wrote you one day this week but cannot say whether I directed it to Olney or Robinson as I intended. I received yours written just before leaving Olney. I hope the children will write often this winter. I shall hope to hear from you in Robinson before many days. The weather has been quite pleasant for the past 4 or 5 days only, or rather too much dust on this bleak hill for pleasure or comfort. Capt. Myers of Co. B thinks of tendering his resignation as he cannot be satisfied in his present position as it is far different from what he expected to occupy and indeed was most faithfully promised that of Chaplain until the day the other was appointed. So you see what comes of promises and must not be surprised if others are used in the same unkind manner. As yet I know nothing of my appointment, have spoken to no one except Dr. Phillips. I shall soon do so though, I assure you. Have seen two or three of the 11th Mo. since I have been here. The regt. is now near Holly Springs which the rebels have evacuated and crossed the Tallahatchie and I think will stop short of Grenada or perhaps Jackson, Tenn., I mean, Miss., the capital of that state, I believe. If so, Memphis will be made the base of operations and this place will be played out as the boys say. But some think we may remain here all winter and I am sorry to say, seem well pleased with the idea. For my part, all my hopes in the maintenance of the Union are based upon the campaign of this winter or of the next six months. For I tell you our traitorous neighbors at home are more to be feared than the open and armed enemies of the country in the southern states. But thank the God of nations, the dark cloud is and must disappear before the energy and bloody sacrifices of an agonized nation in this terrible struggle for life. The Col., adjt. [adjutant] and Dr. Phillips, all left for New Madrid last night and will not return for some days. Two companies F and G are there, are doing well. I attend those in hospital and the companies below on the railroad.

I heard from Hall two days ago, all well and doing well or better. Going to [the] north a more healthy portion of the city. Harry is coming this way and on to Memphis with Col. Bissel. All the friends well.

For the present, good night. Much love to all, Kiss Evie and Rose and Tady for me.

Yours affctly.,

T. S. Hawley

PS

Pa, if you can find a good young horse and can pay in notes, I will pay you the money soon. Soon as the pay master comes this [way]. I must have a horse and I think that would be the best way to get one. Think of it and write soon. Mr. Walker will preach for us today, the Chap[lain] having gone to New Madrid with the Col. & Dr.

Yours,

T. S. Hawley

Thomas Hawley noted in his letter of November 23 the movement of troops as the advance on Vicksburg was proceeding closer to the fortified city on the Mississippi River. Probably the most significant observation Thomas Hawley made in his November 23 letter was in reference to the friction between Ulysses S. Grant and Major General John McClernand. McClernand, a native of Kentucky, grew up in Shawneetown, Illinois. He was a newspaper man, legislator, congressman, and businessman and he was well liked by the soldiers from Illinois. McClernand served under Grant at Belmont, Shiloh and Corinth. In 1862 Lincoln gave McClernand the authority to launch an attack on Vicksburg, but Grant began his campaign before McClernand arrived on the scene. Both men were ambitious and friction was the outcome. In 1863, the situation between the men deteriorated to such a state Grant relieved McClernand of his command because he did not perform well in the assault on Vicksburg and because McClernand so publicly expressed his displeasure with the Union Army and its officers for not supporting his attacks at Vicksburg.

Hawley's letter also described the poor conditions the ex-slaves endured and these people soon found freedom had its price as they struggled to survive.

Head Quarters Medical
Dept. 111th Ills. Vol. Columbus, Ky.
Nov 23rd 1862

Dear Parents and little fokses,

For two long mortal weeks I have no communications from "the dearest spot on earth to me." Surely the Rebels have not cut off our messages. We are not so far away. Persons come from Salem to this place in 12 hours. I am hoping we will be moved farther south. The weather will be more pleasant and we may have a hand in opening up navigation on this river and who could be engaged in a more glorious enterprise?

Gen. Grant has been here for the last two or three days, is amassing a large force at or near Holly Springs and will, I have no doubt, try to pluck the laurels awaiting Gen. McClernand in the capture of Vicksburg. Gen. Grant is jealous of our western Mc. and will keep him down if possible. When will our generals lay aside all political jealousies and advance to deal death blows only for the Union? Never I fear. Such is human frailty and unbounded ambition. The sooner Old Abe cuts off all such heads as do not carry out his orders to the letter, the better for the Union. Blacks are still coming to this place in droves and are living in holes and hollows and vacated secesh houses. They are [moving] that staple to this port in large quantities which made slavery so popular. I saw three steamers laden with it today and lots more on the wharf.

There is quite a flood of passengers on the daily trains at this place and almost every day brings with it 1000 men to do battle for the Union. Today the 126 Ills. Vols. passed this place bound for Jackson. Roads are in fine order and weather pleasant. Push the war into Africa. Maj. Mayberry and Dr. P. [will] send for their ladies soon if we remain. The 72nd Ills. Vols. left this place for LaGrange last week, had been here nearly two months. And the two companies of this Regt. which have been at New Madrid, came back last Friday. Companies D and B still on the railroad and I must go to see them tomorrow. Capt. Myers has his wife here. His resignation was not approved. The Chap. was in camp today but did not preach but got Lieut. Walker to administer the word. We have two very sick men, Mr. Lewis from near Salem and Mr. Smith near Middleton. The rest are able to travel. We expect to occupy a new house soon.

All is bustle and confusion today. No Sunday is known and I think it need not be so. Cannot get late[st] news, a paper today of the 21st. Well, how about your trip to Crawford? How did you all enjoy it enjoy it? And when is Uncle Mathew's folks coming from Columbus, Ohio? And will Florence come back with you? What will Fannie study this winter and what business will you engage in? What do you think, you ens? Please write and give all the news. Speak low, Sis may hear. Mr. Burrows is at this place on a visit to his brother. Only saw him for a short time. Will remain a few days. To all the friends, send love and complements. We are living in a large hospital tent and find it pleasant. Goods of all kinds are enormous[ly] high. Please write immediately.

Your affct. son & bro.,

T. S. Hawley

As the month of December began, Thomas Hawley was lamenting the lack of communication from home and as a result indicated, jokingly, he was considering a "French furlough" which was a term used to describe desertion. His most recent letter from home included Johnny cakes, fried cornmeal bread, and also a newspaper. On December 7, Hawley was still stationed at Columbus, Kentucky, with the 111th Illinois Infantry and he watched the troops move southward. He correctly supposed his regiment would remain throughout the winter garrisoned at Columbus.

Clearly, in Hawley's letter of December 7, he was been promised a place in the regiment, but the promise did not meet his expectations. He stated, "cause to fear, promises with him are worth nothing." This presumably was in reference to Doctor James Phillips, but Hawley didn't elaborate on the issue and continued to discuss the war. However, Thomas Hawley had suddenly found his place within the regiment untenable.

The ever frugal Doctor Hawley avoided the officer's mess because of the charge of $4.00 per week and he and Doctor John K. Rainey began their own private mess which he described in detail, including a recipe for camp hash.

Head Quarters Med. Dept. 111th Ills.
Columbus, Ky. Dec. 7th 1862

Dear Parents,

On this bright Sabbath morning my anxiety was relieved by the arrival of your kind messenger of the 23rd ultimo, the first one for two weeks with the exception of those fine ones written by sister and Coz Sallie which came just in time to prevent my taking a French furlough. Also a small package of Johnny Cakes by mail in a newspaper and I could not think with certainty who it was from but opened it with great care when no one was near, supposing it was a bouquet. You may judge of my surprise when I saw two or three cakes.

Of course long ere this, you are safely housed in our own little home in Olney. Only think what a great pleasure that is, one of which we have been deprived for many years but I hope will not soon again.

I am truly glad to hear that Pa's health is much improving and that Amos is so well and you all had so pleasant a visit to Crawford and among the relatives. Nothing was said of Uncle Mathew's visit or rather intended visit from which I suppose, he did not come out at all. What was the nature of Dora's illness?

Well about that horse. Without [Unless] you find a very good one, young, good riding animal at a fair price, you need not purchase. Use your own good pleasure and all will be well. I think we will remain here until the waters are troubled when we may pass to the sunny South with Gen. McClernand to the tune of Dixie. There is now several regiments at this place and more coming. Some will go on. Gen. Grant, I think, has all the men he wants for present purposes. Negroes are still coming in and are thick all around town. I wish I could send you one. I know you need help.

If you have an opportunity to purchase a good stout horse for family use, I think it a good plan to do it for the pleasure of all the family.

As to my affairs I have said nothing about it to any one except Dr. Phillips, but shall soon. I think you are right in judging that there is reason to fear, promises with him are worth nothing. I shall place no confidence in them hereafter. Dr. Phillips and Maj. Mayberry have sent for wives and are keeping quarters near the regiment. Dr. R. and myself commenced messing at our tents last week and have had so far a pleasant time. We have a good mess chest with teapot and all the necessary [items] for nutrition for cooking. Also stoneware plates & tea cups. All in order. We must purchase all the victuals but can live for $2.00 or $2.50 per week. The mess charges $4.00 for week. Bill of fare for breakfast—coffee, sugar, light bread. Barn or corn fed. No, I mean mast fed. Swine contraband confiscated, found and appropriated and fried down. 2nd course—Hash. Ma would say, and all culinsts, that is wrong, hash last, that should be first. Well so do I and so would all, especially if they had tasted it. None of your boarding house hash, barking and mewing at you all the time you are devouring it until you almost sympathize with those poor unfortunates of the canine & feline race who fell victims to the hash and sausages-makes [-making] knives. But real domestic hash manufactured by Rainey, Hawley and Co. and eaten by the same firm. Ingredients. Contents, Quantities and Qualities of said H A S H—

R_x	fresh beef boiled and chopped (with hatchet)	lbs 1
	Onions strong, sliced with jack knife	lbs 1
	Juice or Grease of wild swine	oz 7
	Bread, dark and dry	gs
	Aqua flunan	PRN

Boil in a frying pan hours, ½ dose ½ at [a] time. Call around same day and take a slice. We have a small sheet iron stove which heats our tent and cooks dinner, all in fine style. Ma, the nice dried fruit is just gone. It was used in hospital and you received many thanks from as many grateful hearts. I assisted to eat to it and enjoyed it much. We now procure fruits, etc., from the Sanitary

Commission as there is a depot here. We now have 32 in hospital and 50 in quarters. No bad cases. Lost one man, Smith, of Co. E. Old Mr. Lewis from near Salem is improving. I did not see Link. Wish I had. Saw Mr. Gosforth of Mt. Carmel and Willie. He is as large as his father. They are in the Sutter tract at Bethel, are doing well. Nothing new in Mt. C.

Ma, have no fears in regard to the Col. keeping me here by retaining my comm[ission]. It is all recorded at Springfield and nothing would be lost if it was burned. They all act friendly enough. I do not go to see any one much but improve my time reading or keeping up the books.

Dr. Rainey prescribes for all sick here. Dr. Phillips for those in hospital and I for those absent. Duties are not arduous but employ most of my time. I also keep up the books. Col. Black is doing well, was unwell last week. I gave him some medicine, is all right. Have said nothing in regard to my commission.

Dick Thatther has the mumps, not bad. Mr. Simmonson is well. Wife unwell ever since he left. The Mores and Ceantine well. All the friends well. Give my compliments to Mr. and Mrs. Gunn and kiss the little girls for me. Respects to Bob and best wishes to Sallie Higgins and Barny. Love to all the family in unbroken doses three times every day. Kisses without wrappers by the doz. And a Merry Christmas (now in time) to all. Please all write soon and often. Is Fannie going to school? Fannie please write.

Your affect son,

T. S. Hawley

Doctor Hawley expressed his increasing unhappiness with 111th Illinois Infantry in his December 12 letter when he wrote, "I am not as well pleased with my associates..." This was in reference of comparing his situation in December 1862 to his situation in 1861. The good-hearted doctor indicated maybe the situation would improve and he might change his opinion. He had just received a visit from Captain and Doctor Charles Carter, Company G, of the 11th Missouri Infantry. Assistant Surgeon Doctor Eli Bowyer, Hawley's old mentor, and Captain Carter were both considered for the rank of major in the 11th Missouri Infantry. During the election, Doctor Eli Bowyer was elected major of the regiment barely nudging Charles Carter by one vote. Thomas Hawley also reflected on the situation in the eastern theatre where there were recent Confederate victories at Second Bull Run and Antietam in 1862. The Battle of Fredericksburg was taking place at the time of this letter, and this battle would also result in a Confederate victory. Hawley also clearly showed his support for the Emancipation Proclamation which would not be officially signed into law until January 1, 1863, but the preliminary announcement was made on September 22, 1862. There was always a risk the proclamation would not be signed on January 1, but Hawley was confident this was the best plan for the country.

Columbus, Ky. December 12, 1862

Dearest Parents, Bro. & Sisters,

The sun rises and sets. The day comes and goes. Mail after mail arrives. Yet the same negative answer to my eager query. No letter. The last received was mailed at Robinson Nov. 23rd. I incidentally heard that you are all well by Mr. Barnes, had just heard from his sister. She from Maner.

I have heard from my other home quite often and from the 11th Mo. Have retained my old custom of writing nearly every, yes every, week and think you must have found quite a batch of letters at Olney upon your return from Crawford. My health that [by] providence remains good and my comforts are not unfurnished or uncared for. Although not as pleasant as last year at this time. I am not as well pleased with my associates as I was at that time and cannot think as much of the regt. as the one I was formerly connected with. But may think better of them in the future. Capt. Carter of the 11th Mo. remained all night with me a day or two ago. From him I got some very interesting news in regard to the regiment and it doings since I left. The capt. was within one vote of being major in opposition to Dr. Bowyer and thinks that Dr. did wrong. I think not. I suppose you have seen the Dr. lately. I heard that he was in Chicago and would be surgeon of the 11th Mo. No, I mean of the 98 Ills. Vols. Have any of the family formed the acquaintance of Dr. Bowyer's family? I think you will find them quite an addition to your circle of friends in Olney. What improvements if any will you make about the little house in Olney? How do you do? And what will you do? What changes in Olney? And if any, are they for the better or worse? How are old acquaintances? You will perceive that I am quizzing you closely. Well, I have not heard since you arrived in Olney how you were all pleased with the change—nor anything about it.

The watery elements are being liberally dispensed in this part of our Union as well as on the Rappanhannock. My hopes are strong that victory will perch upon our banners at all points this winter and fresh and happy spring may usher in an everlasting spring of peace and prosperity to this, our distracted country. If they will only concentrate their forces at Richmond or on Richmond and take it at all hazards with half the rebel army, then we may look for peace. I sincerely hope President Lincoln will stand by his proclamation and see that it is carried out to the letter. I have no fears of the result. Every Negro will assert his freedom and, if necessary, maintain it by force. If pleased with his master, will remain so long as he is remunerated for his labors. I do not anticipate a great uprising on the 1st of January but the dawning only of a new era in this nation's history and in the history of the world. If the authorities have decided upon a winter campaign it will be a severe one to rebeldom. Look out for its overthrow. I want to go to the 11th Mo before long and procure my papers for pay. Hope and think the *paymaster will be around before the end of the year. I want very much to send you a small amount before long but at present am strapped entirely as most men are in the army. Much love to all the family first by wholesale, then by retail. Evie Bell lots, Fannie some, Maria somer, Amos mucher and Ma & Pa musherest because they are biggerest. I wish you all a Merry Christmas. Only wish I had something more substantial. My undying love you have which will neither rust nor discount. Remember me as you affct. son & bro.,*

T. S. Hawley

On December 17, Major General Earl Van Dorn launched a raid against Grant that halted the advancing Union line. Earl Van Dorn's reputation suffered after the Battle of Corinth when Van Dorn's leadership had come under scrutiny, and he even faced a court of inquiry. On December 17, Van Dorn led his force from Grenada, Mississippi, with the intent of capturing and destroying the Union supply depot in Holly Springs. A large Christmas celebration was held in Holly Springs on the evening of December 19 and Van Dorn struck the city early on the morning of December 20. Despite the cold weather, Van Dorn's men overwhelmed the pickets and found most the Union defenders asleep. While skirmishing took place during the capture, virtually the entire garrison of 2,000 men was captured. It was reported the ladies of Holly Springs stood in their yards cheering as Van Dorn's cavalry accomplished their task. The Confederates took advantage of the Union supplies and destroyed the rest. Van Dorn also freed a number of Confederate prisoners. The garrison commander of Holly Springs was Colonel Robert Murphy of the Eighth Wisconsin Infantry. Colonel Murphy was captured while he was still in his nightshirt.[7] Murphy was also in charge of the Union supply depot in Iuka, Mississippi, in September 1862 which Major General Sterling Price overwhelmed and captured prior to the Battle of Iuka. Colonel Murphy had been found not guilty in a court martial for his actions at Iuka when he faced the charges of misbehaving in the face of the enemy. He had been reassigned to duty at Holly Springs under the command of Brigadier General David Stanley. Murphy recorded, "My fate is most mortifying. I have wished a hundred times to-day that I had been killed. I have done all in my power — in truth, my force was inadequate. I have foreseen this and have so advised. No works here, and no force to put in them if they were here, and yet I know General Grant is not to blame; he has done all for the best, and so did I. I have obeyed orders, and have been unfortunate in so doing. The misfortune of war is mine."[8] The unfortunate Colonel Murphy was to be summarily dismissed from the service of the Union Army on January 10, 1863.

By the time of Van Dorn's raid on Holly Springs, Doctor Thomas Hawley was no longer physically serving as part of the 111th Illinois Infantry and he was serving as an assistant surgeon in a hospital in the city the Confederate cavalry targeted. When Doctor Hawley was not tending to his duties at the hospital, he roomed in the residence of Doctor Charles Bonner called Cedarhurst. The residence had been constructed in 1857 and was, no doubt, a pleasant place to reside. In Thomas Hawley's letter, he gave a Union view of Van Dorn's raid into Holly Springs. Hawley was captured by the Confederates and placed under house arrest at Cedarhurst. His captors allowed Hawley to continue with his medical duties, including, treating the Confederate wounded. He was not taken away to a Confederate prisoner-of-war camp but apparently was captured and released as the Confederate cavalry moved northward. In later life, Thomas Hawley stated he was captured seven times by various Confederate soldiers as he worked through the day on wounded and sick soldiers.

As part of the Doctor Bonner's household, Thomas Hawley undoubtedly met Doctor Bonner's daughter, Sherwood, who became a noted author later in life. Katharine Sherwood Bonner became a writer, and authored short fiction and the *Dialect Tales* (1883) and *Suwanee River Tales* (1884). She was particularly noted for her ability to write in Southern dialect. Later in 1878, the yellow fever epidemic struck Holly Springs, Mississippi. She returned there from Boston to care for her family, but her father and brother died in the epidemic. Sherwood died in 1883 at the age of 34 of cancer.[9]

Confederate General Earl Van Dorn's raid on Holly Springs stopped Grant's plan to attack Vicksburg by a land route through Mississippi. Sherman's advance was also halted when his troops were repulsed at the Battle of Chickasaw Bayou on December 29, 1862. As Grant reformulated his plan to capture Vicksburg, these setbacks convinced him that he needed a river based attack. So, by January 30, 1863, he established his headquarters at Milliken's Bend, Louisiana, about 10 miles west of Vicksburg, and decided to use the Mississippi River as the route for concentrating his troops and supplies prior to his attack on Vicksburg.

Holly Springs, Miss.
Dec 24th 1862

Dearest Ones at Home,

How much pleasure it would afford your absent soldier boy to press each one of you to my joyous heart. None can. Language utterly fails and each word would be mere empty sounds in comparison to the unbounded, rapturous joyfulness of a heart and head that knows no greater pleasure than the happiness of those they love and live and fight and if necessary will die for. I wrote you upon my arrival here, dated, I think, the 18th. Was having quite a pleasant time and everything about Holly Springs was going off as merrily as a manger bell until Genl. Van Dorn with his rebel clan saw fit to give us a visit. Since, all has been confusion confounded. I had a pleasant boarding house as I wrote you in my last with Dr. Bonner, a Confederate, a gentleman and a scholar. On the morning of the 20th inst. as I lay in my nice bed thinking of home and my business, then just at daylight, I heard a loud hooping and yelling. I looked out of the window, as soon saw Mr. Butternut riding under a full gallup after blue coats occasionally exchanging a shot but our boys, the brave 29th Ills., was completely surprised. They first captured the picquets [pickets] without a shot, then formed in line near our camp within a quarter of a mile perhaps and came up charging. The Second Ills. Calv. gave a spirited resistance, then being only 2 companies but they soon had to run. The 101 Ills. was taken. 8 cos. of 29 Ills., 100 men of the 62 Ills., 2 cos. 2 Ills. Calv., and stragglers, sick, etc. Not much less than 2,000, 3 or 400 horses, 50 or 60 wagons burned besides 3 or 4 hundred thousand dollars worth of medical, hospital and commissary stores, ammunition, etc. Burned the depot, engines, houses, large hotel, the finest hospital in the west. 4 large rooms all fitted and furnished each with beds, cots, blankets for over 100 men. A steamboat load of medicine & stores. No one can calculate the amount of property destroyed. On the 22nd inst., a large force came up from below and are here at present. The rebels only stayed one day and stragglers part of the night. Many of the citizens were greatly rejoiced and lustily hurrahed for Jeff Davis and their boys and for all this, our boys upon their return had ample revenge. They broke into their houses, took most of their private property in and about the houses and left them almost entirely destitute and every night they burn two or three houses. They set fire to an outhouse belonging to the man I am boarding with but we were just out in [time] to save it. Then some of us were on watch all night.

 The morning the rebels came, I was soon called out with Col. Ferrill of the 29th Ill. They took the col. to Genl. Van Dorn's headquarters and let me off with the promise to come again and that I must remain with Dr. Bonner. Hundreds of them were passing the gate John Gilpin-style hooping and howling like demons incarnate as they saw me with a blue officer's coat on. Some said shoot him. Shoot the d___ rascal, etc. I returned to the house unmolested and remained pretty close for half a day, then I went to attend the wounded. When I was in my room two fellows came up. One with a long saber drawn, the other with a double barrel shotgun, cocked and ready to do execution. I talked quickly with him. He asked about a wounded man on the bed. I told him. [He] Said guessed was all right & left.

 Well another Christmas has come and how my heart burns to be with you and clasp you in affectious warm embrace. Love untold I bear you each one and all. Kiss each other when you shed the loving tears for the absent one and hope this terrible war is for the best. Think of me as trying to do my duty to my country and to my fellow men. And thank the Lord you are as well off as you are. For I have seen families, little children all turned out upon the cold world. I wish you *a happy New Year and may it bear upon its broad bosom the olive branch of peace is my prayer.*

Your affectionate son & bro.,

T. S. Hawley

PS. Please write soon. Direct to me at this place and Genl. hospital.

Yours,

T. S. Hawley

After Van Dorn's raid, Chief Medical Director of the District of West Tennessee for the Union Army, Doctor Horace Wirtz, recorded his attempts to save the hospitals, "As soon as I discovered the enemy were in possession of the place I repaired to the headquarters of the rebel general, near town, and made a formal request that the armory hospital should not be burned, entering an earnest protest on the subject, as the Confederates had already set fire to the railroad depot and commissary storehouse and had declared their intention to destroy all houses occupied by our troops. I received the assurance of General Van Dorn's adjutant that the armory hospital should not be burned, but that it would be protected by a guard. Satisfied with this I returned to my quarters, but had not been there an hour when I was informed the building was on fire, and thus this fine structure, with two thousand bunks, an immense lot of drugs and surgical apparatus, thousands of blankets, sheets, and bed-sacks was soon in ashes."[10]

The December 24 letter was the final letter from Thomas Hawley in 1862 who continued to struggle with finding a suitable position within the Union Army. He had served for a year and a half and now was providing medical care in Union hospitals, no longer assigned to regimental service. This was somewhat due to his own efforts to gain recognition for his experience as a physician. He had served with the 11th Missouri Infantry, the 111th Illinois, and at the Union Hospital at Holly Springs. He had served in the Siege of Island Number Ten and the Siege of Corinth, and received a badge of honor by being captured by the enemy at Holly Springs and he was finally satisfied with his role in the Union medical service. He was wiser and surer of himself at the end of the year than he was at the year's beginning. Despite the events in the war, he still clung to the relationships with his family and even counseled his younger sisters and brother, and served as a source of support for his minister father and his mother. Truly, Thomas Hawley was in a set of circumstances that would define his life, but managed to stay firmly affixed to those values which were important to him, family and friends, and love for his country.

The new year, 1863, loomed, the Emancipation Proclamation was near and the Civil War was ever present.

Three

1863

LaGrange, Vicksburg and Memphis

Confederate General Earl Van Dorn's successful raid on Holly Springs destroyed the Union supply depot and captured the Union garrison including, Thomas Hawley. Next, Van Dorn moved northward advancing on Bolivar, Tennessee, but the Union Army was more prepared after the Confederate success at Holly Springs.

The Southern cavalry were unsuccessful in an encounter with the Union Army at Davis' Mills and then Van Dorn passed around Bolivar, Tennessee. On December 28, 1862, the Confederate cavalry crossed the Tallahatchie River and into the friendly confines of Confederate held territory after a two week foray destroying railroads, destroying between $400,000 and $1,500,000 of supplies at Holly Springs and giving a much needed boost in morale to the Southern troops.

Fortunately for Doctor Thomas Hawley the Confederate cavalry had moved away from Holly Springs leaving him free and it was unclear whether Hawley was considered captured and paroled, or just free of his captors. On January 3, he was boarding at a new location with Doctor B. W. Ross and his family, and although Doctor Ross was a resident of Holly Springs, he was not a supporter of the war. Doctor Ross' home was a fine house in Holly Springs which was built by the doctor in 1857. More importantly Doctor Ross's seventeen year-old daughter, Annie, held the attention of Doctor Thomas Hawley.

In January 1863 Doctor Hawley's responsibility within the army was the medical care of Ward 3 in the Union hospital at Holly Springs. He also included a most eloquent appeal for the end of the war in his January 3 letter.

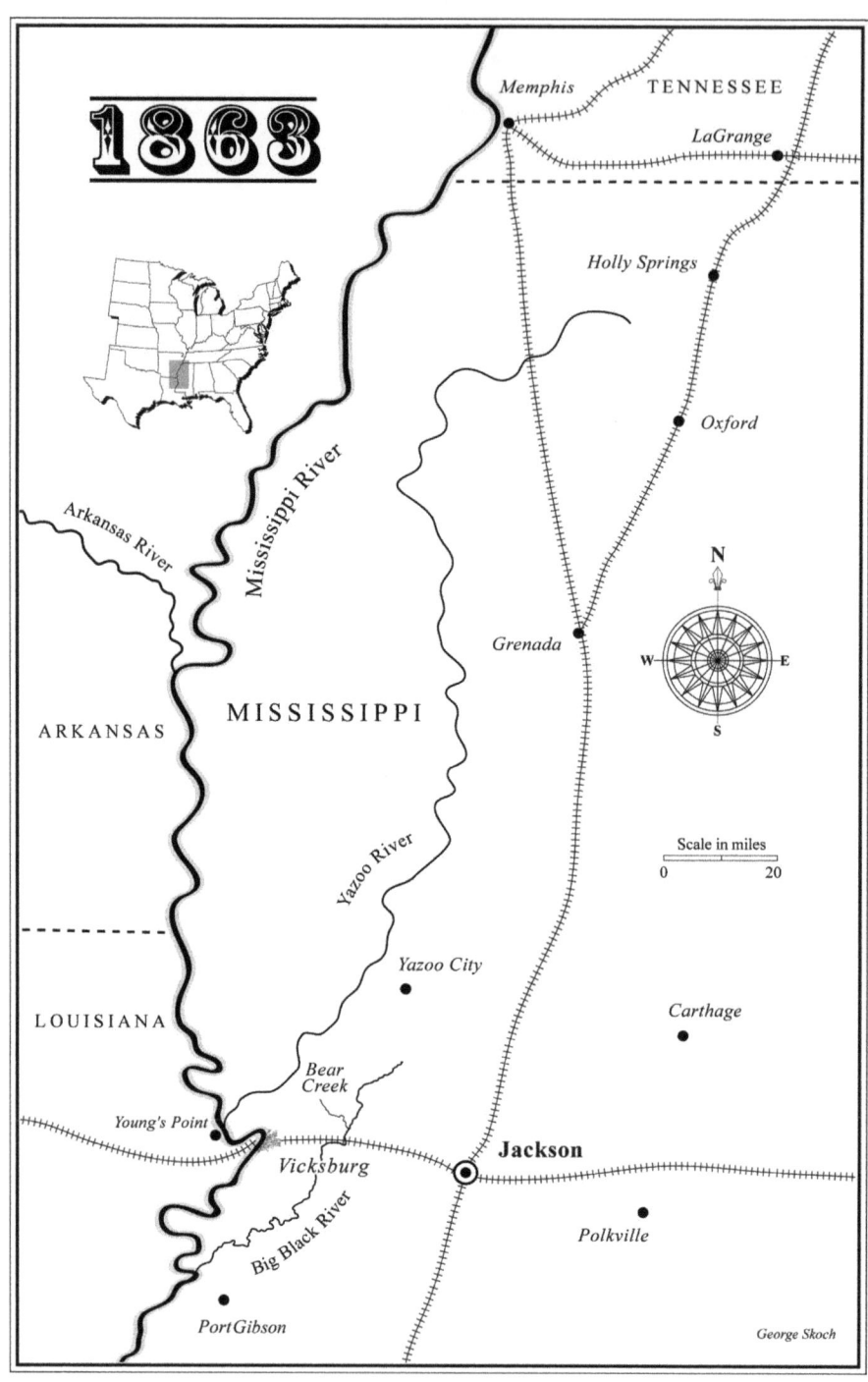

Genl. Hospital
Holly Springs, Miss.
Jan. 3rd 1863
Dear Parents,

Well knowing your anxiety in regard to my fate after hearing and reading the numerous exaggerated statements in regard to the recent raid at this place, I have written just as often as there was any conveyance with the outer world or United States. My health is good for which I am thankful and ever hoping yours may be as good but confess to fears that is not, especially Pa's which I know was feeble and feared that it might be impaired from anxiety and fears. Please be always assured of my welfare and comforts. Trust me in your prayers to the beneficent care of Providence and always hope for the best. The first I well know you always do, the latter you cannot so well, but may try. The weather so far has been unusually pleasant even for this sunny south but the wet weather is now making its appearance, mixed with a little cold. I am boarding with Dr. Ross and find the family very pleasant and they regard me almost as kin. What would you say if I should be? Miss Annie is very pleasant, agreeable young lady, plays and sings finely besides would have graduated last summer if the institute had not been broken up. Writes [in] a fine hand and composes well. Her Ma cried the other [day] because I was going away. They were Union just as long as they could be. The Dr. was opposed to the war and has had nothing to do with it. They are from Penn. or rather he is. They have the most beautiful yard in Holly Springs full of evergreens and hundreds of varieties of flowers, sweet violets on all the borders, now in bloom, which fill the air with sweet fragrance.

Oh how I wish for peace, the end of this terrible war. Who counts the unnumbered tears and groans of a mighty nation mourning for lost brave and dear hearts. But we must have an honorable peace. I am burning with an unquenchable love for the Dear Ones at home. The intense longing desire to see your dear faces again, but rest in peace, all is well. I have the 3rd ward in the Genl. Hospital. Am pleasantly fixed. Please write often. Dr. Elliott is here. Wishes to be remembered. Dr. Green stayed with me one night, is well. Bro. Morrison is here, is well. Bob Friese is here, well. I wish you a happy New Year.

The road will soon be repaired. I will write often.

Your aft. son,
T. S. Hawley

By early January, Thomas Hawley was placed in charge of Union Hospital Number 3 in LaGrange, Tennessee, about 25 miles from Memphis. LaGrange had a population of about 2,000 just prior to the war. Hospital No. 3 was located in the Galt House, one of the local hotels, which served about 160 patients on January 11. The unfortunate residents of LaGrange suffered through some outrages to their domestic tranquility and their possessions as the Union Army used the city as their base. Over forty homes in LaGrange were destroyed or used for firewood during the war. However, as bad as conditions were in LaGrange, Hawley recorded the terrible vengeance unleashed by the Union Army on Holly Springs, including, breaking into private homes and accosting private citizens. It had been recorded during Van Dorn's raid into Holly Springs the local citizens stood in their yards waving and hurrahing for their boys in gray. The Union revenge was cruelly administered to the local citizens. Certainly the Union forces which reclaimed Holly Springs showed little sympathy for the Confederate raiders or those local citizens who supported them. Many citizens were thrown out of their homes and the homes were given to the ex-slaves.

In LaGrange, Thomas Hawley found a position which he was well pleased while working under the command of Doctor Horace Wirtz, Chief Medical Director of the District of West Tennessee. He had worked for Doctor Wirtz in Holly Springs and continued in that capacity in LaGrange.

Thomas Hawley had a strong connection with the chaplain, Reverend Samuel Baldridge, of the 11th Missouri Infantry. Reverend Baldridge resigned his position with the regiment on January 5, 1863, and passed through Holly Springs on his way home. Samuel Coulter Baldridge had taken the spiritual reins of a very difficult regiment, the 11th Missouri Infantry. Baldridge was born on August 6, 1829, in Vermillion County, Indiana, and had graduated from Hanover College in 1849 and then attended the New Albany Presbyterian Theological Seminary until 1852. The Presbyterian Church licensed him to preach in 1853 and he was ordained on October 15, 1854. Baldridge was the minister of the Friendsville, Illinois Presbyterian Church prior to his enlistment.[1] By January 3, Reverend Baldridge's service with the regiment was over and he agreed to deliver Thomas Hawley's January 11 letter to the family.

Also of note in this letter is the fact Thomas Hawley was not officially captured and paroled by the Confederates during the recent raid. Hawley referred to his capture by a fair Southern lady in Holly Springs, presumably Annie Ross.

LaGrange, Tenn.
Jan. 11th 1863
Dear Father and Mother,

It has been so long since I last heard from you that I am almost in despair. You will see by this address that I have moved, am now in charge of Hospital No. 3 at the Gualt House, have over 160 cases, some quite unwell and others convalescent, have plenty of help. I left the city of flowers on last Thursday night

Three. 1863

and almost left my heart there also. I was indeed sorry to leave and they shed tears. Said it was like one of the family leaving. It seemed as though they had always known me, did not know what they would have done without me. That I must come to see them again, etc. There was a fire in town nearly every night, one night a house just across the street. We had to wet the house and pacify the ladys and look out for robbers at once.

Some of the boys broke into private houses, opened all the trunks and boxes, took out money, clothes and all valuables. Destroyed the clothes, ripped them up on the palings, took rings off women's fingers, thrust hands into men's pockets, drove the white folks out and put Negroes in their houses. They have by this time burned every house or nearly so in that beautiful place. It was indeed a lovely place but some bitter rebels have long since repented the raid and destruction of government property.

I must acknowledge I had not seen the horrors of war until quite lately. Hope not to see any more of it soon. The Negroes are filling up the lines most gloriously which I am glad to see. We know what to do with them but what will be done with them? They had better remain with them or their masters for the present. I do not doubt but that they will all be free and are now. But I fear Abraham will be like the Pat that won an elephant at the raffle. What will be done with them!

Oh, if only I knew how you were all prospering. What a lode of anxiety would be removed from my breast and how much smoother would be my rest. Why do not some letters come to hand from home penned by those familiar hands full of kind loving words? Where am I? How will I get away from all these horrors, woes, frustrations and unpleasant associations? I am without money and cannot get away without much trouble but will go to Memphis just as soon as I can and from there to Columbus or some other country not full of trouble. Have my papers from the 11th Mo and can get some pay on them from April 30 to Sept. 18th 1862 as Steward, [$] 30 per month besides clothes dues. Do not think from the tune of this that I am in despair. No, I will keep a bright face and look on the sunny side of all our troubles, just as long as I can.

This is a very pleasant place, larger than I supposed. It has near 3,000 inhabitants, 3 or 4 churches, two fine colleges and many fine buildings. The town is scattered over considerable territory, every dwelling having a large yard almost a park and well decorated with evergreens and fine shrubbery [tear in letter] as Holly Springs [tear in letter] only more so. I wish you could see this country and see and hear the inhabitants. Most that I have met since my tour down the said road have been fine, intelligent, chaste people full of feelings but most of them only for the southern states and for this they should be severely punished and they are being. Not a night passes in this part of the world without being lited up by the flames from two or three houses. Then two or a dozen human beings are turned out in the cold, upon the cold world or upon the colder charity of their former friends without food, money or clothing. This is hard and presents a sad picture but I do earnestly assure you that the half has not been told. There was not half enough red in the brush. I left Columbus on Aug., no Dec. 16, upon the order of Dr. Derby who was ordered by Dr. [Horace] Wirtz, Chief Medical Director, who I got acquainted with at Holly Springs and like him very much. I was in charge of two hospitals there by his direction. He is now in Memphis and I was ordered here, am with Dr. Strode, one of my former classmates at Medical College St. Louis, Mo.

Bro. Baldridge, ex–Chaplain of the 11th Mo., is with me and will return home soon and promises to visit Olney and see you all and will convey this long epistle and a piece of music which I fancied, sent by that Miss Heapsteadler to my sister because I spoke of copying it. But that was nothing like <u>Deal with Me Kindly</u> or <u>Her Bright Smile Haunts Me Still</u> or the <u>Girl I Left Behind Me</u> as sung by my captor. Amos asks if I am still held. I may say that I am not held by parole or by my first captors but by one fair captor. I am still bound although she may not know it. My capture before the order not to exchange prisoners amounts to nothing. But after this, it may. But then I shall not be captured again, as I am still held by my fair one, who if I had remained longer would have sent my sister a fresh bouquet but as it was, gave it to me and I will take pleasure in sending it home as a relic from Holly Springs, also the music. I shall visit the place one of these days if I can. Today it was recaptured by the rebels. One of our soldiers wounded. The Chaplain is in a hurry so I must close. Much love I send you. Kiss all for me. Kiss Eva. I regret to hear Aunt Martha is so unwell. Write soon.

Yours afftly.,
Yours,
T. S. Hawley

The following week, January 17, 1863, Thomas Hawley worked diligently in Hospital Number 3 in LaGrange, Tennessee. His experience in the war provided Hawley with an opportunity to see medical cases he would never have seen in private practice. Being in charge of a general hospital meant he received the worst medical cases from the regiments. Soldiers who could not be serviced by the regimental medical staff went to the general hospitals.

The most significant part of Hawley's letter of January 17 was directed at the status of the war and the need for a proper end of the war. He felt any government which had slavery as its cornerstone was not a suitable form of government. Hawley also remarked a permanent separation between the North and South was equally unsuitable. However, he recorded he had not seen a Southerner who was not fully convinced in the correctness of the Confederate cause. Unfortunately for the Union troops near LaGrange, they received only Southern newspapers which did not help the morale of the troops during the cold and gloomy days and nights of winter.

LaGrange, Tenn.
Genl. Hospital No. 3 Jan 17, 1863
Dear Parents,

    A long period has elapsed since I last heard from you and if you reckon time as I do, you also think the time not short but you may have heard from me much oftener than I have heard from you. Postal facilities have not been very good in this part of the world for the past 30 days with a prospect of so continuing for some time to come. I have not seen a real good Union paper for a month. Nothing but the <u>Chicago Times</u> or <u>Memphis Bulletin</u> find their way to this outpost. I have not heard from the 111 Ills. Vols. since I left them and do not know how soon I will hear from them. I do not like them much, think they will not do much fighting and would not care how soon I was disconnected with it, if I only had a good place in some other regiment and if I find a good opening in this part of the world, may try. As yet I have not and have not mentioned the subject to any person at present. I am very pleasantly situated in a good building, formerly a hotel, just enough to do and all the assistants that is necessary. Have a fine opportunity to see disease in its various forms. Indeed most of my cases have been very bad ones. A larger number than I ever saw before because they are all the worst cases sent in from several regiments. Bro. Morrison is here in charge of the contrabands of which there is a large number and it is still increasing. I have seen them come in with large wagons ladened with all imaginable sort of trumpery, some of their own and some belonging to their former masters. We have 10 or 15 engaged around the hospital, men and women. Chop wood and do washing, carry water and help to cook. I was much surprised and grieved to hear of Aunt Martha's severe illness and can only continue hoping to hear better news next time.

    I wrote you a long letter by Bro. Baldridge formerly Chaplain of the 11 Mo. which he said he would bear to you in person. The envelope contained a nice bouquet from a lady friend in Holly Springs. I send it to you and a piece [of] music which I think you will like especially, one strain on it which I called heavenly. Well, to be honest it does appear to me that this war question is becoming rather uncertain. I cannot say when it will terminate, nor how, but fear we must become still deeper engulfed until it may be necessary to recognize the Southern Confederacy. Our enemys at home are the most to be feared just now. But somehow, I cannot but feel that this war must result in the overthrow of slavery. I cannot think that so heinous a stain upon the world will remain. And if this would-be-called C. S. A is recognized as an independent power with its present *constitution naming for its chief cornerstone, slavery, that [then] will that institution only have received a new impetus with a tendency to engulf the whole west for the great north-west and the south as natural allies bound together by nature's strongest bond, the great rivers. A permanent separation is surely impossible from natures welding together. And looking back upon history we would conclude that the age was rather improving instead of retrograding, that the slaves of nearly every nation had been freed. That despotism was swaying less power over all the world and was destined to be with subject entirely. I cannot see for the life of me how it will be possible for this glorious republic to be put asunder and for the slavocrats become independent. It cannot be done. But I have not found a single individual adhering to the southern cause doubt their ultimate success. And many of our soldiers and officers, at first the most sanguine, are now the most skeptical as to our ultimate power over the rebellious states. Our army is becoming very much demoralized and all from the neglect of their officers to exercise their proper authority. Many scruple not to express their disapproval of the commander-in-chief's order. The right kind of military officers would put such men or officers under arrest. But as it is, they discuss, find fault, get mad, throw down their arms and get 50 others to do the same. Then at that advanced stage all are placed under arrest, and their arms taken from them. Another wrong, nothing but secesh papers are circulated among the United States soldiers. The precious sheets carefully conceal all good news and show up the bad in glowing colors. Well dear friends, enough of this or you will think I am becoming dubious as to the perpetuity of this union of states. My faith is yet unshaken but the time when the olive branch of peace shall wave over this continent is far in [the] dim distance. Well may we say. Tis the nation's severest trial should she pass through successfully, never again will the strength of the Union be so sorely tested. I believe we will be compelled to call up the African citizens for aid.*

How are you prospering financially, socially, politically, etc., etc.? Please write me in full up to date. I am getting along well, just 25 cts. left. No pay since April 30 but have my papers from the 11 Mo. and can draw my pay as soon as I see the paymaster. At present will remain here but cannot say how long. Am comfortable. But sick to hear from home. Love to all. Some 60, some 30, and some a 100 fold, mostly 100. Compliments to all the friends. Love to the relations in Crawford.

Yours affectionately,

T. S. Hawley

On January 26, Doctor Thomas Hawley continued his routine efforts with the Union Army and his letter was primarily devoted to domestic concerns. Aunt Martha, his mother's sister, recently died and he was concerned about the family members who were without a parent and concerned about what would happen to them. His rather sickly brother, Amos, was successful in finding employment but he did not indicate in this letter what work he was doing. He chided his sister, Myra, to write and advised his sister Fannie not to work too hard and to find time for some fun. Another concern for his family was the purchase of the family cow as a source of milk. He received cakes from the family which were delivered on the steamer, *Maria Denning*.

Thomas Hawley continued his connections with the 11th Missouri Infantry remarking he saw his old regiment marching to Germantown, Tennessee, and he looked forward to receiving some letters from his old friends. At LaGrange, the town continued to serve as a Union garrison which contained three or four regiments. Finally, the ever absent paymaster had just arrived at LaGrange which was timely because Doctor Hawley was without funds.

Genl. Hospital No. 3
LaGrange, Tenn. Jan. 26, 1863
Dearest Parents, Bro & Sisters,

Your good, long, kind and affectionate letter came to hand a few days ago. It was written on the 11th inst. and nearly half a month coming. I have written about every week but the mails are now very uncertain. We can get papers from Memphis every morning, but it is so much rebel that one has no satisfaction in reading it. I have heard that Holly Springs has been almost entirely burned up. I am glad to hear that Amos has found some employment.

I mourn with the rest of the family the loss of our dear Aunt Martha. I little thought when I rode over to see them last fall that Dear Aunt would meet me no more on earth. She was always so kind and so glad to see me. The poor little children. I hope they will fall into good hands. Rose and Evie Bell will get along finely I think. But what is to become of Theodocia? How was Grand Pa when you left? I wrote to forward my letters from the regt. sometime ago. I have not heard from them since I left.

Ma wants to know if I want money. I have none but will pretty soon as the paymaster is here and Bro. Morrison also who owes me $70. I think he will pay soon. Saw some of the 11th Mo. They passed through here going to Germantown near Memphis.

Sister M, I will hold you to your promise to write a fools cap sheet for every time I would write to you. Sister F, I am sorry you are not pleased with your teachers. The rules can and will be too strict during school hours, when school is out, then play. I am glad to hear you are improving. I can see that by your letter. Please write more. I have not been very well for a few days but am better today. There is nothing new in this department. No fighting, nor skirmishing but all quiet. I wrote you a long letter and sent it by Bro. Baldridge, formerly Chaplin of the 11th Mo., that with others I suppose you have received long ere this. I do not expect to remain here very long but may go to Memphis or to the regiment.

Sister, I guess I got that paper from some lady. I guess Miss <u>Maria Denning</u>. It contained 3 or 4 of the sweetest cakes you ever saw or tasted. I think some friend will send me the letters due me from the regt. I am very pleasantly fine for one in the army. I have a good boarding house, plenty of music and good things to eat. Occasionally have milk. I hope Pa got a cow for you by this time.

The weather has been rather damp, not much cold but wet. Had a fine snow but that has all disappeared before old Sol's smiling countenance and no merry sound of sleigh bells greet the ear. Army wagons and cotton wagons of which staple article quite a quantity finds a market at this depot. There are a dozen cotton buyers here all the time. There is 3 or 4 regiments at this place. The 26 Illinois are doing provost duty and A. B. Morrison has charge of contrabands and it keeps him busy I guess. Have not heard from Salem since we left. Please write all the news soon. Much love to all, each and every one individually and collectively and specifically. Kisses like drops of rain in April showers, I send you and love as immeasurable as the ocean. Only write oftener.

Yours Affectly.,

T. S. Hawley

On the last Sunday of January 1863, Thomas Hawley recorded as many as 500 men were confined to the general hospitals at LaGrange and he recorded smallpox as one of the more serious problems. Smallpox was a serious disease in the Civil War because it was so contagious and sometimes fatal to those who contracted the disease. The only treatment for smallpox was prevention by quarantining those infected and vaccinating those who had not already contracted the disease. Smallpox patients were isolated, given the best nutrition possible and kept in well-ventilated areas. Although some died, not all cases were fatal and soldiers were treated, and returned to their regiments. One particularly disturbing unsubstantiated allegation in the Civil War was a Southern doctor sold clothes from smallpox infected patients to the Union soldiers in an attempt to infect them.[2] Vaccination was the key to keeping this disease under control and Thomas Hawley wrote he vaccinated some soldiers every day.

In Hawley's January 31 letter, he continued to express his concern for Annie Ross at Holly Springs and the impact the Union Army had on the city. Thomas Hawley recorded he was just getting over an illness. He also described the hospital and staff which he commanded, including a pharmacist, William Lymans, a hospital steward, 11 nurses, a matron, three cooks, P. E. Mott, his clerk, and Jamy, an African-American in charge of the physical condition of the hospital. At the time of this letter, there were about 50 patients in General Hospital Number 3.

Genl. Hospital No. 3
LaGrange, Tenn. Jan. 31 '63

Dear Parents Bro. & Sisters,

 Still tempus fugit and waits for no man but no chronicler of the past events at home reaches my anxious eyes which have become almost tired of gazing into the long mazed distance. Away down in the sunny South away from all near and dear friends among strangers and in a strange land seated here in some man's house or hotel surrounded by sick and trying to write is your son. Yet by an eye of faith I can look from this far off point and see you seated around the sitting room fire, Pa reading, Ma thinking, Amos about to go bed, Evie Bell in bed and Fannie trying to study. I think you have the little house fixed up quite pleasantly. But hope it will suit you better next spring or summer. How are all the old friends in and about Olney? I suppose most of the young men have left but there must be some young ladies. Why not write to one of them? That is always an interesting subject and one that I have not had time to discuss very extensively for some time.

 Tis true, I have been introduced to several in this place but did not spare time to become interested in my subject. Indeed that very interesting case in the city of flowers which I think was rather celestial than terrestrial has rather absorbed my idle moments. The thought that she might be in danger made me nervous and almost sick. Indeed when I wrote you last, I was just recovering from a 4 day sickness and was 3 days confined to my room but was up most of the time, was exposed to the tender care of Wm. Lymans, my druggist, a fine young fellow whose father is surgeon in the 45th Regt. Ill. Vols. and P. E. Mott, my clerk and Jamy our darkee, who brings all the water, builds all the fires, sweeps the floor and runs chores generally. Then I have an orderly to carry dispatches, Hospital Steward to attend to all the food and drawing of rations, have 11 nurses, our matron whose husband is Bandmaster, three cooks, one fine, large stove and furniture and one soup stove, a stove with a large iron boiler especially for soup, 10 or 15 contrabands and one man to attend to them, about 50 sick, all up but for eleven today, a very comfortable office and dispensing room, a fire place in each, bureau, wash stand, maple table on casters, desk for writing, one fine spring skat, sociable, nice bed, a cot, hair mattress, sheets, pillow, blankets, etc. So you see I am for the present very well situated. Could not be more so but how I shall remain is a question of time, but as I said before, think I may go to Memphis soon.

 I need not tell you that my thoughts often recur home. Indeed when I stop to meditate for one moment, home and all the dear ones flies into my mind immediately but during the busy hours my mind remains pretty close to business. It does not take me many hours to go around now as most of the patients are convalescing. There is not more than 500 sick at this place, several cases of smallpox. I am very sorry you have it Olney. It is so unpleasant. All [need to] be well vaccinated with good virus immediately. I vaccinate some almost every day. The weather has been nothing but rain and drizzle and drizzle and rain for the past 3 weeks, instead [of] a cold spell as we used to have up north. Here we have a wet spell and they come so near together that it makes for [a] long wet spell and mud plenty. I think this element, mud, will do as much toward settling up the war as the rebels. But then we must take Vicksburg and will. This place is being strongly fortified and its natural defenses are good of Wolfe River with its high bluffs on two sides and a high hill commanding most of the county back. This place must not be given up for it is on a line with Corinth, Memphis, etc. Consequently you see [it] is of importance. Madam Rumor had it that some rebel general was on the march for this place with 20,000 men but the 6th Ill. Cav. was below Holly Springs the first of this week and saw nothing of them.

You surely must get most of my letters. Remember I still write one every week and shall so long as communication is not broken off. How about the new piano? I hope ere this, its dulcet tones gladden the spirits of all the home friends. If I hear this confirmed, those tones will situate through the air to this place. I will rejoice with you and perhaps [send] a present to each of you. How did you spend New Years, Sister? I know Ma's New Year came in with sadness and it was so to all. I spent it rather pleasantly so far away. Write me all the news. Send my love to Thos. Scott if an opportunity. Remember me to Mr. Mrs. Gunn, to Ada and Fannie. Kiss Evie Bell, Fannie H., Maria D., Amos A. and Ma and Pa for me and with each accept 10,000 loves.

Yours affectionately,

T S. Hawley

While Thomas Hawley labored at General Hospital Number 3 in LaGrange, General Ulysses Grant was preparing his Vicksburg Campaign. In the autumn and early winter of 1862, Grant wanted to send two wings of his army to converge on Vicksburg; but both wings of his army had been stopped. Grant, while stymied, was nonetheless determined to advance and capture Vicksburg in 1863. Thomas Hawley referred to the impending campaign in his February 8 letter. He also made a very strong statement regarding Confederate sympathizers referring, not only to those in the South, but also the Copperheads who opposed the war in Illinois.

Undoubtedly, Thomas Hawley was smitten by Miss Annie Ross of Holly Springs and mentioned her again, as he had in previous letters. The muddy conditions in LaGrange were deplorable and Hawley wrote he had no fear of the enemy because they would not be able to move through the sea of mud in Tennessee. Thomas Hawley mentioned in his February 8 letter he had not been fully discharged from his original regiment, the 11th Missouri Infantry. His friend and mentor, Doctor Eli Bowyer, who was assistant surgeon of the regiment when Thomas Hawley left, had been promoted to the rank of major. Clearly, Thomas Hawley and Eli Bowyer were excellent friends. Finally, Hawley described a "scene of destruction" in a humorous manner, and the event to which he referred was a group of hungry soldiers digging into a hearty breakfast which included a large selection of food.

Genl. Hospital No. 3
LaGrange, Tenn. Feb. 8th 1863

Dear Ma, Pa, Bro. & Sisters (to wit) Maria, Fannie and last but not least Eva Bell. Greeting (If I could) each with an affectionate kiss but as I cannot apply those articles in propria persona you must be content by my dispatching them through love's telegraph. Tis said absence conquers love, But oh, I believe it not. For I find my case is growing more desperate every day and should I not hear from those dear ones soon, shall grow desperater. One letter a month when they use to flock to my standard by the dozens is rather much of a falling off for one poor fellow to bear. When the orderly comes from the P. O. "No letter for you today Doctor," greets my anxious ear, then down goes the corners of a mouth and countenance looks chopfallen. And one soldier looks forlorn. The question is inwardly asked. Why is it? What's the matter? Do they write? Are they sick? Etc., ad infinitum. Now the 111th Ill. may be hording up all these treasures of mine, not know where to send them but I have written them four times and not heard once since I left them. Of course they are yet at Columbus but who knows?

I, as you see by the address of this communication, am still at No. 3 LaGrange and in good quarters. The Paymaster has paid me a visit, that is all as his orders are pay up to August 31st 1862 and I have not been fully discharged from the 11th Mo., must see the Col. at Germantown near Memphis and then Gen. Grant. I understand they will soon pay all the troops up to Jan. 1st. Bro. Morrison paid me $30 which meets my present wants. I purchased a new pr. of boots. The rest of my wearing apparel is as it was when I last saw [you] except a soldier's overcoat I drew from Capt. Carter's co[mpany]. We just had a fine snow last week and today it has dispersed before the warm rays of a southern sun. The citizens all say this winter has been much colder than any in their recollection and more snow. This climate abounds in mud and this country is bounded by mud and the mud blockade is more effectual than the coast embargo. There is no fear of the enemy's approach to this impregnable post because of the mud and we cannot navigate nor perambulate for mud. So you see we are in a fix. But should you see this, mud puddles, during the spring time or clothed in summer's joyous robe, you would be lured and enticed to remain until you was compelled to by the next annual blockade. If sinners entice thee, consent thee not. I was almost tempted to remain in this fair land of orange groves, palm trees and flora gardens and pale girls but neither the orange groves, palm trees, nor flora garden could persuade me but the pale animated roses might. I tell you my dear friends and fellow citizens there is a temptation, especially, Gentle Annie, and such like.

I have formed the acquaintance of a very pleasant lady Mrs. Denman or Denham from Centerville, Ohio, is acquainted with the Swearingens and other friends in Ohio. She was unwell and I cured her. She very cordially invited me to come and see her. Also to bring my sister. I shall call to see her again this afternoon. I have but few patients, 45 and no new ones. Hope to go to Memphis or Vicksburg by or before the great battle. I think the great theatre of war will be transferred to the valley of the Miss. And you have some in Ills. and Ind., if the miserable secesh sympathizers do not stop their demonstrations, I would rather fight them than any southern traitors. I hate them and would shoot them. Hope you will organize companies and hang and drive off all from the legislator to the low Irish Mik. They are all traitors of the deepest dye and richly merit eternal banishment. Don't leave them in the rear but drive them to the front. This rebellion must be put down whether north, east, west or south. All enemys to the Gov[ernment] are traitors.

Monday Morning Feb. 9th 9:30 A.M. 2nd Dispatch.

We have just returned from a scene of destruction. Everything that was of a nourishing character was demolished with a ferocity worthy of a bitter cause. I mean the breakfast scene. We had waffles, toast, steak, coffee, milk, cornbread, light bread none, biscuit[s], etc. They do not use much light bread in this country. Cornbread at every meal. All quiet at this post. Vicksburg not taken but destined to be after a long and severe struggle. Much love to Eva Bell, Fannie and Maria. I want them to write individually, personally and collectively. Lots of fraternal love to Amos A. Would be much pleased to hear from him through the medium of pen & paper. Immeasurable, paternal, unalloyed and double distilled affection for Ma & Pa and would jump up and down to read a letter penned by their hands. It has been nearly two months since such an incident occurred in my presence. Please do write soon and direct as per address of this epistle. Remembering I am in charge of the institution. Heard from Maj. Bowyer, speaks in the warmest terms of friendship and wishes it continued and renewed by correspondence. Compliments to all inquiring friends, especially all the marriageable, handsome, young roses. Yours in the bonds of ever abiding love,

Yours affectionately,

T S. Hawley

P.S. Remember I always write the first of each week. If you have heard from the 111th Ill., please write me of it.

Nelson Hawley, Thomas' father, was a Methodist-Episcopal minister in Illinois and the letter on February 15 is almost entirely devoted to the idea of Nelson joining the 11th Missouri Infantry as chaplain. Thomas Hawley tried to explain in this letter the situation within the 11th Missouri Infantry in regard to spiritual matters. The 11th Missouri Infantry was a difficult regiment and by 1863 had had two chaplains which resigned. The first chaplain was Reverend Joseph Brooks, an ardent abolitionist and an Ohio native, who was forty years-old when he enlisted. He was living in St. Louis at the beginning of the war and was the editor of the *Central Christian Advocate*. In April

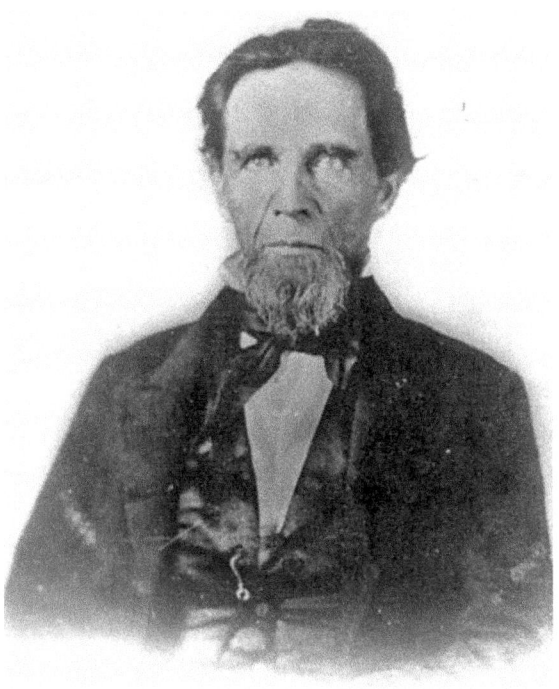

Nelson Hawley, Thomas Hawley's father (courtesy Kathryn Breuer).

1862 Chaplin Joseph Brooks resigned and was replaced by Samuel Baldridge. Reverend Joseph Brooks left the 11th Missouri Infantry to join the 33rd Missouri Infantry which was commanded by his brother. Reverend Brooks left a rather cryptic resignation letter stating, "A condition of things having arisen within this command which will hinder the profitable exercise of the function of my office."[3] Reverend Samuel Baldridge replaced Joseph Brooks as the next chaplain of the regiment in the summer of 1862 and by January 1863, Reverend Baldridge resigned. Reverend Baldridge wrote in his letter of resignation, "Convinced by a long & earnest trial of my inability to work the moral & spiritual welfare of your gallant command in a manner to satisfy my own conscience or the just demands of the government."[4] Hawley recorded in his letter Joseph Brooks and Doctor Thomas Smith were so "mean and professed so much" in their beliefs the command of the regiment was alienated from further religious extremes. Thomas Hawley also advised his father campaigning might be too difficult for him and he might be better suited to be a chaplain in a garrison rather than an active regiment.

Genl. Hospital No. 3
LaGrange, Tenn. Feb. 15th 1863

Dear Pa, Ma and the little folks

Another week has passed without bringing any further intelligence from the magazine of affections. If I could only get off a few days, think all would be well. I could see Dr. Bowyer and settle with the 11th Mo. and perhaps draw some pay extra. The past proposition to the 11th might be considered and put under headway but the 11th are skeptical as to all religious things. The Lt. Col. and others, Mr. Brooks and Dr. Smith acted so mean and professed so much they became disgusted and soon the reigns of passion rent loose and their passage downward has since been rapid. But Pa could do much if his health would permit. For it, I have the greatest solicitation and would earnestly advise that you do not think of living in the tented field until your health is fully restored which I think and hope with proper care and treatment would be good by spring. Pa has devoted too much time housed up for the past 4 or 5 years. Rather a sudden transition from his former mode of living which was overbalanced the other way, too much exposure. The two must counterbalance the other. Let the children have plenty of exercise in the open air. All depends upon that.

The weather for the past few days has been fine speaking jocularly, mud and rain seemed the order of the day, teams stalled and teamsters yelling and cursing. But today all appears fine as a May morn with a fair prospect of it continuing. I strolled about town a short time today and saw hyacinths, almost in bloom, jonquils and rose buds swelling, all the bulbous roots peeping out and I imagined one could almost see them grow. They looked so pretty and flourishing. Then we stepped to the suburbs of the town south where the view is indeed a fine one on the bluff and stretching away down the slope from your feet. Pine[s] are growing luxuriously which the mind keeps a constant rushing through, then dark branches, which sound like the roar of a cascade and you almost look involuntarily to the river winding its way at the foot of the hills but its current flows on undistributed by a rocky bed or of the crashing elements of a Civil War. Your eye can only catch a glimpse occasionally of this winding Wolfe River. I think it must have followed the track of an animal by that name which was trying to evade its pursuers for often you can see it for a short distance then suddenly a pine forest or high hill covers its retreat. Away beyond on the blue ridges of Mississippi 20 miles below, houses and farms are indistinct from the haziness of the air. Houses and fences are knocked down or have been [used] for wood and everything bears the marks of a destroying element. I cannot endorse such measures but to take everything that will support life and that will carry people away gives the citizen ample time to go north or south then leaving nothing behind to support them. In this way and that only can we conjure a peace and I think we will come to this line of policy ere long for I do not now nor never have doubted our ability to conquer the rebellion and once more establish the unity and vindicate the power of this great nation. Which never has, nor never will, be subdued neither by a foreign or internal foe no matter whether he comes from the north, south, east or west. Ultimately all will be well but then how long, oh how long? Are we doomed to go on this way suffering bearing and forbearing.

I recd. a letter or letters from Ma, Pa, Eva Bell and Sister Maria, all of which I acknowledge in my answer to Myra's. They all came to hand the same day. I mailed you a long one last Monday I think. Pa, I have answered part of yours and hardly know what to say about you seeking the chaplaincy of the 11th Mo. I could advise or suggest better if your health was good which hope it may be and think it soon will be.

They, of the gallant Mo 11 who know anything of you, would jump at the idea of your being with them. Dr. B[owyer] will, I know, do all he can for you. Lt. Col. Webber is skeptical, the Col. not now with them is careless about all religious things and so are most of the officers. Bro. Baldridge told me all of his trials but he is not as firm as you are. If you get a post chaplaincy or some other duty at a station it would be much more pleasant and you might stand it better. But if you can contend yourself to remain in Richland and fight the rebels there and occasionally shout at the devil I will most freely send all my extra greenbacks which are now due over $500. Of which I think I can collect over $150 just as soon as I get to Memphis, which I think will be this week or next. I can and will express it just as soon as I get it. You have already done much for your country. But if your health is good and you cannot stay back, go to the 11th Mo if no better place is open and I shall try to be with you. If you must come out to battle, I must be with you. Ma, I have spent all the space on this letter to Pa and filibustering answer. Will try to write you in this week. Love by the thousands I send you. Please write soon and often to your affectionate son and bro.

T. S. Hawley

P. S. I'll answer Eva Bell's letter too soon. Here's a kiss.

On February 20, 1863, Thomas Hawley turned twenty-six years of age and he devoted this letter to his domestic thoughts of the past and future. He wrote, "I have thrown my all upon the altar of my country and shall defend her to the last." At this point in the war, he did not know what this meant because Hawley would fulfill this vow, and remain in the Union Army for another three years during which time he would face some of his greatest challenges. Despite his relatively young age, Thomas Hawley was in charge of a general hospital which the surgeon-in-chief referred to as a "model hospital." Such were the challenges and experience he gained during the Civil War.

Genl. Hospital No. 3
LaGrange, Tenn. Feb 20, 1863

Dear Mother,

 According to [my] promise I select this, my birthday, to pen you a letter. One addressed especially to her who I am indebted for all for I am. My life that dearest boon of all for that tender care during the long period of helpless infancy. Such care and nourishment as only a mother can give. For that careful watchfulness of all my habits and evil tendencies and when I strayed from the path of rectitude, was the first to bring back the little wanderer. For this, Oh how thankful I should be for these and many other unnumbered blessings. I can hardly realize that I am 26 years of age. It seems but yesterday that I was a little boy running after you and asking favors or a little time after drawing, my then, little sister, in the carriage around the suburbs of our little frontier settlement. A few years after my dear bro. & I strolling through the forest ever looking for some curiosity or driving up the good old cows or with an ase and our little pet, Cesar, chasing the cotton tailed rabbits or gathering a bouquet for our watchful and always anxious mother.

 Those were indeed the happy days of my youth. Days long to be remembered and I confess to looking back upon them with feelings of regret, not that I would always be enjoying the springtime of youth. But rather because the precious golden moments were not improved as they might have been. Tis true, my life so far has not been spent without an aim and I think I have realized some at least of my aspirations. That of doing good and alleviating the suffering of my fellow beings and making those with whom I am thrown upon the stage of time happier for having known me.

 This great Civil War has cast a shadow over some of my expectations and aspirations. But has opened a new field for heroism and pure self-sacrificing patriotism which is in my opinion one of the greatest virtues of an honorable citizen of this great free and glorious republic. I have before this intestene strife assumed so hideous a form mapped out for myself a pleasant social life, with those around whom I loved, a life of gratitude and of research into the sciences of nature. The sunny hours of happy youth are past, never to be recalled. The sun advancing rapidly to the zenith of my manhood arouses me from the pleasant fanciful dreaming life of youth and loudly calls to action. The stern battles of life must be fought and won. Yes, and the battles, battles of our country must be fought. Our free institutions handed down by our forefathers, defended & preserved for the benefit of posterity. Truly we live in a great age and should be thankful that we can defend so glorious a cause.

 I have thrown my all upon the altar of my country and shall defend her to the last. Ma, I guess it has been almost a year since I wrote you another letter similar to this in some respects. That year does not seem long although passed mostly upon the tented field. So I am enjoying something of life for I have had witness to the relief of many pains and today have a house full of grateful, good, brave soldiers. Some of them upon their last bed. I wish you could step in and see my hospital. The surgeon-in-chief called it a model hospital the other day in describing it to a surgeon visiting this place. They called in to see a Rebel who we are carefully attending, whose leg was amputated a few days ago.

Dearest Mother, your trials since I left have truly been severe and I only wonder at your powers of endurance both physically and mentally. I feel confident you could not have borne so much but for your great love for a dear and only sister and her poor helpless babes who are now almost orphans. We will do our utmost to protect and care for them. Aunt Martha, who I used to love to write to, has passed away from us forever. But our loss has been her gain. I fear Dear Grandpa will not pass through the winter in safety. I am so glad I took a little time to see them last fall.

Mother in your next, please tell me all about your health and Father's. And also what you think of his joining the army.

Another year, my 27th, is before me. I most sincerely wish to spend in the most profitable way & not let one golden moment pass unimproved. Am making some rules to govern my actions and labors for, especially, those for my improvement. Please advise or suggest any you think best. Or anything I had better do this year or leave off. Your hearty prayers and the rest of the family I know, and feel, I have. My health, thank God, is good, and sincerely hope you are & may continue to enjoy the same great blessing. Nothing new at this post. Has the 111th Ills. gone to Vicksburg? Never have heard. No letters from home since I wrote you last. Please all write soon. Will write you soon as I leave this place. Cannot say when.

Ever your affectionate son,

T. S. Hawley

The letter of February 27 was the last one sent from General Hospital Number 3 which was closed due to the low number of patients to medical staff ratio. There were only fifty patients and more than 20 medical staff. As a result, the staff of General Hospital Number 2 was consolidated with Hospital Number 3, and Thomas Hawley reported for duty in the new hospital. Hospital Number 2 was located in the LaGrange Female College which had been built in 1854 and had contained about 25 rooms. Thomas Hawley was transferred to a hospital with about 150 patients and many in severe condition. Although he was devoted to the medical care of the patients, he had time to reflect on the war. In a very prophetic statement he wrote the fall of Vicksburg must happen and referring to the Mississippi River, he wrote, "although its dark waters may be changed to red by the flow of human blood. It must, shall and will be forever free."

Genl. Hospital No. 3
LaGrange, Tenn. Feb 27th 1863
Dearest Parents, Bro. & Sisters,

Once more the periodical letter writing comes around or within two days of it and anticipating a busy time for the next few days, I thought I would take time by the forelock and write now. My health remains good notwithstanding the very unpleasant weather. And I only lost one case during the past month. They asked what was the reason that I reported no more deaths. Indeed we have had a pleasant time as all the attendants remark and most of the patients wanted to remain with me. But I have not told you, today we concentrated the hospitals, broke up No. Three and I go to No. 2 with Dr. Edwards of the 40th Ill. Vols. The building is only a short distance from here formerly the female seminary. There is about 150 patients and many of them bad. Dr. Edwards has been there some time with Dr. Olnick who now goes to the 26th Ill. regiment. Dr. E. remaining in charge.

I think we can get along pleasantly for the Dr. is disposed to do what's right. I fear I cannot get off from this place very soon for we are scarce of hands now and the doctor wants two or three more men in the surgical department. We were getting along fine in No. 3 and all feel bad to leave. We were like a band of brothers. A Mr. Buitt Whas has been here for some time attending his brother of the 63 Ill., said he had a fine officer's coat that he would give me if he only had it here or if I was near his regiment. His brother died last night and we got him permission to take his body to Memphis but water is so high at Wolf River that the cars cannot pass today and I fear they cannot tomorrow. Today was unusually warm and pleasant. Hyacinths are in bloom. I wish the undersigned could visit that rarest of all roses wasting it sweetness on the desert air near the former city of flowers. I should strive to transplant it in more genial clime, where the miasma of Rebelldom would not wither its opening beauties. But your humble author thinks the climate rather unhealthy much farther south than this and will not gather this bouquet of beauty to place upon the choicest leaf of his herbarium (i.e.) too unhealthy at this present season. Now it may change in that respect. Think it will after Vicksburg falls and the broad bosom of the Father of Waters is no longer tarnished by rebel thralldom and that will come although its dark waters may be changed to red by the flow of human blood. It must, it shall and will be forever free to the whole of the commerce of the wide world and produce for the sustenance of millions of beings shall float on its current. It will indeed be the great artery of the nation, the aorta flowing from the heart of the nation, the mighty Mississippi Valley.

Bro. Morrison is here, all right, well & hearty. I saw Mr. Higgins a few days ago, well, and glad to see us. My compliments to her, Bob and Mrs. M. B. Gunn and the baby. I have not heard from you this month nor from Dr. Bowyer for some days. They are still at Germantown. What does Pa think of the Chaplaincy and what does Dr. Bowyer say about it? I have not heard from him since I wrote him about our positions. Is Mr. Cliff with the 98th Ill.? How does that old secesh Wooley head or Wollard of the 111th Ills. prosper?

By accident I saw Bob Martin at this place last week, had come down on business to Memphis, then to the 40th Ill. below here and on his return trip was waiting for the cars. So I got to see him for a short time. Said the 111 was doing well. His brother was commanding the post. There has been and is plenty of sickness in the regiment. Almost all had had the measles and Dr. Rainey & Philips had their hands full. Said the boys wished I could have remained with them. Promised to write soon. This hospital was broken up because we could not keep enough sick for the number of nurses and attendants. We only had about 50 men sick and over 20 attendants, more than the regulations allow. Dr. Crawford our senior officer is an obliging man. You can direct your letters as formerly only No. 2, for No. 3. And do please send them thick & fast. I want to read them so bad.

My love and complements to all the friends at home. My undivided love you always & hourly have. Your affectionate son & bro.,

T. S. Hawley

By March 7, Thomas Hawley received a large packet of letters which had been held with the 111th Illinois Infantry and he was ecstatic. His letters were delivered by the side-wheel steamboat, the *Belle Memphis*, which was constructed in 1860 and traveled from St. Louis and Memphis. As Hawley wrote his letter he noticed a light on the horizon which he concluded was Union cavalry burning the homes of Southern supporters demonstrating that the war was very difficult for the civilians as well as the soldiers.

Troops were moving toward the Vicksburg area and along with them came the surgeons, quartermasters and others. Grant was massing his army on the western shore of the Mississippi River near Vicksburg. He unsuccessfully attempted during the winter and early spring months to dig a canal to by-pass the guns at Vicksburg. Despite this setback Grant wanted his troops ready to move on the citadel as soon as the weather was suitable. Hawley wrote the 11th Missouri Infantry was scheduled to depart the following week for Vicksburg also. Lieutenant Mark Sappington, a farmer and minister before the war, of the 11th Missouri had recently visited Thomas Hawley.

Genl. Hospital ~~No. 3~~
LaGrange, Tenn. March 7, 1863

Dearest Father, Mother, Bro., Sisters, Myra, Francis, and last but not least Eva Bell.

Your long look[ed] for and precious letters came to hand after so long a delay and your Son & Bro. was overjoyed and jump[ed] up and shouted. Now I have the whole history which was so long broken up. As soon as they came to hand I sit down and keep reading all day and would not stop until all the interesting pieces of history was faithfully perused. I feasted on it, enjoyed them intellectually and physically. They had, as I anticipated, been delayed at the 111th Ills. Vols. and Dr. R. sent them all to me in our big official envelope, postage 18 or 21 cents, 4 from Harry Baker at the same time. He had stopped at Columbus on his way to Memphis, was on the steamer <u>Belle Memphis</u> and could not come up or go up to the regiment, did not ascertain, and I guess does not yet know, that I was away down in Dixie.

This package from the regiment contained the 4 from Hal and two from Myra Dec. 13th & Feb. 27, one from Amos Dec. 24. Sisters, I rather think I have answered by individual letters but will write again and the next will be entirely confidential. Now remember and bear in mind. But Amos I shall answer specifically because he so seldom writes and Fannie I shall lecture for not writing oftener. But then you all wrote such good letters and sent so many nice papers by P. Brillheart that I cannot scold any one very hard. Many thanks for those nice papers and also pretty pictures by Miss Evie Bell Hawley of Olney, Illinois. I do not get to see many little girls but one [day] last week saw one who was a little rebel so her Grandma said. She keeps mum. Once in a while hear some music and occasionally go to church and very seldom sees a handsome young lady. They are a scarce article in this state indeed. I have not seen one.

That nice bunch of letters and papers came to hand by a friend of the 26 Ills. Vols. as he came from Memphis. I very much fear they will be ordered away before I get see them, have not heard from them for some time. The 40 Ills. is still at Davis Mills, 6 miles below Grand Junction. The col. is well as usual and the Dr. has been unwell with chills. Dr. Edwards, the asst. surgeon, is one of my messmates. Dr. Smith of the 6th Iowa has just left as per order to Young's Point, La. Most of the troops are about leaving this point and are filling up the hospitals with their sick. We will be kept very busy for some time under this surplus of patients. We need more help, more surgeons and must have them. About the last of my famous hospital No. 3 left for Memphis today. A few contrabands only remaining and the house is occupied by army quartermasters, telegraph, etc. The secesh, Loggins, who has been under my treatment since his leg was amputated has got along remarkably well and I think will get well. Cotton buyers and other

Copperheads are having a fun time. Now some are getting alarmed. Cotton keeps coming down and the soldiers are down still harder on Copperhead[s].

Sunday evening March 7. Rained hard last night and turned cold this morning. Troops been marching all day. Our brigade left and another came to relieve them, the 26 Ill. left or rather will leave tomorrow. Will go to Collierville between here and Memphis. The fourth division and the 8 [th] division are ordered to Vicksburg and the 11th Missouri will leave next week. And I cannot get to see them. Lieut. Sappington was here a short time ago, but I did not get to see him. He look[ed] for me for some time and had to leave on the train. Only stayed a short time. Heard no particulars from the regiment only that Dr. Bowyer was well and the health generally good. Pa, I think the plan you propose for a house a good one as cannot just now think of any better. The plan I think will economize room and funds. Hope you can make some improvements on the house in the spring. If you can get that school, it will be the next best thing according to my opinion and if well established, will in a few years become a paying institution and the town of Olney will be someday a flourishing little place or rather city. Indeed is that almost now. If we can only put this rebellion down this summer, our northern states will soon recover from the shock and horrors of war and go on in their unequal rate of improvement and unparalleled progress.

But in these southern and border states, 50 years will not erase all the destruction and devastation of the war engine. Indeed some points will forever bear the indelible marks of war's angry strife. Think you this will all come to naught the great sacrifice and loss of blood. A mighty nation will prevail in this cause for the world.

Monday evening. You will think this a journal instead of a letter if I continue it many more days. But just at this time all my time from 8 o'clock until middle of the afternoon is employed at the hospital. I cannot answer letters in detail this time but will try and do so soon, in the meantime continue writing.

I am truly glad to hear that your health is improving and hope Bro. Amos' health will soon be better.

The present you speak of in your last will be magnificent and Sister will be in her element and I hope will coin money and many blessings from dear friends. It will be a household treasure for all while she remains but some Sucor may come and take it and her away. Look out for him.

The 48 & 49 Ills. are coming to this place so I understand and the railroad will be abandoned from Columbus to Jackson. If so, most of the troops stationed at Columbus will be ordered away and 111 may go to Vicksburg. There was quite a light [in the] southwest his evening, cannot say what was the cause but expect the doings of our cavalry burning some secesh domicile. Today there was more rebels in town than soldiers (i. e.) in appearances. Flowers are in bloom and trees begin to clothe themselves in the beautiful verdue of spring yet the nights are quite cold and occasionally some rain. The hospitals are full to overflowing.

Please write soon one and all. Many, many grateful thanks for those nice letters & papers. Remember my inexhaustible love you all have. I send each many unwrapped kisses.

You affect bro. & son,

T. S. Hawley

The letters from home were arriving about three months behind as Thomas Hawley wrote a letter to his younger brother, Amos, on March 13. Amos Hawley was not a healthy person and through the letters Thomas wrote to Amos, it was clear Amos was trying to find some sort of occupation. He had worked on a farm for a while and most recently he worked at the post office which appeared to be unsuccessful. Hawley related in his letter he was called to treat a Union soldier who was guarding a local farmer's property from the ravages of Union troops. The Union soldier was taken with pleurisy which was a painful inflammation of the lungs. Hawley described his treatment which included bleeding the patient, and then administering morphine which helped with the pain and allowed the patient to sleep during the night. Both the patient and Doctor Hawley spent the night at the farmer's house. Meanwhile at the hospital, there were about 150 patients present and several patients suffered from erysipelas. This was a very serious medical problem which was caused by a bacterial infection. If patients suffered from this infection, as many as 40 percent of cases resulted in death. Later in the war, it was discovered iodine applied to the edges of the wounds stopped the further advance of the infection.

Genl. Hospital
LaGrange, Tenn.
March 13, 1863
Dear Brother,

Your kind good letter of last Dec. 24th came to hand a few days ago and was perused with much pleasure. It is so seldom you write. Why cannot you sit down almost any day and pen a few lines to Dixie?

I was in hopes you could find almost constant occupation in the post office if your health would permit. But feared it would not. Am satisfied that your employment must combine more of the outdoor physical exercise which is so essential to every one's health.

The weather is now improving for the past few days has been almost like summer. Indeed today was unpleasant walking during the middle of the day. Wil-

low trees are leafing out and a few other varieties. Also, several kinds of flowers are springing up. Last night I spent outside of our pickets. One of our patients had gone out to guard a planter's property from the depredations of the federal soldiers and was suddenly taken with pleurisy. I found him suffering greatly, took nearly a pint of blood from right arm. This relieved him some but the pains soon returned with all their former severity. Then I cupped on sich and took more blood again. Some relief, administered calomel doses, blister to sich and take two doses of Morphio. Patients sleep heavily all night. But that is half the story. Went out, in the ambulance sat Hospital Steward and teamster. Somebody found the man so bad, the planter, Mr. Lockheart and lady, persuaded me to remain all night. Saw I had plenty to eat, good bed to sleep and young ladies could sing, etc. So I stayed and had a high time. But didn't fall out nor in love with any one of the four. Came out of the skirmish with a whole heart and gizzard. But one could play & sing some. Has sister got the <u>Bonny Blue Flag</u>? My patient is better this morning. Dr. Edwards and myself attend to over 150 patients which keep us with our eyes open. Have had several cases of erysipelas in the hospital. Not so many now. Much love to all the family. I remain, your affct. bro.,

T. S. Hawley

Folks Generally

News from all quarters interesting and think the history of the next few months will tell of the visible beginning of the end of the fall of slavocracy.

Hooker about to strike the head. Rosey & Hunter cutting off either arm and thrusting at the heart. Genl. Grant's gallant western army cutting away with the help of Banks, cutting off each of the lower limbs and shooting at his dinner basket. I think when all the forces begin operating Mr. Rebelldom will be permanently disabled. My health is good. Have not heard from the 111th but once. Saw. Dr. Elliot yesterday, was better, regt. doing well.

I think and hope we will leave here soon. Have not heard from the 11 Mo. lately. All please write soon.

Yours affctly,

T. S. Hawley

Thomas Hawley's letter to his sister, Fannie, of March 15, 1863, was entirely focused on domestic issues, including, valentines, recitation of bible verses, encouragements of lessons, and exercise. Thomas Hawley was still serving as hospital surgeon at LaGrange and he continued in this capacity until May. General Grant and the Union Army were still focused on the Vicksburg campaign. One of operations implemented by Grant was the Yazoo Pass Expedition which was a coordinated effort by Grant's Army of the Tennessee and Admiral David Porter's Mississippi River Squadron. The operation was designed to find a way around the formidable Confederate defenses and artillery at Vicksburg. Grant wanted to find a way to move his army across the Mississippi River and approach Vicksburg from the east. Grant and Porter thought they could use the backwaters of the Mississippi Delta to reach the Yazoo River and once on the Yazoo, the army could approach Vicksburg unopposed from the east. The expedition began in February when a levee on the Mississippi River was broken and the river water flowed into old channels. On March 11, 1863, the Union naval vessels approached a fort which had been constructed to stop the fleet from moving further than Greenwood, Mississippi. Artillery exchanges took place between the fort and the Union vessels over a three day period. In the end, the fort effectively stopped the Union advance which retreated back to the Mississippi River. This delayed Grant's advance on Vicksburg from the east, and although stymied, Grant would not be stopped from his objective.

> *General Hospital*
> *LaGrange, Tenn.*
> *March 15, 1863*
> *Sister Fannie,*
>
> Dear Little Puss. Oh, I want to kiss you so much for that sweet, good, loving letter sent by Mr. Brillheart. It was the best you have written to me yet and I think you might and could do better. You ask if I received a valentine. I answered nary. But should like to know who was the person that would send one to me if I had not been so far off. I think I know a little miss who [would] send one. Myself sure.
>
> I suppose you have numerous correspondence in Salem. Well that's all right. Only keep them up. Florida C. is a pleasant little lady. Almost as ponderous as Miss Myra. I am truly glad to hear you have so fine a Sabbath school in Olney. Hope it may continue. Of the 2,627 bible verses committed to memory, how many did you recite? Eva Bell wants to see me awful bad, does she? Tell her to borrow a pair of wings and fly down here and see me and the pretty flowers, hear the delightful mockingbirds sing and gather bouquets for the sick soldiers. Well little sister, I hear you are going to write me. That will be so nice. Do write soon. I want to get a letter from you very bad.
>
> Fannie, I am so glad to hear that you are progressing well with your studies. Only continue applying your mind closely and you will be amply rewarded in advanced life. You will, my dear. Also train the physical system which is so essential to comfort, usefulness and happiness during our pilgrimage on this mundane shore.
>
> Study hard when you are at it and when playing, go [at] it. You are at that

period of life most interesting and when time well spent, will be most useful. I ardently desire to see you with a complete English education, at least, and shall hope to assist you to the final accomplishment of your education. For I look upon that as the richest inheritance of a daughter or son and replete with the most happiness. But it takes years of ardent and close application. Place your mark high and always look to and aim for it. Think of these things and please write to me some of your thoughts. I send you a few flowers and all the love and pure brotherly affection that [can] be imagined.

T. S. Hawley

Thomas Hawley referred to Sol Street in his March 22, 1863, letter to his family. The 33 year-old Street was a native of Mississippi and had lived near Ripley, Mississippi prior to the war. Street had served in the Army of Virginia, but obtained a discharge and returned to Mississippi in 1862 to defend his home state from the Union Army occupying it. Upon returning to Mississippi, he formed a group of guerrillas to harass the Union occupiers. Captain Sol Street, who operated for 18 months in northern Mississippi, commanded only one company, but his guerrillas usually included support from other irregulars and perhaps another company of cavalry. Street's first clash with the Union Army was on January 5, 1863, when he ambushed the Union cavalry south of Bolivar, Tennessee. From January 5, Street raided along the Mobile and Ohio and Mississippi Central Railroads successfully and was noted for his effective destruction of the railroads. Hawley's letter related the attempt of Street on March 21, 1863, to capture a Union pay train with a force of about 80 men, but instead he derailed a construction train. Sol Street became famous as a notorious guerrilla and later became part of Major General Nathan Bedford Forrest's cavalry. Sol Street was killed by a Confederate soldier, Robert Galloway, on May 2, 1864, in an act of revenge because Street had killed Galloway's father during a robbery in one version of the story.[5]

The threat of guerrillas or spies moving within the Union lines was described in Thomas Hawley's letter. Not only did the Union forces have to fight these irregulars in the countryside, they did not know if citizens were spies or actual combatants. Freemasonry was also mentioned in Hawley's March 22 letter as he described the camaraderie of those soldiers who were part of this organization. Freemasonry was a fraternal, religiously based organization and had particular appeal to some of the soldiers in the Civil War. Although the letter doesn't mention enlisted men as part of the meeting, it does refer to various ranks of officers. Thomas Hawley was very impressed with the military lodge he attended and was favorably inclined to join.

General Hospital LaGrange, Tenn.
March 22nd 1863

Dear Parents, Bro. & Sisters,

 Another Sabbath in the natural course of things has rolled around and spring with all its loveliness has paid us, or is visiting us and is busily engaged in enrobing all nature. The forest trees are putting on their summer dress. Mother earth is being newly carpeted with a finer than your imported Brussles [Brussels lace] and tis just wearing in such beautiful flowers of all tints and shades; and strong for carpet flowers, they are very fragrant. This will indeed soon be to us the "sunny south." But a short time ago twas the rainy south, then the muddy south. The elements appearing to attain the superlative degree in all these qualities. The weather is now indeed pleasant and if your health is not improving, Pa, come down on some mission and recuperate your lost health. But then, some say, the spring is not a good time for a change. I think it is much better than the fall. Peach trees are all in full bloom, grass is growing nicely and these southern mockingbirds do exceed anything I ever heard. I do wish I could send you a pair, shall try it anyhow. When the young birds make their appearance, all say they are the best to sing & train.

 The Order of Free Masons held their anniversary on yesterday, the 1st for their military organization by Gen. Bates at Shawneytown, Ills. Dr. McNeal made quite a speech, had a fine brass band and two guns of the 6 Ills. Calv. Flying Artillery which awakened the southern chivalry from their dreaming musings about 3 o'clock in the afternoon and brought up the northern lights, blue coats, etc. We were united in the surgeon's office (for the meeting was held in front of the 6th Ill. Calv. hospital) and had some beer and introductions to numerous sons of man in the shape of Cols., Drs., surgeons, capts. lieuts., etc., from the far north. All this we enjoyed and the speech afterward, a short exposition of the mystic brotherhood. I long since decided to become a member [at] the first favorable opportunity and may join this military lodge as they are in running order and full of good men.

 There would have been a much larger audience but the 6th Ill. had just been ordered out 3 hours before to capture Sol Street, a notorious guerilla, who it was reported had captured a train of cars a few miles east of Grand Junction and 8 to 10 of this place. I hear this morning the boys returned last night after capturing 3 or 4 men. These infernal rascals attempted to get the pay train and took up a few rails expecting that would come next. But as fortunately for Uncle Sam, an old wood train [was] passing that way and fell into the trap. The villans shot 8 to 10 poor darkies. Burned two or three cars and took a few prisoners. The citizens have free access to all our camps but the guerilla chiefs can come in at any time and get all the information their Black Hearts could wish or the sneaking citizen can get the news for them. They knew exactly when the pay train would come down but did not know of the wood [train] which only thwarted their thieving scheme.

    Harry Baker, I heard from in Memphis, this a few weeks ago, not since. Do not know where he is. Dear Mother, your exceeding good and ever to be remembered letter was read with tears and will be ever cherished and remembered. I received my commission and a pretty good letter from Col. Martin after writing and telegraphing him. Hope to get some pay soon. Mr. Morrison paid me so, I am all right. Bro. M. has had smallpox. I called to see him yesterday and told him it was that disease. Hope and think he will recover. Perhaps you had better not say anything about it. No letter last week. No papers. Two from Maria not long ago, always acceptable, sent you a Memphis Butternut Bulletin last week. Will send more. An ocean full of love to all.

T. S. Hawley

    In Thomas Hawley's March 29 letter, he indicated he continued with his religious activities and attended services performed by Dr. John H. Gray who was the president of the LaGrange Synodical College. Gray became president in 1855 and served until 1878. By Hawley's record the services were attended primarily by the Union soldiers. He also made a few satirical comments about the Southern ladies of LaGrange including a statement about the impact of wind on their "pedal extremities."

    Many times the stress exerted on families separated by absence and war is ignored, but Thomas Hawley mentioned the case of Cal Barney whose wife was living with a Mr. Upton while Barney served in the war. Obviously, as the war approached the conclusion of the second year and there was no end in sight, many families began to crumble. Thomas Hawley's connections with his old regiment, the 11th Missouri Infantry, continued into March, as he encountered his old pharmacist, Zeba French, and met Lieutenant Jacob Blew, who was a married farmer from Claremont, Illinois, before the war. In this letter, Thomas Hawley provided an excellent description of wartime Memphis including the fact a few houses had been burned. He also mentioned a desecration of the monument of Andrew Jackson attributed to Confederate General M. Jeff Thompson who removed the word "federal" from the quote, "The federal union must and shall be preserved."

General Hospital LaGrange, Tenn.
March 29, 1863

Dearest Parents,

    I have just returned from church services by Dr. Gray, Presbyterian. House full but not many citizens out, as the house it is rather cold and some of our boys have taken away the stores. And their March winds play strange feaks with crinolen and ladies pedal extremities. And it would not do for these fair lillies of the sunny south to expose their frail and precious selves to the bleak and chilling winds of March. The weather is more changeable and those changes [more] sudden than the weather a few degrees north. Two weeks ago it was too warm for a woolen coat, today an overcoat is hardly sufficient and old sol's rays cannot penetrate to the "terra firma" because of a strong northwester that makes the windows & doors rattle and drives all the darkies indoors and chills all these merry little flowers until they shake and tremble in their nests. They come springing up and gaily nodding their lovely heads to every passerby that spring was coming. Spring was here they proclaimed but their proclamations proved to be untrue but I think spring will soon be heralded by the proper authorities but this climate cannot be two weeks in advance of your latitude while this all the sudden changes has and that to this highest degree in winter. It is almost as cold and in summer it is much hotter than in the moderate climate of Illinois.

The soil in this part of Tenn. is rather sandy and below the soil is a sticky yellow clay. After the soil is cultivated a year or two, it must be plowed every year and the furrows to run around the hills to prevent washing. Indeed nearly every field is now cut up by gullies and deep ditches so that in a few years of idleness the soil is all washed off and it is impossible to till the soil until [they] are filled up at great trouble and expense.

I took a short respite last week and visited Memphis (would that I could have gone long ago) and saw many old friends. Lt. Col. H. Glaze of the 63 Ills. Jno. Fair, Wolf & Knapp from Olney. Col. Glaze is in his usual good health as are the others. I remained some hours and had a good chat. Stopped at the Gayes, left here at 7 o'clock, landed at M[emphis] about one, stopped at the Officers Hospital and who should I first see but Cal Barney acting as Druggist, has a good place but claims that he was betrayed. Says his wife is in Olney with Mr. Upton, has two small children, has the blues and wishes you if convenient to call. Sends his best respects, as do H. Glaze, etc. Call[ed] and stayed all night with Dr. Friese in charge of contraband hospital in suburbs of Memphis. He has his family there and lives at home. All glad to see me. I also found Dr. French, my old chum and Hospital Steward of the gallant 11th Mo. He was stopping with Mr. Friese, came up from Helena, Ark. where the 11th Mo is stationed. For the present in charge of a few sick and may soon go north in charge of others, will call if he should. Said to me that Pa would most likely be appointed Chaplain of the 11th Mo. which I was glad to hear as Pa has many friends there. I also told him I must be with them if you joined them and that in almost any capacity. Pa, your letter and Bro. Amos' came to hand last week in good time. There has been a great improvement in time. I also saw Wm. Neighbors from Belleville, did not have a very long chat. He is with the 130 Ills. Also saw Col. Niles of the same regt. and Genl. Oglesby looking much better. Hear he will take a command near Vicksburg. Saw Lt. Blew of the 11th Mo., lives near Fairview, not very well, had rheumatism, saw many other army friends and besides that the Elephant. This you know my first visit to Memphis, has a population I should say of near 30,000 when full and now did not notice many vacant houses, has ten business streets running up and down the river banks, plenty high, rather too high when the water is low. I should think a few very good houses for business on these streets. Three or four of them used as hospitals, saw but one or two marble fronts and some iron fronts. Court square is one street from the river and occupies just one solid square. A strong iron fence all around, three gates one each side, two streets from the middle of each side, meet at Jackson's bust in the center.

Then one street from each come to center and one all round with a few cross streets. Jackson's monument, as tis called, but is only a bust mounted on a square pedestal with some few ornaments. In all about four feet high, yes 7 or 8, the features a[re] good and about life size surrounded by an iron fence. The renegade Jeff Thompson disfigured the word federal in Genl. Jackson's immortal saying "The federal union it must and shall be preserved." Magnolias, cedar, pine and spruce and rose trees are growing finely. Also a few forest trees, 15 or 20 perhaps black-jack, on these are placed small boxes for the grey squirrels which are numerous, running and playing on the walks, on the trees, out on the streets, on the iron sentries, skipping along just out of your reach. No dogs are allowed in the square or a fine of five dollars. The streets back from the river are low and dirty. Men are engaged in policing the streets there. The numerous fires have not injured the appearance of the city much. Most of the houses burned being small, old and wooden. Genl. Hamilton and Denser have both left this place while the secesh reigned supreme, had it all their own way but Genl. Smith has changed the status of affairs and meets them all half way. I was in his office and saw a squint eyed, flat headed, drawing with a long parrot beak of a nose. Under it the words "Can I get permit to ship cotton?" and good hit I thought of Mr. Isarealite and traitor.

Ma's dear, good letter was duly received and greatly appreciated. Bro. Morrison is much better, saw him yesterday, will soon leave this place to join his regt. on railroad between here and Memphis. He has paid me up. Please continue writing as often as convenient. They all come I guess, but often behind. Much love to each & all.

Yours,

T. S. Hawley

When the Union Army was successful in forcing Confederate General Pierre Beauregard out of Corinth, Mississippi, in May 1862, the control of two major railroads fell under Union control. Corinth was the junction of the Memphis and Charleston Railroad (east-west) and the Mobile and Ohio Railroad (north-south); and these railroads were critical to the movement of supplies in the mid-south. These railroads were among the longest railroads in the Confederacy. The Memphis and Charleston Railroad was the direct line between the Mississippi River and the Atlantic seaboard. The value of these two railroads was not lost on either side, and because the Union controlled these two rail lines, the railroads were a constant target for Confederate raiders. The Confederates wanted to deny the Union forces a reliable and consistent flow of supplies and reinforcements. Thomas Hawley relayed the story of a Confederate raid on the railroad in his March 29 letter to his sister Fannie. He also wrote disparagingly of the efforts of those on the trains to repel the raiders. Thomas Hawley also wrote that all the hospitals in LaGrange were finally consolidated into one structure and only General Hospital Number 1 remained functioning by the end of March.

Thomas Hawley mentioned his appreciation for the song, *Bonny Blue Flag,* which was a very pro-Southern song and he thought it would be improved if the lyrics could be unionized. Some of the lyrics are:

> We are a band of brothers and native to the soil
> Fighting for our liberty, with treasure, blood and toil
> And when our rights were threatened, the cry rose near and far
> Hurrah for the Bonnie Blue Flag that bears a single star!
>
> Hurrah!
> Hurrah!
> For Southern rights, hurrah!
> Hurrah for the Bonnie Blue Flag that bears a single star.
>
> For Southern rights, hurrah!
> Hurrah for the Bonnie Blue Flag that bears a single star.
>
> Then cheer, boys, cheer, raise a joyous shout
> For Arkansas and North Carolina now have both gone out;
> And let another rousing cheer for Tennessee be given

HdQuats. Med. Dept.
Genl. Hospital LaGrange, Tenn.
The Windy Month of March the 29th
and the year of our Lord 1863

Dear Sister:

Helen Francis, yours of the 22nd inst. is before me and I shall not proceed to analyze it but finish up the news I had not room for on the other four pages addressed to Pa and Ma. Now for fear Sister Myra should become jealous, you must let her claim at least a part of this. I promised her a confidential epistle some time ago but fear I have nothing to give worthy of being locked up in so safe and confiding a bosom. Tell her my heart has lost all its secrets in the last few months. Yet by searching, I might find a few hidden things that by rubbing might appear to be jewels and if she still insists upon holding me to my promise, I shall most cheerfully comply.

Now for the news. The passenger train bound east from Memphis was attacked 40 miles from that point and about 8 west of this by a band of robbers in the service of the United Confederate States of America. They numbered about 8 or 10, had previously placed an iron rail across the track which the engine jumped but became detached from the other cars. The engineer ran to Moscow and brought back some soldiers but the birds had flown, carrying off some 7 or 8 officers, 25 or 30 soldiers and some little baggage. Both parties badly scared. One citizen & Negro shot. Only one shot fired by federals that knocked down a reb—passed through his hat and stunned but did not hurt him. None of our men hurt. They must have all been a pack of cowards. Many of them had arms so to take 40 scoundrels. The rebs fired the cars with turpentine but they did not burn. When the locomotive returned, the train came along all right minus a few passengers. No mail nor express captured. Ma's & Fannie's letter came on same train. I came with Dr. French up on the train [the] evening before.

Peach trees have been in full bloom for some time. Had some lettuce in Memphis and onions. Dr. French and I had our photograph taken together. Tomorrow we consolidate the hospitals at this place. No. 1 into Nos. 2 and 4. No. [Number] One is surrounded by fortifications and would be right in the heart of a fight should that occur. Tell Sister M. I am much obliged for that splendid bouquet so rich, rare and fragrant. Say to Bro. A, many thanks for his good letter. I prize it highly and shall answer soon. Tell Sister Bell I do not doubt that she comes to me on the wings of thought almost every day, that my ears burn lots of times. Then I know she is dreaming of me far away. Tell her I hope she will soon be able to write to me, then I shall jump up and down. Sister M, Frank is near Germantown or between there and Memphis, poor feller. The Sesesh ladies play for us when we ask them and often without, the <u>Bonny Blue Flag</u>. I send sister a copy of a reply written by one of our cols. taken at Shiloh and while in prison at Richmond or south someplace. One officer told me at Charleston. The music is good as sung by the little rebs and if you can unionize it, good. If you have not yet the music, will send it. Much love to all and many thanks for numerous good letters which only [make] this absence endurable. Strive to learn. Will that you do learn, being sure tis worth learning.

Your affct. bro.

T. S. Hawley

Easter arrived on April 5, 1863, with Thomas Hawley writing his weekly letter to his family in Illinois. He lamented the fact the Easter eggs were not to be had and the Union soldiers were probably more effective in catching chickens than subduing the Confederates. He humorously referred to eggs as "henfruit." He again attended church services on that Easter weekend and the homily was offered by the Reverend Simon G. Minor of Seventh Illinois Cavalry. Simon Minor was a 55-year-old Baptist minister and prior to the war he was pastor of the Baptist Church of Canton, Illinois.[6] Hawley wrote although the war around LaGrange was very quiet, there was a rumor of a large Confederate force commanded by General James Chalmers moving toward LaGrange. Finally Thomas Hawley wrote with suggestions of what his father should bring to the 11th Missouri Infantry if he was appointed as regimental chaplain.

Genl. Hospital LaGrange, Tenn.
Sunday April 5th 1863

Dearest

Ones under the Homestead roof,

    Well do I remember the happy Easters we children formerly had at home coloring eggs in a variety of ways and as many fantastic shades with numerous hieroglyphics and names. But today such vegetables as "Henfruit" are not to be had neither for love or money. Indeed that useful piece of furniture to every well regulated barnyard has become extinct in this part of Christendom. One would think in passing through here that the Yankees had been waging a warfare against those bipeds—hens & roosters. That cheerful and timely note from the Ol' Mr. Longs Spurs of Seceshia is played out. Not one is heard at the midnight hour or morning dawn to arouse the drowsey soldier boy as he dreams of fair ones away to the northward.

    Today I attended service twice and we do not have church at night. Once at the Presbyterian Church, sermon by Chaplain of 7 Ills. Calv., house full. At another time, sermon in large ward of our hospital by the Chaplain, Bro. Porter, a private but a very good preacher. The elements appear to have agreed to withhold further demonstrations of a boisterous character and allied to combination the most pleasant, serene and luxuriating, vivifying and ingratiating. Who would not live in this enchanted soil abounding in fine gay and gaudy vegetation of every known variety. Palm trees, oranges and figs, magnolia, cedar, pine, cypress and hollys ever dotting the hills and valleys with their evergreen verdue. The rose in this fair clime has a richer shade, a more delicate tint, a larger developed fullness and form and a sweeter fragrance. Indeed the whole vegetable kingdom appears to have advanced one, yes, 10 degrees higher than your more northern latitude. The nights are deliciously cool and dewy and when the Queen of the Night chooses to grace her throne, all is indeed loneliness for she throws her mazy gossamer veil of all scenery, hiding all the rough angles and corners reminding one of some fairy land where the air is loaded with sweet fragrance and the surrounding gardens of Paradise.

And then occasionally one finds some fairy queen who was born to reign in empires and kingdoms and not preside over the culinary art on [the] wash tub. Tis strange such a beautiful land does not produce more beauties of the fair sex. I have heard one old surgeon describe some of their tallowey skins, towering heads, wasplike waists, languid airs, delicate constitutions, tobacco dippers and Union haters. But there are some bright exceptions to this rule as I have before told you. And there are times when this lovely land loses most of it excellencies.

There is no news of much importance except that Gen. Chalmers is advancing upon the Charleston and Memphis RR someplace between here and Memphis with 6,000 troops. Is now some 20 or 25 miles off but our forces are vigilant and will not be caught napping.

Quite a number of ladies and citizens came out today to hear our northern preacher the first time since we came here. That looks favorable. I will send you my "Carte de Visite." Dr. French wanted mine and I his. So we had them together. It does not do me justice so they all say, and I believe them. We had 6 taken. He was so foolish as to give C. E. Barney one of them and my chum, Dr. Edwards (of whom I have a high opinion) wanted one. The other I send you. I did not succeed in getting any money while at Memphis. They appear determined not to pay me anything but some I will have and that soon. Your letters have been coming very regularly for the past few weeks but none last week which I cannot account for. I have hopes of being relieved from this place soon. Then I will get some pay and will get something else. The rebels are getting rather quiet in this part of Dixie but still express strong hopes of the ultimate success of the rebel cause which I think rather dubious just now and will continue so until their army is played out. All Europe is engaged nearer at home. The rebs can expect no aid from that source. They have conscripted all their able bodied men, from this [time] on their army must decrease, while ours is being augmented all the time and the source not near exhausted yet.

Pa, I would not be surprised to hear that your commission as chaplain of the 11 Mo. had come to hand in the regiment and you recv. official notice to that effect. Take, if you must go, a good substantial trunk, underclothes, blankets, oil cloth, etc. You can purchase any of those necessary articles at Ticnor and Co., St. Louis. It will not be necessary for you to buy a whole military suit now, only a black hat with U. S. in a wreath to designate your rank. Must procure a pass from Gen. Yates, free of charge. I would not be in any great hurry to go after informed or ordered and if your health is not sufficient, so inform them at the regt. You are perhaps surprised to

hear me talk so. I have long thought of this, would not care one half as much if I could only be with you. But Gov. Gamble may not see fit to appoint you. Well, write me or telegraph just as soon as you hear of this matter. Often I think of you all when all around is hushed and still. I run over my past years of unalloyed happiness and wish that I could be with you again and sit and chat away the joyous happy hours. Love I send you unmeasured quantities and 40 kisses apiece.
Your affct. son & brother,
T. S. Hawley

By April 11, the preparatory activities of the Vicksburg campaign were felt in LaGrange. Orders were received directing the remaining patients in General Hospital Number 1 in LaGrange to be transported to Memphis. The failure of the Yazoo Pass Expedition was also publicly announced. Grant's plan to easily and rapidly gain access to the eastern approach to Vicksburg was lost. Next, Grant formulated a more rigorous plan to transport his troops across the Mississippi River south of Vicksburg, then march through the Confederate held Mississippi countryside to Vicksburg. This operation was planned to begin in May. Hawley noted the heavy spring rains and the weather needed to be suitable for a large army to march without being mired in mud.

Thomas Hawley also recorded the presence of a representative of the United States Sanitary Commission at his hospital. He referred to her as a wife of a Union soldier. The United States Sanitary Commission was organized in St. Louis at the beginning of the Civil War. Many regiments suffered severely from poor sanitary conditions as the war began, and poor sanitation and minimal medical supplies often resulted in increased illness and death. The Sanitary Commission's objective was to improve the conditions in the army camps and hospitals. Many of the commission were women who served in various capacities including, nurses, and they were also very effective in obtaining financial support for their activities.

Hawley's April 11 letter noted that ex-slaves struggled in the Civil War. They were caught between freedom from their previous masters and retribution from the Southerners. Hawley related the incident of a guerrilla captain approaching a group of ex-slaves only to be shot through the heart by one the African Americans who, clearly, did not plan to return to the old way of life.

Officers Head Quarters
Genl. Hospital LaGrange, Tenn.
April 11th 1863
Dear Darling Ones at Home,

Another quarter lunar revolution and no greetings messenger from the paternal bosom. Was the communication destroyed or broken up for a time and [if] I

Three. 1863

knew it, the delay would be endurable but as it is my anxiety almost overcomes my sense of propriety. I did tell the orderly I should have him hung if he did not bring me a letter. But the little rascal did not comply with my order. If you should hear of an Israelite being suspended, do not become alarmed, but I think the sentence will be revoked as he has promised to scour my old coat soon. The weather has been fine. And my health good and I can see a general improvement among the soldiers. Our stock is becoming beautifully less and we send one hundred and fifty to Memphis tomorrow and may soon follow with all our forces. If we should advance on Memphis, look out for a desperate affair. But you have heard so much of this, some change of the base of operations, I shall not weary your patience with further details, nor hopes, nor anticipations.

Nothing worthy of note has transpired in this district since my last correspondence. Genl. Smith continues to maintain the same stringent policy that he established on his assuming command of this district. Just at this time there is quite a storm raging among the elements. Aqueous is pouring his forces upon us in innumerable quantities and King Boreus is charging over the plain with the greatest impetuosity bending and bowing trees, shaking windows, scattering tents and frightening contrabands, occasionally the red lightning flashes and the deep toned thunder roars. Hello! What does that mean? Looking below my cot—D. Buninger. Well by George! Where does that come from, looking at same place—a great puddle of water coursing its way out into our room. Not quite sufficient to drown a small man in. Then the supper bell. So I postpone this indefinitely.

After supper, storm abating. We dine in a tent made of flax or hemp. As soon as it gets wet, the rain drives through without the least abstraction down into our tea, on our potatoes, bread, meat, and into the salt & sugar and among the pickles. You see our fare is good or at least a supply of the necessaries of life. I had the pleasure of attending a wedding last week in our hospital. One of the sanitary women from Chicago married a soldier from some other place. The chaplain of the 7 Ills. Calv. performed the interesting ceremony. I thought it good. Not many present, 3 ladies besides the bride, 2 sanitaries, one a major's wife. The minister came in, chatted a while. When all was ready the two joined hands, arose and said yea. Talked a while. The confectionaries were produced, then we attacked those, had another talk and left.

Oh No! The most interesting part I had [al]most forgotten. After the confect[ionaries] had been vanquished, melodious sounds burst upon our astounded ears. The brass band near gave us a fine serenade for which the bridegroom returned thanks and the chaplain spoke in short but sassy notes after which all adjourned. Both, yes, all the parties from the great north. Negroes still occasionally come in to our lines. I saw two large wagons, ladened with boxes of all sizes, trunks, old & fine clothes, old trumpry of all kinds. Negro babies and youngsters, four or five Negro men standing near the wagons, each drawn by their yokes of oxen. *These had not come far. The guerillas got after them, run quite a number off and come back for more. A Negro man anticipating them had procured an old musket secreted behind the fence when the Guerilla Capt. rode up to the house at the head of his company, just going to dismount, the Negro sharpshooter aided him by sending a ball crashing through his rebel heart. The others thought discretion the better part of valor and took to a hasty flight, doubtless supposing a whole brigade of Yankees near. This is the way the Blacks will treat the disolates of this peace, their homes, the robbers of their labor, of their children and their freedom. I hope the execution will permit and insist upon all the able bodied Negro men fighting for their freedom and the unity of this great nation and that soon.*

Latest from all points! All quiet on the Rappahannock. A terrible storm just subsiding, roads in a horrorable condition. Great preparations to attack the doomed city. The gem of secession. Fleet will start in 10 days. Rosecrans on the alert, skirmishing daily, enemy growing bolder and insolent. The Yazoo pass pronounced a failure. Genl. McClernand captures Talamage & some other town in La. The casemounted batteries opposite Vicksburg now ready. Lookout for action soon, "for patient waiting, no loss." There is good news coming. Please tell me in your next how Grandpa and the rest of the family is getting along. I have not heard for a long time. Sister M, I sent you a paper, enclosed a magnolia leaf the other day. Also sent to the family a photograph of self, not unusually good. I shall write to Grand Pa immediately, have not written this winter. Wrote to Sallie a week or two since, sent a paper to Miss Virginia Swearingen. Do not remember whether my name was on it or not.

Received a letter from Harry Baker, not long ago, had a stock of tobacco in Memphis, had almost sold out and would soon return, was in the city when I was there, could not find him. I guess he is at home by this time. I write on this small sheet because I had no news, not because I have no larger, I have. Looking for the pay master soon at this post! 40! Rounds of kisses and three days good hugging for each. I send you by this transport. As ever your affct. son & brother in the bonds of L. R. & F.,

Thomas S. Hawley, MD etc.

At the time of Thomas Hawley's letter of April 24, the preparation for the assault on Vicksburg by Grant's army was in full swing. Grant had moved his army to the west of Vicksburg and he needed to cross the Mississippi River to achieve his desired eastern approach to the city. Because there were no bridges across the Mississippi River, he needed boats and barges to transport his troops to the eastern side of the river before Confederate forces could be moved into position and repulse his landing. The cannons of Vicksburg were positioned so that any vessels passing the city on the Mississippi River were at risk of being shelled. On April 16, Admiral David Dixon Porter successfully moved Union vessels past Vicksburg. He lost only one vessel to the Confederate cannons. On April 17 Brigadier Benjamin Grierson's cavalry began a sixteen day foray through Mississippi. He began his cavalry raid on April 17 from LaGrange, Tennessee, raided through central Mississippi and finally arrived at Baton Rouge, Louisiana, with the objective of drawing Confederate troops away from Vicksburg. On April 22, after his success on April 16, Porter made a second attempt of running the batteries at Vicksburg and successfully passed six gunboats and several barges past the city. Throughout the area, the probing between the Union and Confederate forces was initiated. Something serious was about to happen and each side wanted to keep their respective objectives secret as long as possible.

Thomas Hawley's letter of the April 24 was filled with the anticipation of the Vicksburg campaign and he wrote two sections in his letter on April 24. Hawley's grandfather was seriously ill and his family appealed for him to return home to provide medical care for him. Thomas wrote it was impossible for him to leave and wished the family well.

Genl. Hospital LaGrange, Tenn.
Officers Head Quarters
April 24, 1863
Dearest Parents,

I received yours some time ago saying you would visit Grand Pa in perhaps, and I fear so too, his last sickness. Yesterday a letter from sister saying you had gone and a few days ago, a minder from Ma notified me of your arrival in Robinson. Was pleased to hear you were there to attend and minister to Grandpa's wants. I would only be too happy to come to your relief, but my hands are tied to this place and I cannot leave, hardly get to Memphis. I suppose too, I might get to Memphis but would be at the mercy of an arbitrary medical director who would send me out to some old regiments that I knew nothing of. Or perhaps to attend a Negro hospital. So I preferred to remain at this place as it is [a] more pleasant place.

We have not many patients but I think will have more soon from an expedition that has gone almost to the heart of Dixie and another under Smith below Holly Springs and they have been fighting near Memphis, also at Corinth and from rumors at Vicksburg, too. We will have plenty of news soon. There has been a general strike on the rebel lines of communication which if successful will be a grand victory. As yet we have no special news from any of these, except one was near Columbus 200 miles from here. Dr. Crawford has placed me in charge of No. 4. I hope soon to have a pleasant place.

The weather is quite pleasant. I have been troubled with indigestion for the past few weeks but am better today. As yet no pay. We will send some men to Memphis today or tomorrow for transportation to northern hospitals. The long, good letter from sister with Ma's note to her enclosed, says all well as usual. One from H. C. Baker at St. Louis, all well there, no special news. I have not heard from the 11th Mo. since I last wrote you. We have a very pleasant quiet place here, preaching every Sabbath. But as many of our troops have left and are fighting on both sides of us, I do not know how long it will remain so. We are rather behind in news from all points, plenty of rumors. It says 4 gunboats and two transports ran the batterys at Vicksburg, one transport lost. Grant's Hd. Quarters below.

April 24

We have been looking for an attack upon this place last night and today, are well reinforced and quite well fortified. Have no fears of our success. But may have some heavy skirmishing and perhaps fighting. Genl. Smith is commanding. The 40th Ills. is here, 70 Ohio, 53 Ohio and several detachments. Quartermasters and commissary stores have been removed to fortifications during last night. Feel all right.

If Grandpa is living, assure him of my deep concern and earnest prayers for his recovery. I wrote him a few weeks ago. Words cannot express my warm affections for so exemplary & kind a grandparent.

Love to all. Write soon. Your
Affectionate son,

T. S. Hawley

Thomas Hawley's next letter was written on May 10 after a flurry of action and activity by the Union and Confederate armies. Since his last letter on April 24, the Battle of Grand Gulf was fought on April 29. Grand Gulf is located a few miles south of Vicksburg and Admiral David Porter commanded seven ironclads in an attempt to silence the Confederate guns along the east side of the Mississippi River which was necessary to allow for the safe landing of Major General John McClernand's XIII Corps. Porter was involved in an extensive battle with batteries on land. He silenced a lower battery but failed to silence the upper batteries of Fort Cobun. He was forced to withdraw and the battle was considered a Confederate victory. Grant had his army positioned to the west of Grand Gulf at Hard Times Landing, Louisiana. After the battle, Grant marched his men south of Grand Gulf and transported them successfully onto the Mississippi shore at Bruinsburg. The Union Army began marching overland and successfully drove the Confederate defenders back on May 1 at Port Gibson and on May 3 forced the Confederate evacuation of Grand Gulf.

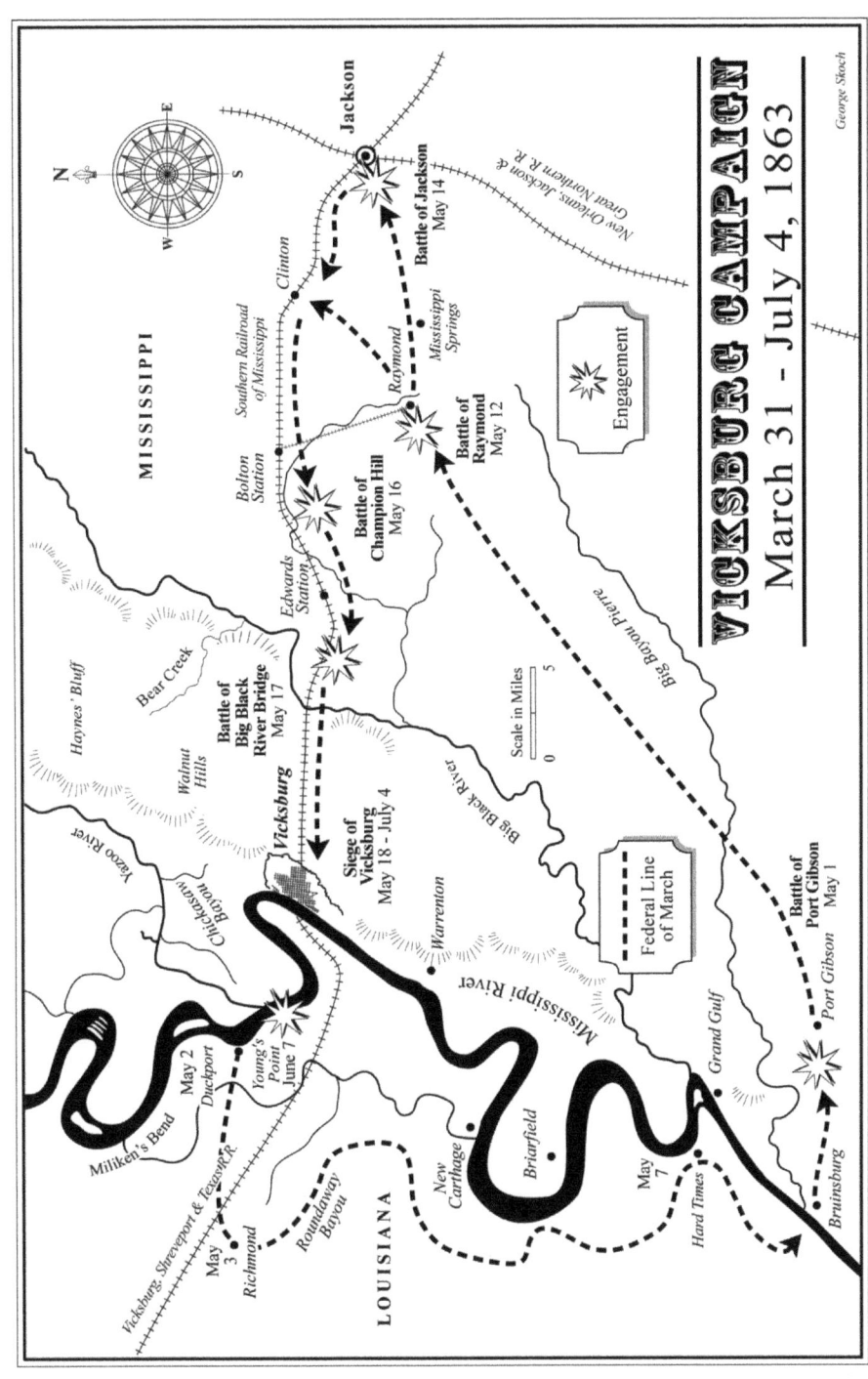

Thomas Hawley was on the move and had progressed to Young's Point which was a few miles south of Milliken's Bend, Louisiana. His trip began on May 3 when he left LaGrange and he traveled to Memphis and stayed there until May 7. Then he traveled south along the Mississippi River on the stern-wheeler, *Sam Young*, and his letter contained descriptions of Helena, Arkansas, Napoleon, Lake Providence, and Greenville, Mississippi. He noted the conditions of the large plantations and slave houses. He related many of the planters' homes had been burnt and the fencing removed. Hawley wrote the trip was pleasant and the scenery was beautiful until he landed at Milliken's Bend where he began his overland trip.

Off Young's Point in View of
Vicksburg on board steamer
<u>Sam Young</u>, *Sunday May 10th 1863*
Dearest Parents, Bro. and Sisters,

Again, I address you from the sunny South. This time indeed for it is uncomfortably warm, yes, I may say hot. I presume and hope ere this, you have heard of my sudden departure for the invulnerable city of the "So called Southern Confederacy." We left LaGrange last Monday at noon, arrived in Memphis about dark, put up at the Green Tree House, saw some old friends, then stopped one night with Dr. R. N. Friese. They are all well. I guess you have heard of the loss of their youngest child, a sweet little fellow died some weeks ago. I saw a man on the cars who lives near Olney. Said he would stop and see you if he had time. We left Memphis. What would [you] give to know who we saw? Well, I will satisfy your curiosity, an MD, of course. Oh well, a special friend Dr. J. K. Wilson, he was with me in Holly Springs, have known him for the last six months and know he will do <u>to tye to</u> *and I've tyed.*

Well, as I was saying, we left Memphis on Thursday evening. No boats had left for the lower river for three or four days and all coming up had been fired into. All by musketry and two or three by cannon and one captured. We came to Helena, Ark. the first night and layed over until morning. Most of us expecting a convoy the shape of a good sized Iron Clad but none honored us so much. At this place I inquired for L. G. Swearengen. Their camp was nearly one mile from the landing and most of the men on a big scout. So I neither got to see nor hear from him. Our trip down the river was indeed pleasant. On Wednesday it was cold and extremely unpleasant and had been for 4 or 5 days. But on Friday, the sun came out. The passengers of whom there was near one hundred officers, soldiers and citizens made themselves comfortable according to their numerous habits and characters. Some lounging in the cabin, in their state rooms, others playing cards, some frequenting the bar which could be told without seeing them there by their actions. A few, we among the others, repaired to the hurricane deck to enjoy the beautiful scenery regardless of the rebel sharpshooters. Indeed we were soon lost in raptures and knew no danger. The mighty, the beautiful Mississippi, after passing Helena, has the appearance of a cluster of gardens surrounded by a chain of silver lakes, the forests and cane brakes are clothed in their richest and fullest verdue. Often we would pass near the shores and could see flowers in endless variety and profuse confusion growing on the banks, and occasionally the winds wafted to us rich fragrance from the magnolia forest sweeter and more delicious than the sweet honey suckle of lilley. We passed numerous large plantations, the Negro houses and building joining it, the appearance of a village. Most of the planters' houses had been burned and the fencing next to the river taken away. The lands and houses back all look lower, and I guess are, than the river. Where ever there is a farm, it must be almost surrounded by a large levee ten or fifteen feet high and most of them have two next to the river and two or three cross lines to prevent washing in case the water should overflow the land. These are built at great expense. The village of Lake Providence is small, 300 inhabitants, I guess. Before the war one or two churches. It was partially bisected by an old bayou running up from the lake about half a mile to the river. It was cut off from the river by two large levies. The great and notorious canal of Lake Providence consisted in its incipiency of two ditches, thirty paces apart, and six or eight feet as deep. These two across the levees and one small ditch 3 or 4 feet deep through the center of the bayou from the line to the lake. The water ran through with great velocity but never was navigable for anything but the small tug boat which was first brought over by land then back through the canal of water and labor. Napoleon, just below the mouth of the Arkansas River, was once, and could soon be made again, a very nice village of 6 or 8 hundred souls but now appears deserted, saw some fine dwellings, a few churches and the marine hospital, a 4 story brick with a nice garden attached. Greenville, near 150 miles below Helena, a small village. We passed about 12 o'clock at night and saw the last of it. They had harbored guerillas and two or three times cannon had fired upon our boats. Then gunboats remained there two or three days, then burned the place. It was on fire as we passed.

We reported at Milliken's Bend 18 miles above this point and the beginning of the main road from above to the rear and below Vicksburg. Carthage 30 miles by wagon train. All had left that place that we wanted to see and the rest were ordered to this point as they were building a new road to Carthage, 10 miles nearer. So we came there and found one or two old transports, some gunboats, a few troops and lots of filth, trash and pestilence.

Monday May 11th

Had not time to close yesterday and today the road will be finished and we will move to the front. Some bombarding yesterday morning and evening and *today no special news yet. Grant near the ridge had sent for another division, will be here today. Provision going to the front, from appearances all quiet in Vicksburg.*

I cannot tell you where to write. I will write soon.

Love to all.

Thomas

By May 18, Thomas Hawley was located at the XVII Corps Hospital near Raymond, Mississippi, where the Battle of Raymond was fought on May 12, 1863. Thomas Hawley's letter of May 18 described in detail his advance from the Mississippi River to Raymond. The supporting medical units were threatened by guerrillas along their march. After Grant moved his army into Mississippi, he began a northeastward march, keeping the Big Black River on his left flank. Grant's three advancing army corps were commanded by William T. Sherman, John McClernand, and James McPherson. McPherson's XVII Corps held the right flank of the Union line and approached Raymond, Mississippi, on May 11. Confederate Brigadier General John Gregg moved his troops from Jackson, Mississippi, and planned to strike hard and swift to surprise and punish the Union right. Gregg's small force of 2,500 men initially surprised the Union XVII Corps, but the odds were clearly in favor of the Union Corps which had 10,000 men in the field. The battle raged until about 2 P.M. when Gregg withdrew. The losses were relatively equal as the Union casualty list totaled 442 men and the Confederates lost 514 killed, missing and wounded. It was this aftermath Thomas Hawley faced as he and his fellow surgeons worked diligently to save lives.

The surgeons and quartermasters of Thomas Hawley's support group landed from the transport ship, *Moderation*, at Carthage, Louisiana, and found a hospital, a few houses, cotton and ex-slaves. Thomas Hawley noticed the wreck of the Union ironclad, *Indianola*, which had been rammed and sunk on February 24, 1863.

On May 16, 1863, the Battle of Champion Hill was fought two days after the mild conflict at the Battle of Jackson. Doctor Hawley's personal description of the battle was included in this letter. Quickly following the Battle of Champion Hill was the Battle of the Big Black River Bridge on May 17, 1863. Thomas Hawley and his medical comrades were assigned duty at Raymond and provided support to Brigadier General Alvin Hovey's division which had fought at the Big Black River. The casualties were high at the Battle of Champion Hill where the Union Army reported casualties of 2,457 and Confederates reported 4,300 killed, wounded and missing. At Champion Hill Lieutenant General John Pemberton was attempting to follow orders to attack the Union supply train when he ran into Grant's main force. The battle was fought until about 1:00 P.M. when the Confederates withdrew moving toward the safety of Vicksburg. On the day following this defeat, the Confederate Army fought a rear-guard action on the east side of the Big Black River Bridge in an attempt to slow the Union pursuit. The Union Army was also successful in this battle but the Confederates were able to burn the bridge over the river slowing the Union advance. By May 18, General Ulysses Grant had masterminded one of the most successful and effective campaigns in history and had thrown the Confederate Army into the confines of the defenses at Vicksburg. By May 18, Grant's three corps were in position to lay siege to Vicksburg.

In Thomas Hawley's May 18 letter, he recorded he was assigned duty under Doctor Madison Mills, who had been appointed Grant's Medical Director in March 1863. Mills was a regular army surgeon and had worked tirelessly to stockpile six months reserves of medical supplies in anticipation of a long and hard-fought campaign. Now that the campaign was underway, Mills had to find a way to care for the wounded soldiers which resulted from Grant's victories. Mills assembled a group of nineteen surgeons (including Thomas Hawley) to accomplish this task and had another four surgeons assigned to care for the Confederate wounded.

Hospital 17 Corps "D" Arrived
6 Miles from Raymond, Miss.
Monday May 18, 1863
Dearest Parents,

It does appear a long, long time since I last heard from you. Yet I know there is a letter or letters at my old station, LaGrange, but I cannot write just now. So as to tell positively where I want them sent as my position is not permanent and would most likely be changed before the letters were sent. I wrote to you from Young's Point about one week ago since that [we] have had rather a rough time. Left there on Monday, I think, with the train for a landing just below and in view of Warrenton, passing in range of their and the Vicksburg guns; but none was fired at the wagons which numbered near 100 ladened with hard tack, sugar, coffee, and salt. These were not placed on board the transport, <u>Moderation,</u> *until next morning when all was ready. Next morning at 10 we steamed down the river sixty miles to Grand Gulf. The morning was fine and river scenery beautiful. The boat was heavily ladened, lots of soldiers and officers aboard. Indeed the old boat was crowded and no accommodations. When she ran the blockade was struck 40 times & you may guess pretty well riddled, had hard work to get anything to eat, which condition has not changed much up to this time nor will until Genl. Grant takes Vicksburg which I think will be soon. We first landed at Carthage 35 miles below Vicksburg, a few houses, a hospital and one regt. and cotton and contrabands in abundance.*

A few miles below we saw the wreck of the ill-fated <u>Indianola</u>. *Some said our men had raised it and we were repairing it. The river is very wide here, could not see her distinctly ten or 15 miles below. We came to Perkins' Landing. One regt. and gunboat at Carthage. I should say one regt. and some quartermaster stores at this place and fine plantations. Down the river 25 miles below, we came to Hard Times, could see but few houses but plenty of Yankees and transportation. When off [at] the last place, Grand Gulf and the Grand Bluffs were plainly seen in the distance. The highest one directly at the bend had the appearance of a mountain almost and ⅓ way up, could see the line of fortifications where the hard fought battle had come off. Big Black [River] coming in just at the base. Well, we remained at this place all night and next day at 10 started for HdQuarters of the Army of the Tennessee, reported to be 25 to thirty miles in the interior and the road infested with guerillas, Genl. Ransom former Col. of the 11th Ill. commanding. Dr. Wilson and I got our baggage in one of the wagons. I had a saddle and bridle, borrowed a little white mule from the wagon master and started, promising to ride part of the time and walk some. I have forgotten to say that the town of Grand Gulf was burned last spring or summer by Com. Farragut because they fired upon his boats after he had warned them of the consequences. We found the road dusty, hilly and the weather hot. For 15 miles from the river, it is a succession of hills and hollows and they at an angle of 45° yet it is cultivated as in Tenn. by ploughing around the hillside. Magnolias grow luxuriously indeed, become so common that they lose their charm. The flowers are larger than a tea cup, pure white cup shaped and very fragrant something like an orange.*

We camped the first night 12 miles from Grand Gulf, rained some next day. Often stopped at houses, found the citizens growling greatly at the treatment of the Yankees. Most of them rather mild, not many with protection papers from the Genl. Provisions rather scarce with the army, had trouble to get any to start with.

The Army must forage, only ⅖ rations, issued. On the evening of the 15th encamped near Raymond, next morning early heard some cannonading. When we got to Raymond, understood that Genl. Grant was driving them toward Vicksburg. We advanced as far as they would let the train, then walked on and soon found the genl. hospital of Genl. Osterhaus' division on the direct road to Vicksburg. We assisted in many operations and at dark went back to our train, eat supper and were soon ordered to move forward that night as Genl. Grant was pushing the enemy over by [Big] Black [River]. Had captured 13 hundred prisoners, 18 pieces of artillery and driven the enemy 5 miles. This was indeed a great battle. The Battle of Champion Hills fought on a succession of steep hills on each side of the main road leading from Raymond to Vicksburg, distant from the latter place about 30 miles and from the former 8 or 9 miles. Genl. Osterhaus'

Hovey's, Logan's, Carr's divisions were the ones engaged principally. The Rebels under Pemberton numbering near 50,000 thousand and all the advantage of position, had skirmished 2 or 3 miles the day before until they knew our force pretty well. The fighting became severe about 10 or 11 o'clock and continued near 6 hours with unabated and almost unparalleled fury. Our brave boys driving them from every chosen position through the woods, charging upon them up the rugged hills, over gullies, cotton & corn fields, capturing batterys in hand to hand engagements and have been capturing prisoners by the thousands and driving them for the last 3 days. Prisoners here say the Rebellion is played out.

Reports came in today that Genl. Grant has driven them across Black River, captured 15 or 20 field pieces and 5 or 6 siege guns and that they did not have time to burn the bridge. We crossed ten divisions and captured 25,000 more prisoners, have seen about that many myself and two batterys. Rode over the battlefield, saw wounded and dead laying in all directions, dead horses, broken guns and gun carriages. Regts. that have been in 3 or 4 battles say it was more terrific than any they had ever before witnessed. Our loss in killed and wounded cannot be less than 2000, perhaps ⅓ killed. The Rebs lost more in killed.

I reported to Chief Medical Director, Madison Mills, was assigned to duty with Dr. Jessup of the 24 Ind. Med. Direct. of Genl. Hovey's division which suffered most of all. This regt. lost in killed and wounded about ½ 200. I cannot say how long I shall remain here. Most of the army will leave tomorrow and we will almost be in the hands of rebels and then rather scarce of provisions and our hands full of prisoners. I mean sick & wounded. My health's good for which I am thankful and I do most sincerely hope you are all well and doing well, will tell you when to write just as soon as I can. In the meantime much love to all. Kiss each other for me and remember I am always thinking of you. I shall try to do my duty to the brave wounded soldiers though it be by suffering privations and hardships. We are thankful for hard crackers and they scarce. One cracker for three men at one meal and some weak soup.

May 24. This letter was written as you see near one week ago. Nothing special of interest has come to pass since. Wounded doing well as could be expected, indeed better. We hear them every day knocking at Vicksburg, some rumors that it is taken. One thing certain they have them in close quarters. Must surrender sooner or later. Most of the army left here soon after this was written. Might have sent it sooner had I known they would open communications by Haynes Bluff & Yazoo River. No regular mail, not even a paper for three weeks. We are getting a better supply of medicine & commissarys. Capt. Geo. Meily is one mile from here at Quimbys Hospt., wounded in knee, badly, doing well.

On May 30, Thomas Hawley was writing from the hospital established following the Battle of Champion Hill fought on May 16 located about twenty miles from the Union line established around Vicksburg. Since the last correspondence, General Grant launched two bloody and unsuccessful attempts to breach the Confederate line at Vicksburg. It is not surprising he felt the Confederate defenders at Vicksburg had lost the will to fight. Grant felt with the series of defeats the Confederate army had just suffered, another strong push could easily break Pemberton's defenses and Vicksburg could be claimed. There was also the need on Grant's part to quickly take the city before he was attacked by Confederate General Joseph Johnston's men out in the countryside. Grant's first attack occurred on May 19 at 9:00 A.M. when the Union artillery began its barrage on the southern defenses, particularly targeting Stockade Redan on the northeastern part of the Confederate line. The assault was carried out by Brigadier General Frank Blair's Second Division which attacked Stockade Redan at 2:00 P.M. Despite the gallant attack, the Confederates were successful in repelling the assault and Sherman's corps lost 134 killed, 571 wounded, and 8 missing. Confederate casualties are not known but probably totaled less than 200 on all parts of the line. McPherson's and McClernand's corps, which launched only limited attacks, suffered a combined total of 23 killed and 206 wounded.

The assault on May 19 was hasty and attempted to capitalize of the Union successes during the campaign. On May 22, Grant decided to launch a full-scale attack on the Confederate defenses with all three corps participating in the assault. The attack on May 22 was particularly important to Thomas Hawley because his old regiment, 11th Missouri Infantry, was selected to lead the afternoon charge on Stockade Redan after the morning assault failed. The 11th Missouri was ordered to advance down the Graveyard Road in column formation and attack Stockade Redan. Stockade Redan was made up of 17 foot high earthen walls and a five foot ditch at the base. The defenders at Stockade Redan were the 36th Mississippi Infantry of General Louis Hébert's Brigade and by the Third Missouri Infantry (CSA) of Colonel Francis Cockrell's Brigade.

At 4:00 P.M., the 11th Missouri Infantry made their assault, yelling as they attacked, but the same wall of musket and artillery fire awaited the regiment that had met the morning's attackers. Of the 325 men of the regiment who made the assault about a third were either killed or wounded and although the regiment reached their objective, the men were not able to break the Confederate line. After dark, the men returned to their line after remaining huddled at the base of the wall throughout the afternoon. Hawley lost many friends in the assault at Stockade Redan. Sherman's XV Corps lost 150 killed, 666 wounded and 42 missing on May 22, and the advantage of the Confederate defensive works was evident in the final tally. Grant's army lost approximately 3,200 men killed, wounded and missing and Pemberton 500.

Three. 1863

In Thomas Hawley's letter of May 30, he referred to flags of truce which were utilized after the conflicts. One of the most graphic incidents regarding flags of truce occurred at Stockade Redan after the assaults on May 19 and May 22 when a truce was declared to remove the dead and wounded three days after the last assault. Some of the dead lay on the battlefield from May 19 until May 25 under the hot Mississippi sun. Although the removal of the casualties was done in cordial manner as the combatants mingled during their labors, soon the soldiers returned to their respective lines and to their deadly tasks.

Doctor Hawley was twenty miles to the rear of the combat but heard the constant cannonading. Pemberton's army was safe behind the formidable defenses, but was also trapped unless Confederate General Joe Johnston could find a way to break the stranglehold Grant had on the city. When Hawley wrote his letter on May 30, he was malnourished and exhausted to the point of being unsure of the date. As the army moved forward, it left the hospitals desperately short of supplies and the main diet of the medical staff consisted of cornbread and meat. Thomas Hawley was in a non-ending cycle of surgery and care for patients severely wounded in the battles. Hawley wrote, "We have some operations every day." His letter also described his living situation and he sketched a drawing of his tent.

Hawley's letter continued with a note made on May 31 and he reported

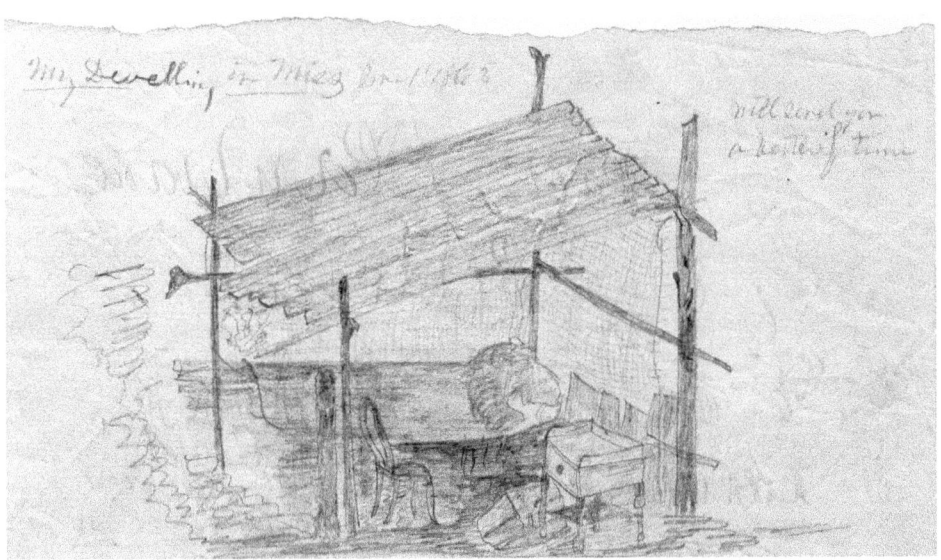

Living quarters of Dr. Thomas Hawley outside Vicksburg, 1863 (Missouri History Museum, St. Louis, Missouri).

the Union cavalry was burning any possible source of supply or support for the Confederate Army in the countryside. Grant was prepared for his siege and he had no intention of allowing the Confederate Army outside of Vicksburg to gain any strength from the local population during the siege. Amid all the death and destruction, Thomas Hawley offered his concern for his family paying their taxes in Illinois. The Union paymaster was not present during such a campaign and Hawley was without any funds to send home. Thomas Hawley wrote of his desire to return to his regiment and to be relieved of the surgical and hospital duties he was performing.

> *Division Hospital Genl. Hovey's Div.*
> *on Battleground of Champion Hills Part of Hospt.*
> *in Champion House the rest under rough sheds*
> *and brush heaps May 30th 1863*
>
> *Dear Parents, Bro. Amos, Sisters, Eva Bell, Fannie, Theo and last but not least, Myra,*
>
> *Your long silent and long absent bro. & son will occasionally be heard from, although not a very big gun. My communications with you are longer than ever before and for the first time during the war are only open to flags of truce which we see quite often as they are by both sides, at least part of the time.*
>
> *The pleasant month of May has almost passed by and still that Gibraltar of the Southern Confeds is not taken although surrounded and set upon by a determined innumerable for who never know failure. The fine May morning just heralded by the triumphant march of the gorgeous orb of day and various joyous and happy carols of a thousand and one feathery songsters (there is one of those ever varying mimicking songs just over my tabernacle trying to attract my attention but he shan't) and as the sun steadily, grandly marches toward the zenith, other sounds come booming to us over the way proclaiming that the beleaguered citadel still holds out with some resistance and that the outside for[ces] are hailing iron and lead into their stronghold. It has been one continual roar since sun up and we are 20 miles from the army. Genl. Grant has been mining and last night some say they heard a terrific explosion which was supposed to be the explosion of the mine. Then there would be a breach in their works and our forces could perhaps effect an entrance which was probably the cause of the heavy firing—this morning and its continuance. Well, I must see the wounded brave until 12 o'clock m. now 7 o'clock A.M.*
>
> *Sunday morning. This, I guess, is May 30th, the first page was written day before yesterday. Everyday we hear the deep thunder tones of our artillery and still word occasionally comes, Vicksburg [is] not ours yet. My health for a few days had been [not] quite as good as usual. Which I must attribute to our rather rough fare for a week or two. It consisted of unsifted, coarse ground cornbread*

Three. 1863

baked without milk, only a little salt and shortening. A few young cabbage plants for greens and fresh beef or pork. The army left us without anything. But for the past week we have been well supplied as the general sent out quite a train. There was a while I would have given 25 cents for a hard cracker. The commissary for hospital will send us a mess chest. We can occasionally buy buttermilk, etc., the cooks can make good salt rising bread. We have ham, fresh beef, occasionally some vegetables, blackberries will soon be ripe and we propose to live better. And I think we will soon leave for the front and as soon as I get there, I hope to be soon ordered to my regiment as I know they want me and are doing me great injustice to retain me here as I cannot draw pay until my return to the regiment. I have not heard from you since I left LaGrange and yet hardly know where to have my letters directed. But better direct them to me care of Maj. Madison Mills, Chief Medical Direct. Army of the Tennessee. This way — T.S.H. asst. Surg. 111 Ills. Vols. care of Maj. Madison Mills, Chief Med Direct. Army Tenn. He has a register of all the surgeons in his department and will know where to send to at any time if he will go to the trouble and I know his chief clerk well. He will do anything for me. I do want to hear from you very much and fear that desire will not be satisfied until it has grown almost too intense to bear. But rest assured, I think of you often, and am doing well for I see more surgery than I have ever seen before. This is as good as a course of lectures. We have some operations every day. Some are rare and important. So you see my time is not thrown away.

Indeed this month had slipped by without my being aware of its hasty flight. The weather is pleasant, a gentle air is stirring all the time. I sleep in an open shed of my own construction. I propose to send you a rough sketch of it some of these times. I tell you, it is pleasant. I pride myself upon its adaptation to my wants, comfort and pleasure. Is situated under a nice tresseled palm tree and numerous, graceful sassafras bushes is quite near. A sturdy old gum whose venerable, mossey, grey beard waves in the air, several feet below each limb. The uppermost one is engaged for the present season by Miss American Nightingale who takes a benefit every day or two and often [at] night. She always has a delighted and full house. We are tolerably well acquainted but she eyes me rather coquettishly sometimes. Just at the foot of this old gray beard flows a cool crystal spring from under the roots of a sassafras tree. Our cooks have guided this fountain into a flour barrel sunk deep in the narrow ravine where cups, canteens, buckets and pots are filled. Still the barrel is full. My residence has four forks at the corners supporting a few planks for a roof is 8 feet square. Sea grass matting from cotton bales hangs on two sides to right and head of bed which is close to one side. Have a seagrass mattress, 1 quilt, double blankets & shawl, have a few boards around lower part of shed, have a stand, supports medicines, books, clothes, etc., a nice parlor, sea moss seated chair. So you see, am well fixed. Two sides of my house are constantly open to admit fresh, pure air, which you know is a fine thing when others are not so abundant. Dr. Taylor talks of going to the front today. But I guess he will not. So I will not finish this yet, will but send a later dispatch. Affectionately, etc.

2nd Dispatch. Yesterday was May 31, I guess. If so, today Monday June 1st. This morning the air is filled with smoke like Indian summer. I hardly know how to account for it except that our cavalry are burning depots. What's that depots, corn mills and other property. You must know nearly every planter has a corn mill attached to the cotton gin and with two or 4 mules soon prepares enough corn meal for his negroes. Dr. Taylor thinks of going at least part of the way to Vicksburg and may go all the way. I cannot think we will remain more than 10 days longer in this place. Dr. wants to get an ambulance train to remove most of the sick. 2 or 3 hundred conveyed. I am getting along finely. But Pa, the most I regret that I have not been able to send you any money which I hoped to do long ago. I have spent but little. How will you pay your taxes and mine? But I suppose you have found some way ere this, for June 1st is the last day of grace. Well, I hope you have not been put to much trouble and are doing well. Oh, how much I wish that I knew you were. I do not doubt you all suffer privations and that without mumurring as you always have done. I shall do all in my power to send you some before long. But how poor promises seem and are. Tell me your plans and just how you are all doing. In every letter I have sent you love but with each sending it increases, if possible, the store on hand for you all. The longer I am from home the greater the desire to be with you. Absence increases instead of decreasing the family ties. If this comes to hand in due time, you may write as directed in this letter. I shall try and write you oftener. With each, a sweet kiss I greet you

Your affect bro. & son,

T. S. Hawley

As Thomas Hawley gathered his thoughts on June 7, 1863, the siege of Vicksburg continued; but the doctor was reflective in this letter and offered an insightful look at the aftermath of the battles in a sad and thoughtful manner. He did not want to linger near the battlefield, "where the ground was saturated with the life current of our fellow men." Both sides fought well, but the battles were terrible, particularly for those charged with dealing with the human results. The medical professionals in the Civil War were faced with situations modern medicine would consider barbaric, but they worked with the tools they had. The large bore musket balls were particularly effective in inflicting massive damage on the human body and those who survived often found they were amputees. Hawley also described the mass graves and the aftermath of soldiers buried in shallow graves.

On June 7, Thomas Hawley offered medical care to the wounded and as he served in the hospital, he mentioned Confederates were allowed to enter the camp. Presumably, this was allowed so care could be provided to those Confederates patients in the Union hospital. While this was occurring, the noise of battle carried to the hospital bearing the reminder of the ever present siege. Hawley recorded an ambulance train brought in more wounded the evening before.

Genl. Hospital 12th Divs. Army Tenn.
20 miles east of Vicksburg on the road
from that place to Jackson or rather between
the railroad and common road
June 7th 1863 Sunday

Dear Parents,

When I last had the exquisite pleasure of perusing one of your interesting epistles, I was quietly perusing my vocation as asst. surgeon in Genl. Hospital at the pleasant village of LaGrange which now seems far removed from the seat of war. That has been over one long month and now this Sabbath morning finds me over two hundred miles south away from the haunts of men, in appearance, at least, for who cares to linger or live near the scene of bloody carnage where the ground is saturated with the life current of our fellow men, where every hill is a cemetery and every gully becomes a receptacle of 10s or hundreds bearing once the grace of vigorous manhood, but now their limbs devoid of flesh refused a covering of mother earth protrude as if they would fain be monuments of fallen heroes who died victims to a false idea. Long mounds on the hills with a single board bearing these inscriptions 25 or 100 Union soldiers buried here or Sergt. ___ of Co. Regt. or Lt. ___ Regt., etc., or 117 Rebs here at the head of some deep gully. These often meet the eye and the trees, those silent but living witnesses of war's terribleness, bearing testimony when the tide of war raged hottest. This battle ground was too broken to use artillery much, so that more destructive weapon, the musket, came into full play. All around, the trees bear marks of small balls and what is rather unusual, these are but seldom higher than a man's head recording distinctly the sure aim and unflinching carnage of the men engaged. Ours were mostly old veterans and I think the enemy fought well. They say we fought well but outgeneraled them. They also blame their Georgia regts. for not fighting better. Most of our prisoners were from that state and she held out Union as long as possible from the outside pressure.

June 9, 2nd Dispatch.

Later. All quiet. We have had frequent visits from our rebel friends. Col. Lyon came in yesterday and had a long conversation, is a strong rebel and holds *many erroneous views. While here, a dispatch came asking him permission to let our ambulance train advance and bring away our wounded, was granted and late last night, they came on from Big Black, near Genl. Osterhaus' Divs. They have been there 4 days attacking. We may all leave today. If so, shall be in the light of freedom & Christendom.*

We have had a weary time here but it has been very profitable to me. More soon, I hear that Grant will not permit any letters to go north of our lines. If so, I may not hear from you for some time to come. What shall I do? Still they boom, boom from Vicksburg and I think they must give up soon.

On June 16, Thomas Hawley reported interesting and remarkable developments in his military career. He was appointed assistant surgeon of the 11th Missouri Infantry, his original regiment, where his old friend and mentor, Doctor Eli Bowyer, had been promoted to the rank of major. As recorded in his letters, Hawley was officially a member of the 111th Illinois Infantry, but he held no allegiance to that regiment and needed to resign. Since he departed the 11th Missouri, he had constant communication and interaction with the men of the regiment. Since he left the regiment, the 11th Missouri Infantry had obtained quite a reputation as a fighting regiment and had won recognition and accolades in several battles. They performed notable service in the Battle of Iuka on September 19, 1862, when they surprised the 37th Alabama and 36th Mississippi infantries and withstood three charges from these regiments. Next, the 11th Missouri was noted for their action at the Battle of Corinth on October 3–4. On October 4, when the Confederates had broken the Union line, the 11th Missouri and 27th Ohio infantries made a gallant charge and stopped the Confederates, thus securing a Union victory. Most recently, the 11th Missouri was chosen to lead Sherman's afternoon attack on Stockade Redan on May 22. These battles had taken their toll on the regiment; but Thomas Hawley was glad to be back with the regiment and received a "hearty welcome" from the men of the regiment.

Young's Point June 16, 1863

Dear Parents,

I mailed a letter to sister Myra a few days ago giving a short history of my journeys and the cause of my visit to the camp of the 11th Mo. I found them absent yesterday upon my arrival but they returned today from the capture of Richmond [Louisiana] driving a larger number of the enemy before them. I found a hearty welcome and a commission as first asst. surg. I guess I shall resign as 2 asst. surg. 111 Ill., hope to get my pay, then be fully reinstated as asst. surg. 11 Mo. Vols. I was ordered to report here to Dr. Mills, Chief Med. Direct. Please write to me at this point and regt., Genl. Mower's Brigade.

Give all news. I cannot say yet what will be the result of this change or if it can be effected. Ten thousand loves to all, each and every one. Health improving. Siege continues.

Your afft. Son,

T. S. Hawley

After the assault on Stockade Redan on May 22, the 11th Missouri Infantry participated in two expeditions into the Mississippi countryside to keep General Joe Johnston at bay and away from the Union siege at Vicksburg. On June 15, the regiment was involved in action on the western side of the Mississippi River, near Richmond, Louisiana.

Sergeant William Notestine wrote a letter to his family on June 12 describing the regiment's activities and results of the Vicksburg campaign of the 11th Missouri, "The campaign is one of extraordinary interest and also of unparalleled hardship.... The dust was suffocating and the heat was intolerable. We also had to do on half rations until the evacuation of Haines Bluff. Yet in compensation for all this we expect a great & glorius victory. We willingly endure the many privations of the campaign life when a great deal can be accomplished. Our Brigade which is the 2nd Brigade of Tuttle's Division & Sherman's Army Corps has been detached since the 23rd of May and we have had more than our share of marching. The Brid. is wore out and run down and we were sent here for rest and to protect this side of the river which was threatened a few days ago. They had quite a fight up at Miliken Bend and a negro regiment saved the day driving off the rebels with great slaughter and saving our camp."[7]

Doctor Thomas Hawley while looking over the morning reports reflected on the situation of the regiment. "I was looking over one of the company report books and find it numbered just over one year ago, 84 ... now 17." Hawley continued to reflect on his condition and the condition of the men in the regiment, "I am not sick, but emaciated from defective nutrition and want of proper diet."

Certainly the past year had a significant toll on the regiment as noted by Hawley's examination of men able to report for duty. As assistant surgeon, Thomas Hawley worked under the command of Doctor Melancthon Fish and unlike Doctor Thomas Smith, the previous regimental surgeon, Hawley worked well with Fish. Hawley recorded Doctor Fish was ill, but his old friend Zeba French was present and gladly welcomed his old comrade. Finally, Hawley was welcomed back by Major Eli Bowyer, probably his most close and intimate friend.

His last administrative detail was the submission of his resignation to the 111th Illinois Infantry which he did without regret. The 111th Illinois

Infantry was still in Kentucky and since Hawley left the regiment, he had worked in a hospital in Holly Springs, been captured by Confederate raiders, fallen in love with Annie Ross, commanded his own hospital in LaGrange, participated in the medical support of one of America's greatest military campaigns and finally, been appointed as assistant surgeon in one of the Civil War's premier fighting regiments. If Thomas Hawley was seeking adventure, he had found it.

Young's Point, La.
Camp 11th Mo. Vols.
June 21, 1863

Dear Parents,

Another Sabbath has dawned upon us and finds me among my old, tried friends of the gallant 11 Mo. which has made so many successful charges upon the enemys of our country. It is fearful to think of the great ravages of war. I was just looking over one of the company report books and find it numbered just one year ago 84, today less one half, had 42 men able for duty last June, now 17. I have been with the regiment nearly one week, have done all the prescribing since my arrival, Dr. Fish being unwell. He and I so far get along well. I am rather pleased with his appearance. Dr. French is well. He and I are doing well. My health is improving since my arrival inside our lines. Well indeed. I am not sick, but emaciated from defective nutrition and want of proper diet while out in the rebel lines. Beside the unusual amount of labor and impure air which we were compelled to suffer the greater part of the day, I was indeed glad to get among old friends and out of that pest hole. All the surgeons and medical attendants were sick and some not well yet. I began to improve the moment I landed on the banks of the mighty Mississippi.

Monday Morning June 22, 1863
Second dispatch latest from all points

Thank kind providence. I saw a courier directly from your midst, Jas. Palmsteer. Dr. French and I called on Col. Glaze and Capt. McClure of the 63 Ills., had a pleasant chat, saw the newly appointed Chaplain, just from Mt. Carmel, then I ascertained that the sutler, Jas., was on hand, just from the land of liberty. The Col. and I immediately hastened to his tent. He said had no idea of seeing me but had a request from you to see me if he could. I shall call to see them often as they promised to do with me. Dr. French and I walked into a grove near to hear a Mr. Van Meter from New York connected with the Sanitary Commission. He gave us a very pleasant talk. It could not be called a sermon but a good, social, friendly chat for the benefit of the brothers in arms.

He is a fine singer and very pleasant speaker. After the talk, we all returned to our quarters in better spirits and feeling friendly in good humor with everyone. I heard some scoffing and others, speaking, desiring of hearing such every week. Yesterday the weather was unusually cool but today is warmer. The health of the regiment is not improving but rather getting worse. Maj. Bowyer is the same old intimate, confidential friend as I know he always will be. The more I know him, the better I feel towards him. Jas. P. told me, Uncle Goodale, he said but I guess meant, Gooding, had paid you a visit, that Grand Pa was safe in Olney and you had had a general family reunion.

I doubt not you all enjoyed this more than words can express. I shall wait, perhaps not too patiently, for the details as I have not heard for 40 or 50 days, but I reckon it almost half a life time but will not tell you the full events of that time just now. I suppose you felt bad about the small house but that could not be avoided just then but may be in the future. Yet that should not mar your pleasure. Such reunions are as living, vibrant oasis's in the voyage of life but few yet ever to be remembered and looked back on with pleasure. It is not necessary for me to wish I had been with you, that would do no good. But if it could have been so, can you guess at half the unbounded happiness I should have enjoyed during my stay? It is beyond human conception. I would have felt freer than the wild bird just set at liberty. It would have been like the sudden recovery of paradise lost. But this war must be fought out to a successful issue. I shall tender my resignation as second assistant surg. of the 111 Ills. Vols in a day or two and forward that to Col. Martin at Paducah. I shall also write to Col. Black and tell him my position. Please write soon and specify all important events and write. I shall not be satisfied with one letter a week, but will rather want one from each member of the family per week. Then I shall have all the details. Give my love to all inquiring friends and bear in mind you always bear precedence in that current article. Kiss E. Bell, Fannie & Myra & hug the rest for me 3 times per day.
Yours affctly.,
T. S. Hawley

On June 25 Grant made a desperate attempt to breach the Confederate line when his men placed 2,200 pounds of black powder near the Confederate line and exploded this mine. Regiment after regiment assailed the Confederate defenders; but 26 hours later the battle was over and the Confederates had stopped the assault. Grant had another mine detonated on July 1, but it was not followed with an infantry assault. Confederate General John Pemberton surrendered Vicksburg on July 4, 1863, and on that day 2,166 officers and 27,230 enlisted men surrendered. General Ulysses Grant granted parole to all the Confederate soldiers at Vicksburg and at long last the mighty Confederate citadel fell under Union control.

Thomas Hawley celebrated the surrender of Vicksburg in his July 5 letter but also lamented the death of Colonel Andrew J. Weber of the 11th Missouri Infantry. On June 29, the Confederates shelled the regiment as it guarded the brigade's supplies and a shell fragment struck Colonel Andrew Weber in the head. It was thought he had a concussion as a result of the wound, but Weber died on the morning of June 30. The medical report stated Colonel Weber died of compression of the brain. This was the final blow to a costly campaign for the regiment. Duncan McCall, a member of the 11th Missouri Infantry, wrote of Andrew Weber, "He filled every place with honor to himself and with the esteem and friendship of his brother officers; a sober officer, taking pride in seeing his men appear well, the first to face danger; always kind and obliging, and never resorting to extreme measures, he won the good will of his men, who would follow him wherever he saw fit to lead them."[8] Thomas Hawley wrote Andrew Weber, while a brave and honorable man, disavowed any belief in God.

After the numerous miles marched, the poor nutrition, many operations and medical duties, Hawley was elated in the outcome of the siege of Vicksburg. He also captured a Confederate signal flag and proudly sent it to his family in Illinois.

Young's Point, La.
July 5th 1863
Dear Parents,

Glad tidings of great joy to you and all the great northwest. Yesterday, the 88 anniversary of our grand nation's birth has been doubly consecrated by the fall of the rebel forlorn hope, the last stronghold of the so called southern Confederacy, Vicksburg, the Great, the Mighty, has indeed fallen as I myself can bear testimony. My old friend, Jms. Palmsteer, sent me word that Col. Glaze was on the point of leaving this sunny south for the family circle at the land of prairie flowers, pretty girls and pleasant homes. He is no longer a soldier but a citizen of the U. S. of America.

He was very unpleasantly situated so I learn. The staff officers being a mean, unprincipled, licentious lot. I hear other rumors but cannot say for the foundation. I shall send this letter by him if the boat does not leave too soon. Dr. French, Mr. DeWitt and myself rode opposite Vicksburg, got a skiff and crossed into the city, had a chat with some of the soldiers of whom we saw more than our own. They all seemed anxious to be paroled and sent home, had become tired of fighting. Said they rather take the oath of allegiance to the USA than be sent into their army. The place looks much battered down and demolished. All the fences down and the citizens say their own soldiers treat them worse than ours do. They lost all their fine gardens because the stock must live. So it was turned out for them to graze in. Looks odd to see their fancy officers gaily dressed, riding old skeletons of horses.

We passed some of their camps. Many of them in the railroad yard cuts, had caves dug to hide in and in the hills back of the first line of hills of the rise the city, inside of the work, was very uneven. They could camp inside those works with impunity or in the hollows from danger. Our sick list is increasing but not many fatal so far. Col. A. J. Weber was killed on the 30th of June. Pa, I suppose you remember him. He was our major when you saw the regt., a young man only 19 when he entered the service 2 years ago as capt. Co. B. from Springfield, Ills. By his bravery and gentlemanly conduct, won the esteem and confidence of all his officers & men. They elected him major last spring. Lt. Col. Panabaker resigned. He was appointed Lt. Col. in the fall, Col. Mower apptd. as Brig. Genl., Col. Weber became Col. by promotion only a few months ago after many hair's breath's escapes. He alone was hurt by a shell of the whole regt. close together. He died 20 hours after injury. The fragment took affect directly on the crown of the head, concussing the brain. He never uttered a rational word after being hurt. He always, or rather for the past year, expressed his unbelief in a God or Christianity. They all say had it not been for him and Dr. Fish, Pa would have been Chaplain of the 11th Mo. sometime ago.

Just 2 months after hearing from you, about July 2nd I received a letter from Pa, June 12th, was truly glad to hear of your prosperity and probable success with the school and social affairs. Grandpa is among you safe, the rest well. All good news.

Geo. E. Meily died as I feared he would near our hospital at Champion Hills, Miss. I just learned from J. Palmsteer that our mutual friend Jas. Jann died a few days ago. He in the regt. and I, ¼ miles away, knew nothing of it. I guess it must have been congestive chill. We lost one more man before I got to see him. I captured a signal flag on the highest pinnacle in Vicksburg on the 4th of July 1863. Shall I send it to you as a trophy? If I can by Col. G., send also much love and kind wishes. Write soon to your aff. son & bro.,

T. S. Hawley

As assistant surgeon of the 11th Missouri Infantry, Thomas Hawley was heavily involved in treating the soldiers who remained with the regiment. However, as a prolific letter writer, he continued to communicate with the men of the 111th Illinois Infantry and gossip was rampant. It was reported the chaplain of the regiment, Reverend James Wollard, had lost his congregation because the soldiers thought he was a rebel sympathizer. Also, in a cryptic statement Doctor Hawley related Doctor James Phillips "lost his wife and his reputation." Thomas Hawley felt he was ill-used by the 111th Illinois and there was some satisfaction on his part when things did not go well for some of his old comrades. Doctor Phillips reportedly was withholding too many discharges and to his detriment, some notice had been drawn to this. Hawley was perfectly happy in his new role with the 11th Missouri and referred to his new comrades as "old, true and tried friends." Thomas Hawley revealed he had petitioned to join the regiment in the spring when Major Eli Bowyer was promoted from assistant surgeon to regimental staff with the rank of major. This left only one physician in the regiment, Doctor Melancthon Fish, who did all the work and was ill by the time Thomas Hawley arrived. After his arrival, the sick list began to grow smaller being reduced from 70 to 48. There were only fourteen men in the hospital on July 12.

Back home in Olney, Illinois, Reverend Nelson Hawley gave up his interest in the chaplaincy in the 11th Missouri Infantry and was elected as the president of the Olney Male and Female College. Hawley addressed various sections of his July 12 letter to the different family members. He wished his father success in his new post and hoped his health improved. To sister Fannie, he encouraged exercise and success in her studies. To his mother, he related his general physical condition and wrote the duties of a Civil War surgeon were "onerous duties and constant exposure." He lost much weight during the campaign and was suffering from scurvy. Finally, he reported the regiment was moved to garrison duty near the Big Black River Bridge.

Young's Point, La.
HdQrs. Med. Dept. 11th Mo. Regt.
July 12th 1863
Sunday
Dear Father and Mother,

During the past week I have been highly favored with messages from home and elsewhere. One was from Mr. Simmonson, he gives me quite a history of the regt. Dr. Phillips, poor man lost his wife and his reputation with the regt. Mr. S. said he would not give certificates for leaves or discharges until the men were almost dead. Some had talked of petitioning Dr. R. to leave the regt. said his medicine done them no good. Old Pap Wollard associated with the rebels, some thought he was a rebel sympathizer and would not go to hear him preach. Some of the officers had resigned because this was becoming too much of a war to free the Nigger. Quite a number of desertions. The regt. was very much reduced at that time. Some of them at Ft. Nieman Ky. was anxious for me to return to the regt., said I have many friends, inquired particularly about all the family, said would be pleased to hear from you.

I recd. Myra's letter of July 1st and wrote to her at St. Louis. Ma's good long letter from Robinson and one from Myra at the same time. All tarried a while at LaGrange, Tenn. Another which I now propose to answer from Ma, Pa & Fannie, date June 27. I am pleased to hear you speak favorable of my change from the 111 Ills. to the 11 Mo. Infty. for here I know of whom I have to deal, old, true and tried friends. I resolved to leave the 111th Ills. as soon as I found how they had treated me and made no effort to have that changed. I had some correspondence with Maj. Bowyer and found they had no assistant, told them [I] would accept the appointment if he could get it. This was early last spring, was recommended. So after my commission dates May 14, 1863. Dr. French and I have had a busy time since Dr. Fish left. Indeed done all the work before but since he left the sickness has greatly increased besides we have all the business to attend. I do now three times as much work as Dr. Fish done when he was here. Have worked every way to keep the men in good health. Procured ten barrels of whiskey and made it strong and bitter, gave this to the companies for 6 or 8 days. And reduced the list from 70 to 48. That has been gone for two or three days. Now we have 14 in hospital and 64 in quarters.

All this country is low and was submerged this spring after troops had encamped on the ground all winter. Now the very soil stinks after a little rain and warm [sun] shine. The air is filled with horrorable odors. One will take short breaths to avoid breathing so much of it but amen, all this, no sick. We have only lost two men. One came here entirely disabled, the other I did not see at all, died of congestive chill. Jasper Jann of the 63 Ills. died a few weeks ago of some disease.

I am truly gratified to hear of your unanimous election to the presidency of the Olney Male & Female College. It is no more than I expected when you gave your consent and I know they were glad of the chance. I hope you can get Mary Scott. With her, Myra, yourself and one or two others, you will have a complete faculty. Indeed you must not do much yourself but have plenty of teachers. I cannot see why that school should not be the best in southern Ills. and I firmly believe it will under your guidance and with such teachers as you get to assist.

I knew you would all enjoy a visit from Uncle Matthew and lady. Hope Grand Pa's health will improve this summer. [I] know he must feel much better being where everything moves off quietly. Do hope some of you return the visit of Uncle and see Columbus. Myra should go anyhow. She will learn so much. I wish and think two of three might go. But then I suppose when it would be pleasant to be on a visit, it will be time for your school to commence. Then you will be confined closely but I cannot think of any more useful, profitable occupation or one of a higher calling. Yes Pa, I got your letter in regard to the changes & purchases you had been making and contemplating. Your purchase of town lots, I think a good investment. Another thing, your conclusion not to build additions or improvements to the old house suits me exactly. I think that unprofitable business, with not be best satisfaction for after numerous outlays enough to build a new [one], you still have an old house. Except to paint & some slight repairs I would not do much.

Dear Sister Fannie,

Your letters are somewhat like angels visits, few and far between and good when they do come. I wish I could step in and enjoy vacation with you a few days. Take plenty of recreation, outdoor exercise. I wish you had a pony that I have here to ride. He is such a nice little fellow, not higher than your head but they will not let us send horses north. I would certainly have sent him to you. He was a present from a friend of mine. I heard something about that nice paper you had at the exhibition. Was highly pleased to hear so good a report. I know you will always be at the head of your class. I hope to see you graduate at some fine college with honor. I know you can if you will set your foot down and say I will, then you will.

Dear Mother,

Although your letter richly merits a separate answer from all the rest but as there are so many on hand at the same time, I'll answer this here and the one from Robinson separately. Tis true, the place I occupied for a while was dangerous but then bullets are not so deleterious to the health of surgeons as the wear and tear to the constitution by onerous duties and constant exposure. While in the rebel territory my health was very much impaired by the lack of variety in diet and constant attention to the sick or wounded. I was reduced to a mere skeleton and had symptoms of scurvy, gums coming loose from my teeth, constant irritation of the lower limbs, etc. Irritation of the stomach, everything I eat would disagree with me. Constant eructation from stomach, etc. But since my arrival at this place, there has been a general improvement and I have regained flesh & health. Appetite good, got some dried fruit, not much fresh vegetables. Some canned fruit.

Just now, Dr. Hoffman, the other assistant surgeon, came to hand and I will not have so much to do. I find he is an old schoolmate of mine but I do not remember much about him. Hope he is a pleasant fellow. We move to the vicinity of Vicksburg today sometime. F. Notestine is well. E. Ridgley goes home on leave of absence or wants to, as do many of the officers. Saml. Donald was wounded May 22. H. Kalz & Saml. Conrad here, well.

Much love to all the family hearts held.

Your affctly.,

T. S. Hawley

July 14th Left Sunday for rear of Vicksburg, first to by steamer, then back by car, next day, all pulled off pretty quietly. News still good from east. We are now encamped near the famous Black River Bridge and expect to remain some time. Direct to same brigade at this place. Health improving. Yours,

T. S. Hawley

As announced in Thomas Hawley's previous letter, the 11th Missouri Infantry had moved from the Louisiana side of the Mississippi River to outpost duty near the Big Black River Bridge about fifteen miles east of Vicksburg. In Hawley's July 17 letter, he wrote that 1st Lieutenant Elmore Ridgely was on a medical leave of absence after the Vicksburg Campaign. Hawley wanted the thirty-one year old Ridgely to hand deliver this letter but Ridgely left before it was completed. In December 1863, Elmore Ridgely, Company E, resigned due to an infection of the lungs. The regimental pharmacist and Thomas Hawley's good friend, Zeba French, was also granted a medical furlough. This was accomplished by a personal intercession on the part of Thomas Hawley. It was also evident from the letter that Doctor Melancthon Fish's illness had resulted in a deterioration of the medical support for the regiment. Thomas Hawley's experience managing the hospital in LaGrange served the regiment well as he acquired new hospital tents, medicines and improved the medical department's mess—all of which were desperately needed.

Despite the success at Vicksburg and relative inactivity of the 11th Missouri Infantry performing the outpost duties of protecting the Big Black River Bridge, the war continued. Grant captured the capital of one of the most staunchly supportive states in the Confederacy when he captured Jackson on May 14, but since that time, the Confederates had retaken and fortified the city. During the first Battle of Jackson, Confederate General Joe Johnston had just arrived prior to the Union advance on the city and lamented, "I am too late."[9] Now he was more prepared for his Union adversaries. From July 9 until July 16, Major General William Sherman battled for the city of Jackson, until General Johnston ordered his troops to evacuate the city. When Sherman advanced into the city, he brought flour and pork for the starving civilians. Sherman lost 129 men killed, 752 wounded, and 231 missing during the battle.

Thomas Hawley also reported the "rebels still wander about" and this presumably referred to the large number of Confederate soldiers who were paroled after the capture of Vicksburg. It has been suggested one of Grant's objectives was these displaced men might cause enough mischief in the countryside to draw resources from the Confederate government to deal with them. Some of the Confederate soldiers who were captured in the recent battle of Jackson were soldiers who were paroled at Vicksburg and Thomas Hawley wrote of his disapproval of their actions to take up arms during their parole.

The 11th Missouri still suffered from the effects of the long and arduous campaign and over 100 men were still sick, mostly with malaria, typhoid fever, and congestive chills. Hawley tried to treat these with quinine and bitters, treatments derived from barks of various plants. Finally, Captain Modesta Green, Company C, waited for Thomas Hawley to complete his letter to transport it to Vicksburg so it could be sent home.

Black River Bridge Mills
HdQuarters. Med. Dept.
11th Mo. Inft.
July 17, 1863

Dear Parents, Bro. and Sisters,

My last forwarded from this point I fear will be sometime reaching you. So I concluded to begin before the first of the week that I might be enabled to mail this early. Since I last wrote you, I have seen 4 or 5 persons that I might have sent letters by hand. They [had] just been written. Lieut. Ridgley procured his leave on my certification and left almost before I knew it. Jas. Palmsteer, I saw in Vicksburg was going north, may not visit Olney. Bro A. B. Morrison will leave or has with the body of his brother Charley. He was having plenty of trouble and Dr. French left for Sumner today. I wrote out his request for leave and took it to Genl. Grant's Headquarters and it was approved by Maj. Bowers of the Mt. Carmel Register but now Asst. Adj. Genl. of the Army of the Tenn. After most arduous labors I procured two new hospital tents for the 11th Mo. Inft., a thing they greatly needed and could not procure. Our regiment is now better supplied than any I know of. So most of them say and most of these things have been procured since your most O. B. D. S. took charge of the medical department. Oh what a boasting, you say. Our medical dispensing wagon is a complete success- mess, chest & stove. Hospital stores & medicines for 3 months.

Second dispatch—One day later

Jackson has for the second time surrendered to the superior strength and skill of the Yankee armies. Johnson left night before last in hot haste for the inaccessible swamps of the sea coast or interior of Georgia but not without some show of resistance. Our "brave boys" fell, many of them during the last day's engagement which was a hot one as far as I can gather from the meager news at present. The rebels still wander about and many will not go out of our lines but I hear that some took up arms at Jackson before they had been exchanged and many of them were taken prisoners. Is it a question in your mind what should be their doom? Hang many by the neck until dead. They have been dealing like savages with our government during this whole rebellion and we have always treated them as an indulgent parent treats a wayward child, all the while sparing the rod. It should now begin to smart and burn that its admonitions may be more indelible.

I am fully convinced that the Confederate States of America will be among the things that were, and will not her short history be a dark one? What punishment is ample enough? I think his satanic majesty has prepared a warmer department in his domains for their special accommodation.

They have the presumption to call upon our officers for medicine and commissary supplies. Many of the citizens live exclusively upon that government which they have spent their all in trying to destroy, have daily exhausted the English vocabulary in apply[ing] epithets to it and its advocates.

Regiment still at Champion Hills, Miss. They left here on the 17th on the evening before my return from Vicksburg. I found over one hundred sick and immediately made accommodation for their better care and treatment. I prescribed for them this morning and pop up our new hospital tents and they are doing fine. Dr. Hoffman is with the regt. If they stay long, I shall go out and send him in but I hear they will likely return in a few days. I have just been looking over some of your old letters. It does me so much good to read and peruse their loving contents. It enlivens heart, body & soul.

Still later from all points. Sunday July 19th. Regt. still absent. Mercury 102° in the shade and 122° in sun. Iron becomes so hot you cannot touch it and will soon seek the shade. Sick and wounded are all the time coming in from the front, that's Jackson. Here they are transferred from the ambulances to the cars and sent to Vicksburg from there to permanent hospitals or steamboats for a trip north and many are there who would give treasures for the change. Indeed if it was not for the pleasant winds during the heat of the day, we would be compelled to remain under shelter but as it is, men stir around as they would a thousand miles north. But indeed I do not think they suffer any more than honest hands at home. You know often there it is 104° in sun and sometimes in shade besides the change is greater. Our men, all Yankee soldiers I mean, suffer from malaria, the amount of intermittents is truly astonishing. I do not know of one who escaped if he has used no prophylactic bitters, quinine, etc. I have felt preemptory symptoms often and once had a slight chill but none since and I take two or three grains every day or two. A few days ago we had over one hundred sick. Out of all that number there was not more than six who were not complaining of chills or chills and fever. Intermittents, remittents, congestion and typho malaraial fevers. Several cases of congestion. You know the nearer we approach the equator, the more common and malignant becomes the congestive fevers. We lost one man with it last night after 24 hours illness. It was more melancholy as his brother died of the same disease not more than 10 days ago at Young's Point, La.

We have several cases more on hand. Maj. Bowyer's health is good. I saw Isaac Man, Jno. Bussard, N. Shours, P. Seiler and some others yesterday in the 30th Ills. They guarded a train up from near Jackson and reported its evacuation. I have not heard the program to be inaugurated now but feel assured it will be *all right and will all [be] home before another 4th of July. Capt. Green is on the tender not 50 feet from my tent and will take this to Vicksburg and there comes the locomotive. Much love to all. Grand Pa, Pa & Ma, Rosa, Eva Bell, Fannie, Myra I suppose in St. Louis. Amos, tell him to write and all inquiring friends. Direct as usual to me 11th Mo. Inft. Genl. Mowers Brig., etc.*

Your affct. Son,

T. S. Hawley

Thomas Hawley began his narration in the letter written on July 26 along the Big Black River and he ended the letter on July 29 at Bear Creek, Mississippi. The regiment made five moves over a ten-day period. He was very eloquent in his initial remarks about the war and he felt the fall of the Confederacy had begun. The Confederate defeats at Gettysburg and Vicksburg, as well as the notable but unsuccessful cavalry raid of General John Hunt Morgan into Ohio, resulted in less than a favorable outlook for the South. After serving in the surgeon's role in the Vicksburg campaign, Hawley had earned the right to remark on the "terribleness of the horrors of war."

General John Hunt Morgan's 2500 cavalry and artillery left Sparta, Tennessee, on June 11, 1863, on a notorious raid into the Union controlled Kentucky and the northern states of Indiana and Ohio. This followed his successful Christmas Raid of December 1862. For 46 days he covered about 1000 miles destroying property and putting fear into the citizens of the north. Morgan was successful in many respects in his "Great Raid of 1863" and captured about 6000 Union soldiers, destroyed numerous bridges and railroads and produced terror and fear in the Northern civilians. However, in the end most of Morgan's troops were captured, but Morgan was able to escape. Thomas Hawley reported in his letter a planter felt the raid caused "more good than harm" to the Union, because the raid into Northern soil made the war more real to the Northern population and increased the resolve to continue the war with the South.

Thomas Hawley mentioned the diet for the soldiers in the regiment and stressed the need for vegetables which were expensive and hard to find. The continued diet of meat, hardtack and cornbread was leading to scurvy and general malnutrition. The overall health of the regiment continued to improve from a medical standpoint despite the regimental surgeon's absence due to his illness. Hawley reported Samuel Conrad and Samuel Mann were seriously ill and fortunately for these two farmers from Sumner, Illinois, they were able to regain their health and finish the war.

Hd Quarters Med. Dept.
11th Mo. Inft. Camp near
Missingers Ferry Black River
Miss. 15 miles Rear of Vicksburg
July 26th 1863

Dearest Parents, Bro. and Sisters,

Time still rolls on and we may feel assured is developing the beginning of the end of this rebellion. God grant we may never have another and hasten the downfall of the present. The fine independent people of the northern states cannot have an idea of the terribleness, the horrors of war. We all think Morgan's raid will do some northern dead heads and Copperheads a vast amount of good and I have heard numbers say they hoped a "raid" would visit southern Ills. I have expressed the same wish but always let Olney out. An old planter not 3 miles from here told me he was satisfied all those invasions of northern soil done our cause more good than harm as it always aroused the people to arms and was as good as enforcing a draft. Since our arrival at Young's Point our regt. has suffered terribly.

Camp Sherman, Bear Creek, Miss. July 29, 1863

We have moved 5 times in ten days expecting every camp would be a permanent one. [We] have as high as 200 sick which there [is] a great deal of labor on the surgeons. My health has been somewhat impaired but is a little better today. I shall get a few days of rest if possible and may come home. I need rest more than anything else, no fever or special disease. Many of our men are procuring furloughs.

I just received the <u>W. C. Advocate</u> of the 15 sent by Bro. Amos for which I am much obliged. I saw Bro. Massey's of same date but had not much time to read. Only saw him a few days, did not get to see Dr. Elliott, nor Col. Hicks. They are both commanding the brigade. His health is good I believe.

We are on beach ridges near the road from Jackson to Hayne's Bluffs and I think in a healthy location. Hope soon to have the regt. in better health. We need vegetables. I need them more than anything else. I bought two cans of tomatoes and small bottle [of] pickles for $3.00. Since using them, I feel better. Maj. Bowyer well. McCoy is back. Dr. Fish's time is out but not comeback yet. I have not heard from him. I know nothing special to write you. Only write a little oftener. I have not heard for some time and my anxiety makes it much longer.

Saml. Conrad's almost dying.

Saml. Mann is unwell.

Our regiment has not suffered as much as others of the same brigade. There is some talk of our going to Natchez, Miss. It may be "all talk and no Cider" but I think it quite probable. I came near seeing Link a few days ago. He passed our regt. and some of the boys saw him. Nearly all Grant's army will be encamped between Big Black River and Vicksburg or the Miss.

Well, it's mail time. Our regt. has joined the Division & Corps. Direct to me—Camp Sherman this way:

T. S. H.

11th Mo. Inft.
2nd Brigade 3rd Divis. 15th A. C.
Camp Sherman, Bear Creek, Miss.

Much love to each one and all. Kiss Eva Bell, Fannie, Rosa, Ma, Pa, Myra, Amos & Grandpa for me.

Your most respectful obt. servt. and affct. son & bro.,

T. S. Hawley, MD, etc.

In early August, Thomas Hawley and the 11th Missouri Infantry were camped at Camp Sherman near Bear Creek, Mississippi, which was described as being about 15 miles from Vicksburg. Hawley began and ended his letter of August 2 deriding the Copperheads in Illinois. He even offered the assistance of the regiment to stabilize the situation at home. Richland County, Illinois, where the Hawley family lived was far enough south in Illinois to have a group of people with Southern leanings. These Southern transplants were organized enough to be vocal about their opposition to the war. Some members of this group would later in the war form the Knights of the Golden Circle and the Sons of Liberty, pro-Southern organizations in northern states. The situation in Richland County would eventually deteriorate to such a condition the provost-marshal in Illinois would call for troops to stabilize the area.

Thomas Hawley struggled to regain his health and was instrumental in obtaining medical furloughs for many of the men in regiment. These furloughs were very important because recuperating at home was often more successful than staying in the regiment. Even though it was suggested Doctor Hawley should obtain a furlough for himself, he remained at his post and cared for the soldiers in the regiment. Hawley, again, recorded the poor condition of the 11th Missouri in his August letter stating only 100 men of a 1,000 man regiment were able to march. So bad were the conditions, the command planned the drastic step to consolidate the ten companies into five.

Despite the conditions in Mississippi, Doctor Hawley had time to enter two humorous sections to his letter. The first section was a reflection on "old maids," and the second humorous story related to his interaction with a Southern lady and her uncle who was suffering from bilious fever. Hawley also recorded he was visited by cousin, Lincoln "Link" Swearingen, of the 5th Illinois Cavalry

> All well Aug. 4th 1863. If you want us to assist in the cleaning out of Copperheads of Olney, just send for the 11th Mo.
>
> HdQarts. 11th Mo. Vol. Inft.
> Camp Sherman, Bear Creek, Miss.
> Aug 2nd 1863
>
> Dear Mother & Father,
>
> I guess I will be compelled to rehearse the usual story of no letter for a long period with all the anxious longings and lookings, only to be disappointed. Our mails do not as yet come to us daily but at any and [all] times and it is an interesting period not quite so much noise and bustle as there used to be at San Francisco at the arrivals of the first steamers after 4 or 5 anxious months away from home. But there are many anxious inquiries for letters from home or friends in the north. It has been some time since I heard from you. Nothing was said of Col. Glaze. Did he bring the trophy that I captured in Vicksburg, the signal flag? Quite a number of our men have gone home on furlough. I suppose you will see some of them. I thought some of applying but so long as my health is tolerable good, I will continue in the path of duty. I was advised a week ago to ask leave but could not leave poor, sick soldiers when there was not help enough. Then I had been doing the duty of four men, now some of them have returned and my duties are less arduous. Dr. Fish is still in New York. Dr. Hoffman goes to Vicksburg today to be mustered. There is some fear that he cannot be mustered since there is an order to muster out the Col., one asst. surg., and the major and half the other officers and consolidate the ten companies into five. The others to be made up of old troops or conscripts. Our regiment is far below the minimum. They have started on the march with 90 or 100 men, one tenth of what they should have or are being paid for or rather paying the officers for. I was discharged from the 111th Ills. June 24 by order Genl. Grant in order to accept a commission in the 11th Mo. Vols. and was mustered in to date from June 25, 1863. Lincoln G. Swearingen surprised me the other day by a call when I was not looking for him. His health is good and is getting along fine still with the 5th Ill. Calv. He surely deserves a promotion and but for the dastardly meanness of Mumford, would have received one long ago. Lincoln is I think in every way a worthy young man. I always did like him better than any others of the family; however, Mr. L. S. and I have always been on the best of terms. Link showed me his mother's photograph taken at Chillicothe. She has improved some I think. He says her health is much better.
>
> May we not attribute her peculiar manners for the last few years to poor

health rather than to any real evil intentions? Coz. Sallie still remains in the state of single blessedness, better so than marry as some do. The honors of an old maid's life is all a chimera of the brain conceived in the fertile brain of some well-to-do matrons who think the one great aim of women is to teach her own offspring the ways of the world and the round about way to heaven, not so intentionally but by neglect. The best relation that man or woman can sustain to their fellow mortals is that which will procure the greatest amount of happiness to the largest number of human beings. No two have the same tastes, acquaintances or desires. What is one's standard of earthly bliss might not be another's. Therefore let us honor the old maids for there must, of necessity, be an increase of that unfortunate class. I may make some old maid or somebody else blissfully happy or miserably miserable after this horrible war is over.

A lady, fair, fat and not forty, called upon your most obedient and asked a professional visit to her Secesh uncle who was sick as she thought of the bilious fever, inquired very innocently if I had had much experience in that disease or if I gave much quinine. I replied with some sarcasm that my experience had been amply sufficient to treat the case, perhaps as scientifically as most of their resident physicians. She had just spoken rather disparagingly of some of them. Well, she wanted me to come right away. I declined giving a posture of business as the cause but promised to come at the earliest period. I called a few days after, found Mr. Secesh much better so that I feared he might recover. I gave nothing, advised many things, had quite a chat. My young lady was at Vicksburg during the siege, lived most of the time in a cave, dining room in a little arbor in front. Said she had got up as often as 6 times before drinking one cup of tea to run in[to a] cave from the bomb shells, rather unpleasant tea parties, spoke of many young friends, ladies wounded by shells, etc.

We are encamped about 15 miles from Vicksburg on the high beach ridges undulating between the two rivers, the Mississippi and the Big Black, water good. We use in the hospital cistern water but are encamped in the woods. I am looking for Coz. Link again today. They are camped about 8 miles from here. My best regards to Grand Pa and all the folks. I love you, one and all, immeasurably. I hear rumors of trouble in Olney with the vile, slimy, Copperheads. Crush them. I could, would and will if they cross my path.

Your most affectionately,

T. S. Hawley

I am about well. Less to do. Have no fears.

On August 11 and 13, Thomas Hawley wrote two hasty letters to the family in Illinois. On August 11, he was on a 40 mile round trip to Vicksburg to pick up medical supplies for the regiment. He reported about the health of individual officers in the regiment and received a surprise of ginger cookies sent to him from his sister Fannie. He was also attempting to receive his pay as part of the 11th Missouri Infantry. Finally, he related the citizens of Vicksburg were taking the oath of allegiance to the United States government insuring their loyalty and no longer being loyal to the Confederate States of America.

Near Genl. Grants HdQrs.
Vicksburg, Miss. Aug 11th 1863

Dearest Parent, Bro. and Sisters,

I did not get to write on the first part of the week as we were on our way from Bear Creek to this place on business to procure medicine and see the paymaster. I will return to the regiment today. My health is better and duties not so arduous. I heard from Sister Myra last week dated St. Louis, Mo. July 25. I have not heard from home for several weeks. I do not doubt your writing often and cannot see why I cannot get them. Our mails are very irregular arriving at any and all times. Mr. Notestine, I saw on Sunday at the regt. He is doing business at this post as carpenter. His health is good. Finley has had the chills.

Maj. Bowyer is still somewhat unwell, rather of the intermittent form of fever, not bad. Talks some of coming home. I cannot possibly leave now but should Dr. Fish return, then I will apply for a leave of absence. Link visited me often in the last few weeks which I enjoyed. He is the same, looks well, but complains occasionally. Capt. McClure of the 63 Ills. handed me 3 ginger snaps, a present, he said, from Sister Fannie. Geo. Memsser, the bearer. I hastily opened the pckg. for a note or some clue to them but found nothing but 3 sweet morsels which I shall enjoy in the future. I am in great haste, must draw medicines, a few sanitary goods from our kind friends in the U. S., see the paymaster and go to the 11th Mo., 20 miles from this place through the hot sun & dust. I hardly expect to get any money now, but will get all the necessary papers.

No news of importance at this post. Only they are cleaning up, policing and building government storehouses. The citizens are flocking in and taking the oath. There is a great change in this state and may we hope that all the wandering states will soon follow the example of Mr. Tenn, etc. I have heard of the raid at Olney but had not many fears from such dastardly cowards. I think there is plenty at home for them. But if not, we are ready, willing, would be glad to come and fix 'em. Have sent some home on furlough which will well give them a taste of war. Well, breakfast is ready. So I must stop this. Much love to all, Grandpa, Pa & Ma and all the dear little folks.

Write soon. Write often from your,

Affct. son,

T. S. Hawley

Bear Creek, Miss. Aug. 13

    I am truly sorry. I did not get to send this note at the city but I was sorely pressed for time and could not put it in the [post] office, and here it is yet when it should have gone at the first of the week my usual time of writing you. When I returned I found a note from Bro., Fannie and Pa, July 19. Nearly a month coming. Some get letters 6 and 7 days old. My health is much better indeed. I am doing well and the health of the men is improving. I did not get my pay as usual. But think I will before a great while. Had a chat with Maj. Bowyers, formerly of the Mt. Carmel Register. He inquired after the family, etc. Saw Mr. Goforth and Jonny. Both well. Lieut. John Myers going home on leave. I saw Genl. Grant and Sherman in Vicksburg, both looking well. Bro. Amos, I will answer yours & Fannie['s] letters in my next (i.e.) in two or three days. I was glad to hear from you. Hope you passed through the raid at Olney without any foreboding as to the result. My love to Grand Pa, Pa, Ma, Amos, Myra, Fannie, Evie Bell, Cousins and the other little chicks.

From you affect. Sojer,

T. S. Hawley

    Thomas Hawley wrote letters to his family on sequential days of August 16 and August 17. The first letter was written to Fannie which contained an interesting description of the social interactions between the Union soldiers and the women in Mississippi. Hawley referred to the pseudo- and true widows who sought aid from the occupation army as a method of securing protection, rations and supplies for their families. There was also another reference to the unrest in Illinois due to the Copperheads' activities. Finally, Thomas Hawley provided a description of the diet of the soldiers of the 11th Missouri Infantry, including boiled beef steak which was humorously estimated to be 40 years-old.

Med. Dept. 11th Mo.
Camp Sherman, Bear Creek, Miss.
August 16, 1863
Dear Sister Fannie,

    It would give me, your older brother, infinite joy and unbounded pleasure, to bestow a long lingering kiss upon those ruby lips of yours and you know if I should have the chance of stealing one, I would take two, three, 4, 5, 6 and so, ad infinitum, then if I could buss you so often I might hug you awhile. Besides we might hold a chat, a tete a tete, etc. (is that spelt right?) to do all that I must visit Olney, must travel over one week, must have a leave of absence from our Pa, Genl. Grant, for he does not permit any of his sojer boys to leave home with-

Three. 1863

out asking . Then they must have a good and sufficient reason. So I will not bestow that kiss until I have a good reason.

Maj. Bowyer is going home soon and I shall send one by him if you want it second handed. Now we gents do not often have the exquisite pleasure of kissing young ladies although we sometimes go to see them. Nearly all the officers here go occasionally to see the "wider" [widow]. Everybody has a wider that they visit because at every house you find two, three, or half a dozen. The truth is their husbands are in the Rebel army but they all claim our protections as good loyal citizens and draw rations from Uncle Samuel's storehouse. We have got some peaches and apples in the country but they all gone now. Sometimes the boys bring in vegetables, milk & chickens by riding 20 or 25 miles. We have a cow that gives two quarts of milk per day.

Now my dear Sister, that last messenger of yours was the best of all. I was a little surprised at the composition, yet I could see by it that that was not your best, that you could do better. Such letters truly does my soul good. I see Pa's envelope and circular all very nice and good but do not you think Mr. Shaw can spell Pa's name right? I showed it to Maj. Bowyer, Jim Notestine, Lieut. Sappington and other friends. Are you and Eva Bell both going? Guess so. I hope you will make rapid progress. Can you ride the pony Pa has? If so, try him occasionally and do not fear the Copperheads for they do not look just like other snakes and we boys will be home one of these days to attend to their snakeships. Supper, Supper. Henry Kaley says. So I attend the call. Well supper over. Perhaps my general Miss, you would like to see our bill of fare. Well, here tis.

Broiled beef steak, 40 years old.

Light bread with holes in big enough to hide a toad, 40 years bake in a clay oven. I mean the bread, not the toad. I took my share of the bread, mind you toasted. For toad toasted, is not a fashionable dish. Then we had potatoes, boiled and some more not in the barrel and fresh milk from Boss or Brindle. I don't know which one or tuther. Beside dried apples stewed in a tin pan, sugar sweet & brown from the Indies, I guess. Salt, saltish from Kanawa or old ocean. Pepper, black from the West Indies or East I. Tea, green from China.

Besides tin plates, pans, knives & forks, Britannica mugs or cups, etc., et cetera. I took bread and milk for desert. Yes, and we had a strong smell of cod fish from off the coast of Newfoundland or New England. Good smellers, you think, but now in the mess chest. Well my dear Sis, I have made lots of errors in this short epistle. I wish you would correct them and write your criticisms to me, immediately without delay and in post haste if you please. Or write what you please, if you please. But at least write soon and please remember me as always your affectionate

Bro. Tommy

Hd. Quarters under a Beech nut tree
Med. Dept. 11th Mo. I.
[August 16, 1863]

Thomas Hawley to his Dear Little Sister Evie Bell H.,

 with fourteen kisses greeting and much love sending hopes to see her bright smiling face one of these days. Then we will talk this matter [over]. [We] will have a good long chat. I know you are quite a good little girl and intend to be better to run, romp & play than to study your lessons. Is Fannie a funny teacher? Learn you [to] play on the pandorder. I want to hear you play and sing so much. You must be good to your Cozen Rosa, and when I come home we will have lots of fun, won't we though? Write soon. You affectionate bro.,

Tommy

Is good bye just now.

 On August 17, 1863, the letter was addressed to his brother, Amos, who struggled with his health and Hawley referred to a weak heart and neuralgia. The August 17 letter was devoted to medical advice for Amos and suggested ways to care for himself. Thomas Hawley reported 100 to 110 soldiers of the regiment were still sick, either in their quarters or in the hospital with chills, diarrhea and fevers being the primary causes of the illnesses.

 The letter was written on poorer quality paper than normal and it was noted the paper was obtained from the Confederate supplies at Vicksburg. Thomas Hawley also noted in this letter the Confederates were seeking assistance from the government of Mexico in their cause against the Union. He also mentioned a few names from the regiment, including, Henry Kaley, the hospital clerk. Kaley, a twenty-year-old soldier in Company H, had been wounded in the battle of Iuka on September 19, 1862. Hawley also referred to Samuel Donnell who had been recently wounded at Vicksburg and had previously been wounded during the Battle of Iuka. He mentioned Samuel Mann and Samuel Conrad who he had described as being ill in previous letters. Certainly, the condition of the 11th Missouri Infantry was poor and it was planned for furloughs to begin for 40–50 of those under medical care as a way to improve the health of these men.

Hd. Qtrs. Med. Dept. 11th Mo. Inft.
Camp Sherman, Bear Creek, Miss.
Aug. 17, 1863

Dear Brother,

 Amos, your kind favor of the 20th ultimo came to hand in due time which with us is about two weeks. I was gratified to hear from you as the family had not written special of your health. I think you did right in not engaging in any special business during the warm months, for any excitement of the mind or acceleration of the heart action may do injury. From what the family sometimes writes I am led to believe that you need tonics. Tonic bitters, some preparation of iron and quinine or either alone. Your frequent attacks of neuralgia indicate that and you may have some decayed teeth which are the exciting cause. If so, do not stop a moment until they are extracted or filled for I am fully persuaded that one or two decayed teeth if left to annoy and irritate the nervous system may and will injure one's health for years. I am glad to hear you had the pleasure of visiting Mt. Carmel. I know you all enjoyed it hugely. I received a long letter from Rud Stuz, he says he paid you a visit in Olney and had a fine time. I suppose you found many changes in our old associates but not so much in the town. Rudolph is a good and pious young man. Wrote me an excellent letter, is in the Post Office. I saw Ingersoll. He was just on the point of starting for home on leave of 20 days. He is the second Lieut. in the 48 Ills. Mr. Goforth is sutler. I saw him last week, well. The reg. is 4 or 5 miles from here on Oak Ridge. I will see them some of these days if I have time. Henry Kaley is cooking for us now but is not well. Saml. Conrad has been sick a long time in hospital. He is now some better. I shall send him home for a time if I can. Saml. Mann is unwell and wants a furlough. Saml. Donnell was badly wounded at Vicksburg on the 22nd of May and lost an arm. I believe I have not seen him since. Many of our men are still unwell. Chills and fever and some diarrhea. We have about 70 or 80 sick in quarters and 25 or 30 in hospital and if we can send 40 or 50 men north on furlough to northern hospitals or to the Invalid Corps which is an organization for those who are not able to march or do active duty in the field and we will discharge a few. I suppose Dr. French told you what the flag I sent was used for. Anything Ma sends or any of the rest will be acceptable. I do assure you Ma spoke about sending some fruit by Dr. F.

I write you this on a secesh sheet captured in Vicksburg. Don't you think they must have been hard up? You should see some of their paper printed on old brown paper. Do not be impatient about the war ending. It will close when this rebellion and its cause are settled beyond care and I think not before. I do not doubt that the Rebels have made overtures to the French Emperor and if he sees fit to accept them, then we must thrash him and drive him from Mexico. Coz Mollie S. gives me good news. Says Grand Pa has given you the farm Link lived on. I am truly glad you are so fortunate. Hope you can soon bring it to good account. Write soon and give all the news. Love to all from your affct. brother,

Thomas

In the letter Thomas Hawley wrote on August 20, 1863, he recorded Major Eli Bowyer of the 11th Missouri Infantry was scheduled to begin his furlough soon and Thomas Hawley wanted Major Bowyer to take his letters home rather than trust the mail system. Lieutenant John Finley began his furlough first and the letters were sent with him. Lieutenant John Finley was a twenty-nine-year-old officer of Company F and had been a teacher from Xenia, Illinois. Thomas Hawley wrote that the widow he had been visiting was over her illness and he would no longer be visiting her.

The regimental medical list was reviewed and organized when the medical examining board visited the regiment. Seventy-seven men were discharged, furloughed, or transferred. Thomas Hawley wrote some of the men had been absent for almost two years. Overwhelmingly, those men who were transferred were sent to the Veteran Reserve Corps which was organized by the Union Army to allow soldiers who were infirmed or partially disabled to continue to serve in the army but perform light duties. This allowed the regiment to perform their duties in a regular manner without the burden of partially disabled men. Doctor F. H. Hoffman worked with the regiment and Thomas Hawley during this time of convalescence, but the only reference to Doctor Hoffman in the regimental records was he was transferred to the 31st Infantry in September 1863. By all indications, Doctor Hoffman provided invaluable expertise for the regiment during his time with it.

Thomas Hawley referred to the incident which involved the explosion on the *City of Madison* at Vicksburg. The *City of Madison* was a private service, side-wheel riverboat which had been contracted to serve as a supply and transport vessel. It was originally used for the United States Mail Line, but by August 1863, it was hauling supplies and on August 19 it was docked at Vicksburg with a load of gunpowder and percussion shells. As the riverboat engines were fired and preparation was underway for movement on the river, an explosion resulted. By all accounts the explosion was terrific and it was reported men were thrown as far as a hundred yards from the boat. Accounts vary to the cause of the disaster from a careless person dropping a box of percussion shells to sabotage by a local Southern sympathizer.

The account of the explosion of the *City of Madison* was recorded in the *New York Times*.

> Another Disaster on the Mississippi; Explosion of the Ammunition Steamer *City of Madison*. Over One Hundred and Fifty Lives Believed to Have Been Lost.
>
> Cincinnati, Friday, Aug. 21.
>
> Some particulars of the explosion of the steamer *City of Madison* at Vicksburgh were received here last night. The steamer was being loaded with ammunition, and had received nearly her full load when a negro carrying a percussion shell on board let it fall, causing an instant explosion. The boat took fire, and the fire communicated to the ammunition on board, blowing the steamer to pieces. Out of one hundred and sixty men

on board, only four are known to have escaped. The *City of Madison* was a large side-wheel steamer, owned by Capt. J. S. Neal, of Madison, Ind. She was worth about $40,000."[10]

Finally the friendship between Thomas Hawley and Eli Bowyer was made evident as Hawley stated in the letter, "He is my best friend." Bowyer supported Hawley in his new role and gave credibility to him with the regiment. When the army paymaster was late, Bowyer loaned Thomas Hawley money he needed. Although Eli Bowyer may have been one of the most unmilitary appearing majors in the Union Army, it was clear he was an exemplary individual.

Med. Dept 11th Mo. Inf. Vol.
Bear Creek, Miss.
Aug 20, 1863

Dearest Parents, Bro. & Sisters,

Maj. Bowyer has just received his leave which I had prepared a heavy mail for but Lieut. Finley of Co. F was starting yesterday bound for Olney so I concluded to avail myself of the first steamer and sent by him. I have no news of importance besides what that mail contained, except that Coz Link is here, was too unwell for that expedition into the interior and remained in camp. Today was well enough to call over and will stay all night. My health is improving, at least I feel better. Take a ride every day. Went out 5 or 6 miles this evening. The widow is almost well. So I shall have to look for a new patient.

Since I last wrote, the examining board has been round. We recommended about 80 men for furloughing, discharges and transfers to the Invalid Corps. They discharged or furloughed 33 & transferred over 20, in all about 77. So our sick lists will be materially decreased. Some of these cases have been on the sick list for the last two years. Many of our men are yet sick but majority of them convalescent.

Dr. Hoffman goes to Vicksburg tomorrow after medicines and sanitary stores. A sad accident occurred there [Vicksburg] today so I learn from Capt. Henry of this regt. The <u>Madison</u>, a large side wheel steamer was being loaded with munitions of war and some of the men let a box of percussion shells fall. It exploded and the boiler exploded and some more ammunition, so that many lives were lost and much property, but you will hear the full details before this can reach you. I have already told you much of Maj. Bowyer. He is my best friend. I see him every day. To him I owe a large share of the confidence of the men & officers of this command.

Day before yesterday he opened a well filled purse and offered all I wanted of its contents. I finally took 25 because I knew I was welcome to it. I owe him

3 times that and do not know what I should have done sometimes if he had not offered it. I am glad Dr. French called to see you. He could give you lots of news and is a good social fellow, is one of my confidential friends. I presented him with some good music if he would call and see you. I have asked quite a number to stop and pay you a visit. So if you have an influx of army men, officers & soldiers, charge it to my account. You know how dear you, each and all, are to me. But how much I would endure, or give, to see your bright faces, you cannot guess. I need not assure you of my fixed purpose if the opportunity presents itself to see you this fall. Cannot say when. Link has written.

Love to Grand Pa, Pa, Ma, Fannie, Amos, Rose, and last but not least Eva Bell and secondly, but not leastly, yet lastly send. Give Myra baskets of love from you affct.,

Bub,

T. S. Hawley

From the time of Thomas Hawley's last letter, he had traveled to Memphis and on October 6, 1863, he was aboard the steamer, *Metropolitan*, destined for a four-day trip to Vicksburg.

After the fall of Vicksburg, Grant's army remained in place and awaited the next opportunity to engage its Southern foes. It wasn't until October when Grant had the opportunity to move when he was given command of the Union forces around Chattanooga, Tennessee. Along the Chickamauga Creek in northern Georgia, for three days in September, the fury of General Braxton Bragg's Confederate Army was unleashed and soundly defeated the Union forces which had been stalking him since he left Perryville, Kentucky, in October 1862. At the Battle of Chickamauga on September 18–20, Southern forces capitalized on an errant order issued by Major General William Rosecrans to withdraw Brigadier General Thomas Wood's division out of the Union line, just as 10,000 Confederate soldiers were preparing to attack that very position. The result was the Union line rolled up around the breech and Rosecrans' army was forced to retreat to Chattanooga where they were besieged to the point of starvation. On September 23, Grant received a message ordering him to dispatch as many men as possible to the assistance of General William Rosecrans in Chattanooga. Grant immediately sent Major General William Sherman with part of two corps toward the east. General Grant was then ordered to Louisville, Kentucky, where he met with Secretary of War, Edwin Stanton, and was made commander of the newly formed Military Division of Mississippi which gave Grant control of most of the Union forces in the western theatre. Rosecrans was removed as commander of the Union forces in Chattanooga when Grant arrived there. Grant made known his objective in Chattanooga and it was, "Hold Chattanooga at all hazards."[11] On October

23, 1863, Major General Ulysses Grant arrived at Chattanooga and began his personal command of the Union Military Division of the Mississippi. While the active theatre of the war was moving eastward, the men of the 11th Missouri remained in Mississippi and Tennessee.

While Sherman marched to Chattanooga, Thomas Hawley correctly predicted the regiment would remain in Mississippi throughout the winter. The regiment was still trying to regain its strength.

Memphis
October 6th 1863
Dearest Parents,

After rather a pleasant but slow trip we have arrived in safety and are on board the steamer, <u>Metropolitan</u>, bound for Vicksburg and it will take us at least four days as the capt. says. We will have to remain anchored each night as the river is so low. We did so coming down.

We understand from Genl. Sherman's officers that our army corps will remain near Vicksburg this winter but that you know is very uncertain. The 4th Divis. Genl. Smith's is all that has been removed. That has the 26th Ills., 40th Ills., 6th Iowa and there I see many good friends coming down and at Memphis. Some of our same Divis. Lt. Jones is all right. Boat's going. Love to all. Write soon as usual. 40 bushels of love and loving kindness.

On November 14, Thomas Hawley and the 11th Missouri Infantry were assigned to garrison duty and railroad protection duty at LaGrange, Tennessee. About twelve months earlier, Hawley was commanding his first hospital in the war at this location, but LaGrange was in deplorable condition and had been ill-used by the occupying force. Many of the citizens were dependent upon the Union Army and planned to stay away if the Union didn't occupy the town. Even the colleges and seminaries in the town were "destroyed." The regimental hospital was located in Emmanuel Episcopal Church.

The regiment traveled from Memphis to LaGrange and the train the regiment used as transportation was fired upon by guerrillas killing and wounding some of the men. At LaGrange Thomas Hawley was sharing a room with his close friend, Major Eli Bowyer, and the 11th Missouri Infantry's colonel, William Barnum, and his wife roomed across the hall. William Barnum had been a married merchant living in Springfield, Illinois, prior to the war. Barnum was born in New Jersey and had immigrated to Illinois. William Barnum worked in the wholesale grocery business in the 1850s. He also studied law and was admitted to the Illinois bar in 1859. At the beginning of the war he organized a company of sharpshooters which became Company I, and the marksmanship of the company proved to be a valuable skill as the company faced the war ahead. In the spring of 1863, William Barnum was promoted from the rank of captain in Company I to lieutenant colonel and upon the death of Colonel A. J. Weber, he assumed command of the regiment.

Hd. Quarters Med. Dept. 11th Mo. Infт. Vols.
Roomed with Maj. Bowyer in
Ward G of my Old Hospital No. 4
LaGrange, Tenn. Nov. 14th 1863
Dear Parents, Bro. & Sisters,

Truth is stranger than fiction after passing through the many vicissitudes incident to an active camp life, I again find myself stationed in this once pretty village but now rendered desolate by the demon of war. Its colleges and seminary building destroyed, its churches desecrated, private dwellings ravaged until all of the former inhabitants have removed to more genial society. During the last two or three weeks almost every soldier left, nearly all of the citizens were dependent upon them for support and many of them left, some removed to Memphis, others went north. But now so many of Uncle Sam's boys have returned, the citizens will return and live in peace and harmony. Some will and are living in the new bonds of love and matrimony. I know of three or four officers who have married in this town and cannot say how many others, some for three months or during the war. I shall not enter in those indissoluble bonds for any time in this town, but if I should by chance find my way to Holly Springs and all parties willing, I shall not vouch for all ceremonies that I might be accessory to. You will remember the City of Flowers is only 20 miles south of this place and I may remark a good road. Since my arrival I have seen several citizens of my acquaintance but I regret to say my old boarding house friends have removed to Memphis. I am pleased to hear they will most likely be back soon.

There is a strong probability of our going, or rather of our remaining at this post all winter. Gen. Mower will be near here. Also, Gen. Tuttle, Comdg. Division, for he sent word for me to give up the hospital I was then, or am now, occupying as he wants the house for headquarters. I mailed you a letter at Memphis yesterday, Nov. 12. We left that city about dark. Our brigade on one train. 8 miles from the city, a band of miserable, sneaking guerillas fired upon the boys as they were crowded in and on top of the cars. They wounded two of the 5th Minnesota and killed a Negro on top of the cars. The cars were struck in numerous places. Some of our boys were prepared and returned the fire, giving them more than they sent. I have not heard whether any Rebs were killed or not. Some of the boys said they heard groaning.

Mrs. Barnum and Col. have a room directly opposite ours in the second story. The building is fine, large and pleasantly situated. Dr. French remained in

Memphis to bring up the rest of the camp and garrison equippage and our hospital stores. If you are at leisure any pleasant afternoon, give us a call. I may take the Episcopal Church for a hospital but would prefer a private dwelling if one can be procured.

Give my love to you know who and my compliments to all inquiring friends. I do hope letters will reach your most obedient [servant] more frequently, or my health will not improve as rapidly as it should. Tell Bro. Amos to please write soon and Sister Myra or Coz Sallie, I have not yet heard from. If they write, they have the faculty of sending them on slow moles.

Good-bye for today. Your affect. son,

Thos. S. Hawley

Direct it to the Regt., Brigade to as usual and LaGrange, Tenn.

The regiment settled into the winter quarters in November at LaGrange, Tennessee. The letter of November 22 was filled with more familial issues and references to Hawley's social interactions with those in the regiment. He referred to George Gaddy as the bearer of letters. Corporal George Gaddy was twenty-two years old and had been a resident Olney, Illinois. Gaddy was wounded in the 11th Missouri Infantry's bloody assault on Stockade Redan on May 22, 1863, and had been subsequently captured and released.[12] Early in the letter, Thomas Hawley made his first reference to Miss Carrie. It is unknown which Miss Carrie he referred, but in less than two years, he would marry Miss Caroline Joy. Caroline Joy, M. L. A., was a Preceptress of Southern Illinois Female College from 1862 to 1863 and was a Preceptress of the Olney Female College from 1863 to 1864. She graduated from Ohio Wesleyan

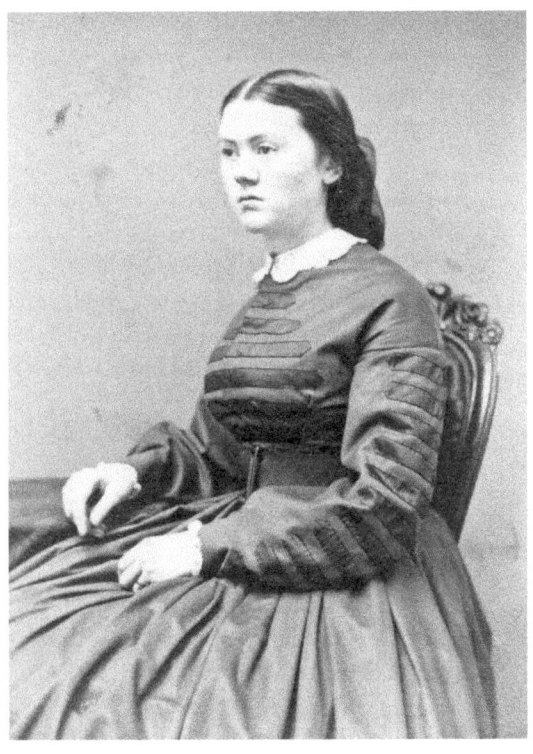

Caroline Joy Hawley, ca. 1860s (Missouri History Museum, St. Louis, Missouri).

in 1861.[13] She taught French, Latin, and mathematics. She was the youngest daughter of Captain Wilder Joy of Delaware County, Ohio. She met Thomas Hawley during one of his furloughs through his sisters, Myra and Fannie, who were both instructors at the Olney Female College.

The paymaster had finally arrived to pay the regiment for its time of service and Thomas Hawley received pay of over $600 for an unspecified period of time. Ever the son of a minister, Hawley and Eli Bowyer made two attempts to attend church services without success but made a vow to lead a "moral, religious and useful life." He wrote the regiment had no religious life and had been without a chaplain for almost a year. Others mentioned in the letter were Doctor Augustus Hoffmiester of the 8th Iowa Infantry and Corporal John "Dock" Wilson, regimental clerk, who had resided in Fairview, Illinois. As Hawley wrote his letter, he had to tolerate the very human and playful actions of Eli Bowyer. After Major Bowyer left him, his thoughts drifted to life after the war and he wrote of a possible place to live with the qualities he sought for a pleasant and useful life.

HdQtrs. Med. Dept. 11th Mo. Inft. Vols.
LaGrange, Tenn. Nov. 22, 1863
Sunday
Dear Parents, Bro, Sisters and Coz,

For the last few days letters have been coming about right, only sometime on the way. The pckg. by Mr. Eckley with its precious love messages written Nov. 8 arrived safe Nov. 17th, over it I had quite a love feast with nuts for desert. I went to Memphis Nov. 19, returned on the 21st, had quite a pleasant time. On my return found Geo. Gaddy and the fine bundle of papers, a good letter from Bro. also his and Coz Sallie's "Photos," both of which I think are good, as do my friends. Sister M., many thanks for Miss Carrie's which everybody admires and especially your most obdt. Today my little friend, Dock Wilson, Regimental Clerk gave me the sweet message from Sis in return for which favor I gave him a sound hugging as he was about the right size. Now to answer the interrogations of each. I shall try to answer each one individually but it will take some time. I must acknowledge the receipt of my photos safe and better ones than I expected. As for these, then do as you see fit and I am satisfied, yes, pleased. You have not yet to acknowledge the receipt of an express pkg [of] $110 from me, to do as you please with and $50 from Link to Molley expressed from Black River, Miss. Oct. 30, 1863. I have the receipt. I recd. at that time—$415. Took most to pay debts and buy some supplies of clothing, etc. Yesterday I recd. $223 more. All of which I now have in my possession and will send you $100 more as soon as I hear from the other.

Sunday evening. Just returned from seeing my friend Surg. Hiefmeister of the 8 Iowa, an intelligent, warm and worthy German. Major and I called twice at the church but found no preacher. Then attend[ed] a short rehearsal at the lodge under the sipher of the L & A [masonic symbols], had rather a pleasant time. Pa, I think it is a good organization and feel under renewed vows and obligation to lead a moral, religious and useful life.

You may say to Coz. Sallie I will send her letter to Coz Link as soon as I hear where he is. I understood they would be ordered to this Department by land. Come up near Holly Springs & Grenada. I hardly think they will come that route. Dr. French is slightly unwell today but nothing serious. The Quartermaster, Ed Applegate, and I called on a lady to see about boarding. She invited me to call and take lessons that Sallie would teach me. You may hear of my taking lessons, but whether I shall learn much music is a question. I have not heard from the 111th Ills. Regt. since I left. Amos says you sent some letters to me from Col. Black & they have not come to hand. But I must write to them soon any how. My health is good. Excuse this style. Maj. Bowyer has been pulling my hair, smiting me on the cheek and I did not according to orders, turn the other. So he renewed his slapping, pulling, cuffing, etc. I pleaded sick & then he left me alone. So I will with this interlude continue.

That family letter was indeed a source of real pleasure and happiness to me. I have found one has much more anxiety just after returning from home to hear often from the friends that after remaining away some time, but for the first few weeks and is almost distracted if he does not hear every 8 or 10 days. And I am so yet. We now begin to count the time by months when we shall leave the service and return to peace, home & dear friends. Then I may seek a home of my own and where will that be? Olney is a pleasant flourishing place but there I will always be a boy. Now confidentially, I have often thought of a place near St. Louis, Mo. that I might ultimately gain an honorable entrance to that city, a point 8 or 10 miles this side on or near the Ohio & Miss R. R. is a rich, fertile country, good market, good to pay up, sufficiently sickly, near enough to derive some benefits from the city in the way of lectures reporting interesting cases, cultivating the acquaintances of influential medical men of whom I now have served and among them strong friends. I have thought of many places and this appears to me in the most favorable light, yet it may not under a stronger light. The major thinks favorable of it. What do you ens? We know it's hardly worthwhile to think much of it yet. We will send some men and officers to Missouri for recruits as they have a chance to volunteer before Jan. or run the risk of being conscripted. We hope to fill up the regiment and do some good service yet.

I like the "photos" very well. If you want more of that class, say so and I will send you the money. I intend to take some opportunity soon to go to Memphis and will have it [photograph] taken in full length and in complete uniform and send you some. I shall answer Ma's good letter soon and sister's loving letter, also Coz Sallie's. Yes, and I may add Bro. Amos, sister Fannie, Bell's and Coz

Dora's. All of which I think excellently good. I must write to Col. Black, Coz Link and various others. I cannot mention all of them just now.

 I am most assuredly favored above many others in having so many near and dear friends. All of which pray for me almost daily in which I have much faith and trust and pray that the divine Father will care for and provide for us all as seeing right in His divine wisdom. I have and am trying to improve in the way to holiness, must and will read the scriptures more. If we remain here, I shall have some time to study and read and may, and I hope, will have frequent opportunities to attend preaching. We have no worship in the brigade. No chaplain except a universalist and I will not go to hear him. Language can't describe my intense desire to be with the dear ones at home, to hear your pleasant, kind voices, see your smiling countenances, to embrace each most lovingly. Tis said that absence conquers love, But Oh! I believe it not. I know it's a yarn. Write soon. Write often. Write one. Write all to your affectionate son, brother & coz,

Thos S. Hawley

Quite an extensive relationship.

 At the end of November, Thomas Hawley wrote a letter to his younger cousin, Theadora, "Dora," with several items of advice. He first related the regiment was scheduled to spend the winter in LaGrange, Tennessee, and the 11th Missouri Infantry was well fortified and prepared for any Confederate threat. Then, he humorously recommended to Dora the best way to be a soldier was to remain in school, study hard and become a congressman. Certainly, by this stage of war the glamour of the military service had worn thin and Thomas Hawley suggested to his cousin it was easier to fight the war from congress than in the field. He also advised him to study hard, get plenty of exercise and live a moral life.

 Just prior to this letter, the Battle of Missionary Ridge was fought near Chattanooga. The beginning of the battle began with the Battle of Lookout Mountain which was fought on November 24, 1863, and concluded with the Battle of Missionary Ridge on November 25, 1863. In September 1863, Major General William Rosecrans' Union Army was defeated by Braxton Bragg at the Battle of Chickamauga. The Union Army retreated to Chattanooga and was besieged to the point of starvation. Grant was able to break the blockade surrounding Chattanooga and concentrate reinforcements. Once his forces were in position he fought his way out of the Confederate encirclement with decisive victories at the Battle of Lookout Mountain and the Battle of Missionary Ridge. In both battles, Grant's attacks did not work as he had planned but the victories were secured. The Confederate Army was pushed off the ridges around Chattanooga opening the way for a major campaign in 1864 with Atlanta as the objective.

HdQtrs. Med. Dept. 11*th* Mo. Vols.
LaGrange, Tenn. Nov. 28, 1863

Dear Coz Theadora,

Many thanks for your letter which was received in due time and read with much pleasure. I was gratified to know that you were now able to correspond with. It appears but a few short years since I could carry you in my arms and now you are almost old enough to trounce a small boy. But what pleases me most of all is your well manifested interest in the studies of school. Soon you will be able to study the sciences and, I hope, languages, also the higher branches in mathematics, all of which I feel confident you will have a great interest in. I most sincerely hope the day is not far distant when I shall hear of your graduating with honors in some western college. You can do it, my boy. Only set you mark high and you can do it. When there is a will, there is a way. Remember the care of your smaller sisters may devolve upon you some day and the best treasure you can lay up is first a good and liberal education for yourself, then to see to their welfare. And Dora, as you love them, keep yourself clean from the vices of this sinful world. They will soon look up to you as an example and for protection. Guard them well. Please think often of this.

But my Larkie, you must jump, hop, skip, play ball and ride, just as often as all the lessons are learned and all the chores attended to. And see here, if you sell me on another great long story about some chap going to cut his throat, I'll pound you most beautifully.

Now if you want to be a good soldier boy and serve your country, enlist to stay at home and study your lessons, then some day run for congressman and get badly—ahead of your competition. Why, my lad, you can and are running for congress now (i. e.) if you are studying closely and I wager a small pile of green backs that you will win. Then you can make a speech without almost cutting a poor fellow's throat. The soldiers in camp are all doing well. We are building a great fort at this place and hope to stay all winter. There are pine trees growing around. The weather is quite warm and pleasant. No Rebels near I guess, but all the soldiers are up at 4 ½ o'clock with their guns prepared for all the Rebs. Much love home, when you write and know me as ever your affct. Coz,

Thos. S. Hawley

Thomas Hawley's letter of December 5 began as a tranquil and domestic scene with family sitting around a fire enjoying popcorn and newspapers, but the letter revealed the regiment, and their surgeon, had the unpleasant tasks of trying to guard the railroads from marauding Confederates determined to disrupt Union supplies and reinforcements. The greatest threat appeared to be from the Confederate cavalry of Major General Nathan Bedford Forrest who William Sherman referred to as "that devil" because of his effectiveness in dealing with his Union adversaries. The other Confederate mentioned was Lieutenant General Stephen Dill Lee who commanded troops in Mississippi in 1863. An example of the difficulty of guarding the railroad was described by Thomas Hawley as the 11th Missouri Infantry marched 22 miles one day and then counter-marched because the Confederates had cut communications and attacked a camp, destroying rail cars, a store house, rails and forcing the defending Union cavalry to retreat. As the Union infantry approached the raiders, the Confederates retreated to fight another day. As the Union infantry was settling into camp, there was an alarm that the Confederates had attacked another location eight miles away and again the infantry marched to the new point of attack. The result of these actions was a stalemate for both sides. The damage was quickly repaired, and both sides lost a few men but were weary for their efforts.

The state of the 11th Missouri Infantry's hospital was acceptable with about 25 men as patients and Hawley proudly reported he had not lost any patients during the preceding month. He found the men had a better chance of survival under his care than under the care of the larger hospitals in Memphis which "kill nearly all the bad cases." Thomas Hawley concluded his December 5 letter referring to the Sucker State, which was a nickname for Illinois in the nineteenth century. This name had several possible origins, including, the sucker part of tobacco plants which were grown in the state and possibly a reference to crayfish which lived in the lower and soggy portions of land. Hawley was successful in attending church and concluded his letter by wishing the family a Merry Christmas and Happy New Year.

HdQuarters. Med. Dept. 11th Mo. Inf.
LaGrange, Tenn. Dec. 5th 1863
Dear Parents, Honored and Beloved,

The chilling winds of December are around us again and the pleasant social circle is nightly formed near the family hearthstone or enclosing the little stove. Merry jokes or kind and loving words are telegraphed around. The nuts are cracked, corn popped, the news read, and war items discussed, hopes and wishes for the safe return of some absent one, at the family altar supplications ascend for his safe return. How great a blessing to be the object of so many earnest prayers and we should never cease returning thanks.

Your kind messages by the politeness of Mrs. Finley came to hand yesterday all safe. I owe you much for the good papers you send. Maj. Bower, the Col. and lady read them. Then I will send some to the boys in hospital of whom we now have from 18 to 25. All doing well, did not lose a man last month, nor send any to Genl. Hospital. I shall keep all, so long as we remain at a station. I cannot trust the hospital at Memphis. They kill nearly all the bad cases. I have one man, Jno. Kern, who has had chronic dysentery for 10 months. If he cannot get home, will not last long. I made out his certificate for furlough and hope he will get it soon. In these diseases of a miasmatic character, a change of location and climate is the first, all important step. To send such a case home is of more benefit to the sick soldier than all the drugs that can be stuffed down his throat. This fully proven this summer and fall when we sent nearly all the sick men and officers home on leave and furlough with but few exceptions, their improvement was miraculous. It is not so necessary now but in the intestinal disorders will, I think, be beneficial.

Just after dinner, feel refreshed, for the last two or three days the boom of cannons has not been uncommon. On the 3rd it was reported that Genl. Forest or Lee was meditating an attack on the railroad between here and Corinth. I mean that this was rumored on the second and known on the 3rd at 4 o'clock of that day. We were preparing to move at daylight, started for Pocohantas 27 miles east, marched until near dark, came to a halt as our train and artillery was fast in the rear and in a swamp, bivouacked for the night, having gone 22 miles and tired and foot sore. Up the next morning at 4 and counter march to the rear as the Rebs had cut off our communications, burned some camp and garrison equippage, two cars, one Union house, tore up the railroad track, scared our cavalry, etc. After marching back 3 or 4 miles, heard the booming of cannon, then ordered to load but not cap the guns except the company in the rear. They must be always ready and stay back from the others two or three hundred yards. Then we all marched fast before the sound of cannon. All were languid, sore, and many stragglers stopping by the way but at the prospect of a brush with the Rebs, every boy was up and eager for the fray. But Mr. Scary Butternut heard of our coming and came to the conclusion that discretion was the better part of valor and [with the] shining light had left for the deep fastinesses of Dixie where the slimey Rattle Snake hiss and the poor down trodden Negro moans and groans. We returned to this camp the same day with sore muscles, blistered feet and knawing appetites. Sleep well only to be early aroused for Mr. Reb was on hand again. This time toward Memphis near the ancient city of Moscow. 8 miles west some troops went down on [the] train. A Negro regt. kept them off the bridge until other troops arrived. The 6th Ill. Cav. pitched in and killed and wounded several, but lost some among them, I hear, their col., no the col. of 3rd Iowa, comdg. Cavl. Brigade. Col. Hatch, a brave and gallant officer would have been a Brig. Genl.

No news from Memphis for 3 days, no mail sent out. Rebs not heard from today. I will finish tomorrow and send by first mail.

Sunday evening Dec. 6. All quiet and pleasant. No enemy in unpleasant proximity. The weather unusually salubrious today, was like a May morning in the Sucer State. I have just learned that Col. Hatch was not killed. The Rebs have surely left. I heard preaching today by Dr. Gray and it was an excellent sermon. I also attend Sabbath School. Most of the scholars, soldiers, a few citizens & children. The fort is almost done. So we did not work on it today. I shall go to Memphis if possible and will express you some money. I wish you, I pray you, a Merry, Merry Christmas and Happy New Year. What intense pleasure and happiness it would afford me to spend these hallmark days under the homestead roof where Father, Mother, bro. & sisters meet in the family circle. But for the present it remains for me to kiss, hug and look deep in the windows of your soul as it were by faith. And write often, hoping to hear from you. Kiss Eva Bell, Fannie, Dora, Bro. A., Sister Myra, Ma & Pa. All for you 50 times each, a small squeeze thrown in.

Your most affectionately,

Thos. S. Hawley, MD

The final letter written in 1863 dated December 13, 1863, and Thomas Hawley was concluding another year in his room looking over the correspondence in his portfolio. In a time of limited communications, the letters to and from Doctor Hawley were informational and emotional ties to his family. He had just returned to his room from attending a bell ringing and from a sermon encouraging the soldiers to endure challenges in a Christian manner. Getting to and from church was a challenge in itself as the ever present mud made perambulation difficult and often soiled clothes.

Thomas Hawley mentioned his communication with Miss Carrie Anderson. The letter included the story of the unfortunate Captain Robert Affleck whose foot was amputated as a result of an accident which occurred as he was trying to get into an army wagon. The activities in the war effort and the injuries which resulted were not all caused on the battlefield. Hawley had just returned from Memphis where he had acquired medical supplies and religious materials which he distributed to his friends and patients. He also wrote he had sent $100 as a Christmas present to the family. Finally, he wished his father success in his efforts to improve the school he was managing.

Thomas Hawley also wrote of the appointment of 1st Lieutenant Lewis Gray as recruiting officer for the 11th Missouri Veteran Infantry. Lieutenant Gray was one of the regiment who had been wounded in the assault on Stockade Redan at Vicksburg on May 22, 1863. He had recovered enough to assume this role, but he would resign his commission in the spring of 1864 as result of his wound. It should be noted the men of the 11th Missouri Infantry enlisted for a period of three years and the term of enlistment expired in August 1864. Colonel William Barnum began efforts to ensure the identity of the regiment by organizing a veteran regiment, a regiment in which soldiers whose term of enlistment had expired and then reenlisted. Despite orders which prevented regiments from recruiting more than ninety days prior to the expiration of the term of enlistment, many regiments, including the 11th Missouri Infantry, actively recruited soldiers. The 11th Missouri successfully accomplished the enlistment of a veteran regiment and extended the term of service from August 1864 to January 1866 for about three hundred of the soldiers of the regiment including Thomas Hawley. The veteran regiment would not be formally organized until the summer of 1864.

My Room nice & comfortable
LaGrange, Tenn. Dec. 13th 1863
Sunday P.M.
Dearest Parents, Bro. and Sisters,

Looking over a pkg. of letters in my nice portfolio, I find quite a number in the pocket marked unanswered. All from home but one. Now I am confident that I have written one letter for each of these but those sent were usually addressed as this one is. So if I do not always answer individually, please do not stop for I could not endure this life of a soldier without your kind, good, advising letters. I am fully persuaded they are the main means of keeping me to what I am. I am truly thankful it is no worse than it is. Hope and pray that it may be better with me than it is. Your good letters in a measure make up for the pious example and daily precepts that I have always been accustomed to at home and the many blessed privileges I had there.

Today Maj. B. and I attended the ringing of the bell and found a house full of soldiers and the chaplain of the 7th Ills. Calv. about to address them. We enjoyed the sermon a great deal. He is an earnest and pleasant speaker. The text was "Then therefore endure hardness as a good soldier of Jesus Christ." The southern winter has set in with all its variableness. A May day followed by a cold December one, then April showers, no, dreary heavy drenching rains until the mud becomes intolerable. You become dull and stupid indoors, have an attack of the blues. This drives you into the open air when you stick fast in the Sacred Soil of Dixie, get mad, fall down and soil your brass, coat and blue buttons, poor feller. I have not got the Blues but would have if I had just not received two letters and I would feel Oh So Much better if one of them was from home but not one for the last 10 days. Please do write as often as any one of you can spare a half an hour and not interfere with your necessary duties. One of my letters was all the way from New Orleans. Who from do you think? Not from any of Dixie's fair "little rebels." Oh No, from Dr. Israel B. Washburn, surg. of the 46 Ind., one of my Champion Hill chums. He's all right and will do <u>to tye too</u>. He wants notes from the cases we had in Champion Hills Hospital and will have some of them to their termination. The men were of his Divs.

The other was from Miss Carrie Anderson. I wrote to her just for fun and she answered, I guess in the same way, besides giving me much news and asked for my opinion of the war. She heard Capt. Robt. Affleck had his foot amputated. He was unwell and in getting into an army wagon, fell and the heavy wheel crushed it to pieces. Spoke of four contemplated weddings to Miss Prinns, Miss Emma Best, Mr. Schell and Miss Josie Kircher, [I] don't know them. Wrote of her Grand Pa's disease, Nov. 16. No other news. I was in the city of Memphis last week procuring medical supplies, sanitary goods and also got a small library of religious books, tracks and papers for the boys. I distributed the papers, one to each tent. The boys were anxious to read them, asked me if I was acting chaplain. The books I shall keep as a hospital library for the sick and convalescent. While in Memphis, I expressed home, one hundred dollars. Fifty dollars I gave you, my dear parents, as a Christmas gift. I would rather have purchased presents separately and sent but could not do it here. So please accept this little token as a free will offering to these I hold dearer than life itself. To whom I owe so much that can never be paid. Now accept it, you must and I trust will. My health is good and I have some time to devote to study and reading. Maj. B. is well and doing well, Lieut. Gray has been appointed recruiting officer for the veterans of this command. Not much of an office though. I have taken no lessons from Miss Sallie, only called once or twice. She regards me as too much of a Yankee or abolitionist. Well I am glad of it for I am both until this war is ended. Sisters, I purchased five pieces of music for you and will mail them this week, will send the Atlantic Monthly to Amos. Please send me the Journal occasionally. I have not heard from the 111th Ills. for a long time. Pa, I am glad to hear that your school is progressing so well. I regard it is quite an undertaking to build up a school after such an antecedent or predecessor in such war times and with such a wiley opponent. You and your valuable auxiliaries have great reason to feel confident of success in the establishment of a good high school in the west and who can tell of its future renown or wide spread influence as such it will be the seed of great good. I wish you had the magnificent college building that is here rapidly going to ruin from the ravages of war. Surely the war is going to last until every southern lord will be shorn of his ill gotten treasures that they may feel the bitings of poverty.

Much love to each precious member of the dear family circle. A real Christmas Holiday. Love as a present to all from the absent,

Thomas Hawley

So ended the year of 1863 for Thomas Hawley. He began the year a recent prisoner of General Earl Van Dorn's Confederates in Holly Springs, Mississippi, and soon moved to LaGrange, Tennessee, and was in charge of a hospital. He began and ended the year in the same spot — LaGrange, but so much had changed during the year. From his hospital duty, he participated in the Vicksburg Campaign, one of history's most exciting stories. For 45 days he worked in conditions which defy description as a Union Army surgeon offering assistance to the soldiers who were wounded in the numerous battles in May and June 1863. He performed operations daily and then tried to preserve the lives of those who suffered so much. He also re-joined the 11th Missouri Infantry as assistant surgeon and he was content for the first time in the war. The remainder of the year he tended to the decimated regiment and strove to bring the number of effective soldiers to a level to maintain the regiment's integrity, all without the assistance of the regimental surgeon who was absent most of the second half of the year.

Thomas Hawley's family continued to write supportive letters. Not all was pleasant at home as the Southern-supporting Copperheads made life difficult for the citizens of Richland County, Illinois. His father abandoned thoughts of becoming a Union chaplain and instead took control of a school. His mother continued to care and support the family. His sisters were in school and Fannie and Myra were teaching. Brother Amos continued in his frail condition and stoutly tried to find suitable employment. Finally, Thomas Hawley was introduced to Miss Carrie Joy who taught at the school his father supervised and who would later become his wife. Despite the ravages of war, life moved ahead and Thomas Hawley even gave thoughts of where he would like to live and what qualities of a community were important to him. The happiness of a war-free America would have to wait, because for Thomas Hawley, the Union needed to be preserved and he was willing to sacrifice everything to accomplish this. He wanted a peace which guaranteed human rights and supported the constitution. He wanted a peace which would last for ever and ever.

Four

1864

LaGrange, Tupelo, Oxford, Missouri and Nashville

On January 1, 1864, Thomas Hawley and the 11th Missouri were tucked away in winter quarters in LaGrange, Tennessee. The regiment was healing and regaining many of the wounded and sick soldiers back into service. The regiment, now well supplied and well fed, was gaining the strength lost during the Vicksburg Campaign which had taken such a devastating toll. Although the active, large campaigns were in the east with the objectives being Atlanta and Richmond, the 11th Missouri Infantry was faced with many possible sites for campaigning in the west. Although 1863 was a devastating year for the Confederacy, the new year found the South resolved to keep the Northern armies off the sacred soil of the South. Numerous Confederate forces continued to operate in Tennessee, Mississippi and Arkansas, and new challenges faced the 11th Missouri Infantry and their surgeon, Doctor Thomas Hawley.

On January 24, 1864, Thomas Hawley wrote his sister, Fannie, from LaGrange. He mentioned the regiment was on the move and would soon pass through Memphis. Regimental records show the regiment left LaGrange, Tennessee, on January 26 and moved to Memphis and then to Vicksburg until February 5. Hawley wrote there were several possible locations where he might travel, including, Texas, Red River Valley in Louisiana, St. Louis or possibly home. The letters from home continued to be salve for his soul and his hospital steward and friend, Zeba French, picked up the mail for Thomas. While his sister thought her life mundane and without interest, Thomas Hawley wrote that her bits of news were wonderful for his well-being. Hawley chided his sister about her position as a teacher and the type of discipline she might use. Thomas Hawley and Fannie reviewed each other's letters throughout the

Four. 1864

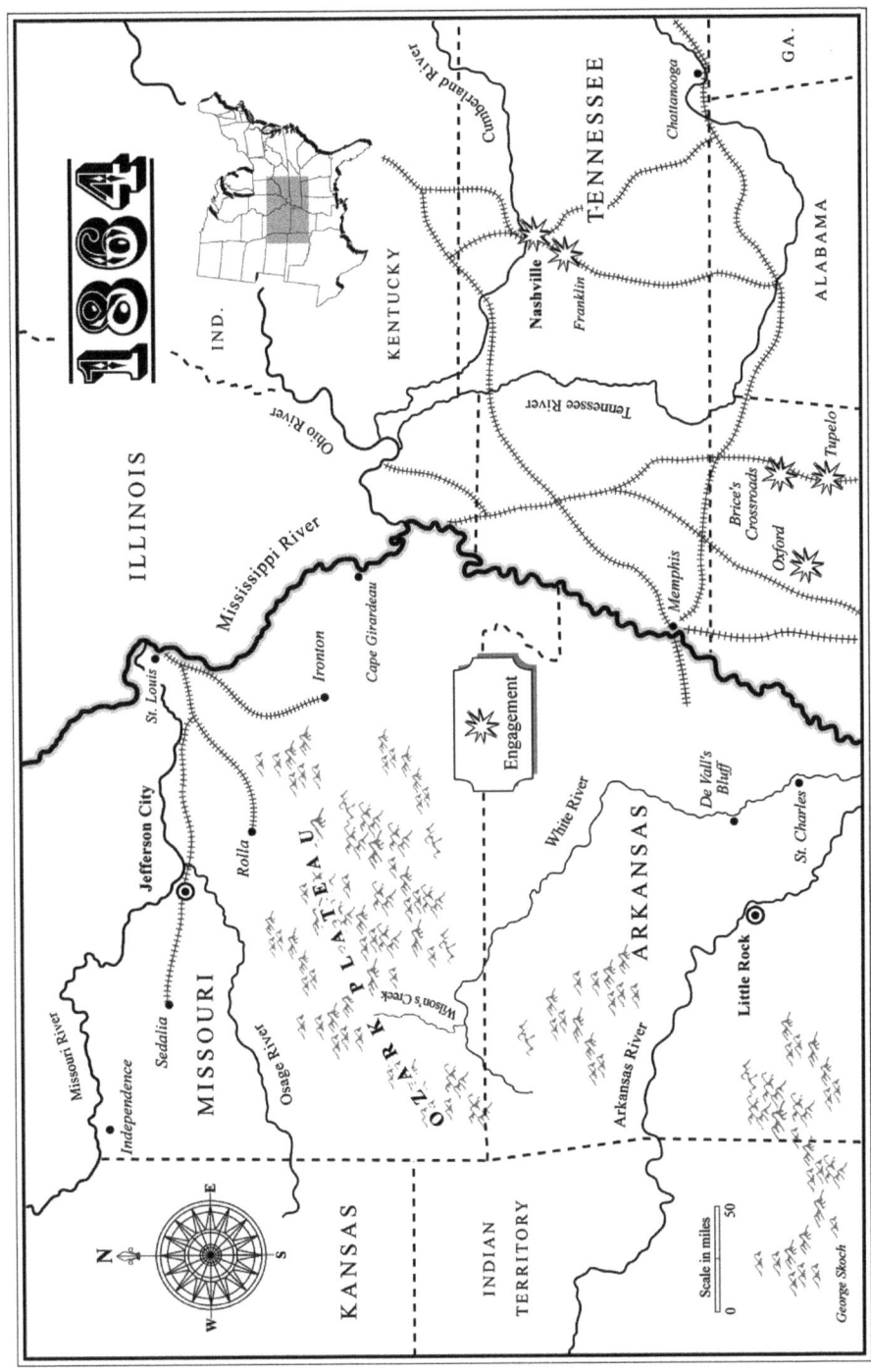

war for grammatical errors and composition and routinely criticized each other, in a friendly way.

Room Office of Surg.
11th Mo. Infty. Veterans
Jan 23rd 64
Darling Sister

Your precious love missels [missiles] have been raining down upon me like shells upon a beleaguered city but with far different effect, instead of disaffection, they have increased the distance love, if they could be. The first unanswered mailed Dec. 28th recd. Jan. 9th stopped in Memphis & Mr. Postmaster sent me a polite note saying he had a letter for me. I sent down Dr. French. He brought it. I have read it & reread it. It is no trouble for me to read your letters. I suppose not half as it is for you to read mine for I wrote a good deal and have not always time to spare. So I write in haste. The weather today is lovely, the sun is throwing its warm genial rays upon this note making it appear lighter than the ideas contained therein to you, I think. Well, now to answer the questions beginning at the first. We will soon pass through Memphis. I will call on Mr. Frank if I have time. I am truly glad you got so much music on Christmas. Yes, Harry is a good fellow. I suppose to you at least. You did right to send one of my photos to the Miss McNelley. I know them well but would like to have Jos. or Jms. No, I would not receive any young gents as scholars. They are always green and will not stick to their lessons. Yours of Jan. 5, I did not think you wrote so often. How I love you. Oh no, you are not neglectful, any of you ens.

You may think your long letter to me for leisure reading when I tell you I read that long one three times and I find [it] and others good, nourishing mental diet. So please to continue to send you[r] <u>So Much of Nothings</u>*. I'll digest and feast on them. Fully installed as school Teacher or Mame, eh? Good for you sis. Now bluster around, look cross, scold, pull hair, clap hands, box ears, etc., etc. Let 'em know you are [boss] soon, or will you try the milk and water sugar and candy treatment? Oh No, I know you will do neither but act consistent and have, oh so many boys & girls in love with you and their lessons. Study the character of each closely, then train it gently as you would the tender plant or flower. Sorry you was unwell during the holidays. When I come up there we will have a sleigh ride. So don't cry, nor put finger in your eye. So Mrs. A. Brainard has changed her companion, poor girl!*

Criticize you, you say, well to begin, you yourself are too fat, too short, too good and love too much and sing. It will break your heart, Sis. Well, I cannot criticize you now. I have just been reading too many of your good long letters. So please wait until I get mad then look out, my daughter of Zion. It will be more than the bombardment of Charleston. Well, all the letters answered I believe.

Four. 1864 169

Now Sis, can you read this? I fear it will trouble you and take you sometime. Well [we] are all the time talking about going home or to Red River or Texas. We are under orders but cannot say where we will have to go to. Some think we will have to go to St. Louis soon. But most concerns is saying we will first go to Red River first but not be gone long. There is no doubt about our going home soon, at least this Spring.

My health is better but a trip home or to some riding expedition will help me. I need more exercising in the open air. We had a pleasant time conferring two or three degrees upon ladies and gents last night in our town. The degree of master masons daughter.

The health is tolerable good. Major is well and in a good humor. We have pleasant times. Please give my best compliments to your associates in school and all my old friends, generally. Write soon, much love to all, Pa, Ma, Amos, Fannie, Bell and remember me as ever your affct. brother through thick & thin.

Thos. S. Hawley

On January 29, the letter from Thomas Hawley to his sister began by outlining the preparation of the regiment's movement south, but the exact destination was unknown. One possible destination was Mobile, Alabama, but the second part of the letter written on the *St. Florence* with 790 officers and soldiers on January 31 indicated the likely destination as Vicksburg, Mississippi. Hawley humorously speculated about the young women in Illinois trying to find husbands.

Camp Near Memphis, Tenn
January 29, 1864

Dearest Sister

Here we are in the suburbs of the once Dixie City but now partially unionized by the persuasive influence of Federal bayonets and the foaming argument of a few hundred dark throated stern iron looking orators. Memphis is called a gay city but is full of dark deeds. Its record was always stained, war's contagion has not cleansed its appearance. Since our arrival Uncle Samuel with his usual promptness has sent among us one of his disbursing agents who left us all with a flush hand. I saw Adams agent and by a small deposit received a small receipt which was this rec[eived] of Mr. So & So $100 directed to Rev. N. Hawley, Olney, Ills. Then comes a long rigma role, but uninteresting, this leaves me on hand $140, or near, but I fear it will go almost as fast as some of their predecessors. We soon expect to embark on steamer for the lower river, have been here ten days with tents and in light fitting trim. We will march with but three wagons to the regt., three small tents but few blankets and indeed almost destitute of the *necessarys of life but shall depend in a measure on the residents of the country. Where will we go? Oh, what a question for a lady to ask a military man. Do you suppose he would tell if he knew; if he didn't, would he? Well to guess, say near the Gulf of Mexico. How would Mobile do?*

A pretty gracefully ringleted miss of an uncertain age from 16 to 19 said to me half sorrowfully, half mischievously, "Oh, it would be too bad for you to go to Mobile." I carelessly said "Well, I don't know." She explained and said for us, as I was leaving. Her mother and [she her]self advanced in a friendly manner as much as said you['re] a good feller and thank you humble [sir]. I am trouble for some but medicine sent to them. Miss Mattie said she was so much afraid it was for her, that she would not take anything but whiskey, that was her medicine, etc., etc.

The 49th Illinois with which you associate so much----------------------I find has left to new parts unknown. The 117th I cannot find indeed. Almost every regt. has left and I think we will leave in the morning and shall probably land at Vicksburg, Miss. Our contemplated promised furlough home will necessarily be postponed for an indefinite period. But when this Spartan band reaches their homes, there will be rejoicing. The Adjt. General of Missouri has telegraphed us to let him know when we will come and as near as possible the time, route, etc., etc. His inferences is we are to be received with the honors of war by a grand oration, magnificent reception, luxurious luxuries, etc.

They are looking for books, Oh, boats to carry us south. Books can carry the mind but not the body.

Finley Mrs. will leave for Olney and can tell you some things that I cannot write. We have had a pleasant time while she was with us and will miss her from our table. While there are some we would not weep much to miss for some time. Now Sis, you must not work too hard with your music, living, correspondence & church, domestic affairs etc. But do your duty toward yourself, your maker & your friends. You write well, spell better than I do or any, no, many others. Since you might deal more in principles or arguments and descriptive accounts of men, ladies, and things. The best mode of teaching you will think of often. The weather for the last two weeks has been unusually fine, not much rain, not very cold but now some appearance of rain just as we must embark on crowded transports. It is now thundering, mercury near 60°. Well my dear Sis, what naughty sprite prompted you to write me no more of your companion of her journeying. I have not heard from her I regret to say for a long, long time. Well I bid you a good night. While I make my bed on mother earth to dream of you, of loved ones at home and not at home. Good night. A kiss.

Jan 31 '64

On board <u>St. Florence</u> *bound south. Will leave at all hours if you take the word of men and officers. But if you wait for the order [of] a slow old general as* we must, you'll say we leave Feb 1st. We will not be much crowded. I think our regt. near 400. Pioneer Corps 350, General Tuttle and staff. Hangers on 40. 790. Pretty full.

Health and spirits good for the circumstances, in rain night before last. Regt. ordered to river, layed all night on open levee (it rained torrents), new tents, mud bad, cold supper, officers absent, men drunk, cursing & moaning which made it an unmilitary step for some to purgatory. If the brave suffering men could have consigned the generals & quartermasters to a warmer place than the pope's summer residence. Mrs. Finley will be the bearer of this probably (i.e.) if I can get it to her. Today is Sunday but it appears like anything else here. Yet I must say most of the stores are closed uptown. I intended to purchase some more music for you but could not for time. Sis I cannot answer all you[r] questions because the letters are not censurable. So you must be content to wait for "you know patient waiting, no loss." I presume you young ladies will improve the time this year and pop the question to some poor unsuspecting stay-at-home gent. Poor Chaps. If they cannot stand the charges of the Rebs, how much less can they bear, the winning fascinating smiles of the fair maidens of "God's Country" (i. e.) according to the war vocabulary [of] the Free North. Well we boys almost envy them the trying ordeal. Well, give my best complements to your friends and my friends and Uncle Sam's best friends only and unconditionally. Love more than language can express to the loved ones at home. You may write to me as usual. Directing 1st Division, 16 Army Corps. You may say Army in field near Vicksburg.

Love to you

Thomas
Your brother

Since Thomas Hawley's last letter in January the regiment moved from Vicksburg to outpost duty again guarding the supply and communication system along the Big Black River until February 27. Then the regiment returned to Vicksburg until March 4 and then part of the regiment traveled to St. Louis from March 10 to 16. For those soldiers in the 11th Missouri who chose to re-enlist to become veterans, they were offered furloughs before they started serving their new tour of duty. Special Field Order No. 14 issued on March 6, 1864, stated the 11th Missouri soldiers who re-enlisted were "hereby ordered to proceed to Memphis, Tenn. where the arms, ordnance stores and other property excepting necessary cooking utensil, will be turned over when the Regiments will proceed with their officers to their respective states ... the 11th Missouri to St. Louis Mo.... The men who have not re-enlisted as Veterans will be assigned temporarily to other Regiments of the same states and will be provided with Descriptive Rolls."[1]

Thomas Hawley chose to re-enlist in the new veteran regiment and his happiness and lightheartedness was evident in his letter on March 14 to an unidentified group of friends. He even went as far as to write a false set of orders directing him to have fun for the next 30 to 40 days in St. Louis and in Olney, Illinois. As he wrote this letter, he was aboard the paddle-wheeler, *Emma Boyd*, two days away from St. Louis. All was not happiness for Thomas Hawley because he wrote of a severe illness of his frail younger brother, Amos.

For those who chose not to re-enlist, or the non-veterans, their lot was to continue the war effort within other regiments. There were approximately 100 soldiers of the 11th Missouri Infantry who became non-veterans and were transferred to the 33rd Missouri Infantry. These men were soon marching as part of the 1,300 men of the 33rd Missouri Infantry in the Red River Campaign in Louisiana. In fact, the Union Army needed all the soldiers possible and made sure these excellent soldiers were part of the Red River Campaign while their enlistment continued. This campaign was one of the grandest defeats for the Union in the Civil War. The campaign began on March 10 and lasted until May 22, 1864, and while Thomas Hawley and the veteran soldiers of the 11th Missouri Infantry enjoyed their furlough, the non-veteran 11th Missouri Infantry served under the command of Union General Nathaniel Banks who, clearly, was not the man to lead this expedition. There were several battles in which the non-veterans participated, including, the capture of Fort DeRussey, Battle of Mansfield, Battle of Pleasant Hill and the Battle of Yellow Bayou. When the campaign was over, the war was still not over for the non-veteran soldiers of the 11th Missouri Infantry as they campaigned throughout the term of enlistment which ended in August.

11th *Mo. Infty. Vet. Vols.*
On steamer <u>Emma Boyd</u>
below Memphis, Tenn.
*March 14*th *64*
Dear Friends,

Many thanks for your kind letter written about the 1st inst. I had been exceedingly anxious not having heard for a long time, nearly one month and Bro. A. so sick on the same day. I wrote you a letter, had just mailed it and returned to the regt. when two was handed me. One from home by Ma & Myra. I shall kiss 40 times in or about three weeks if all goes well, providence favoring us, most likely summer. We will arrive in Memphis this afternoon, turn over all [to] regimental quartermaster and ordinance stores, then proceed direct to St. Louis, transact some business, then disperse to visit our respective "Dear Ones" two, threes and half dozs. as the case may be. Remain 30 or 40 days and nights to return to the field of strife. To me these visits appear more like a transfer from earth's tempestuous sea to a paradise of love, sunshine & flowers.

I have just reread your loving letters but cannot answer them in detail now. I am writing in our state room, i. e., the Major & I. Soldiers and officers playing cards with (the usual slang accompanying it) at my right and left. Boys dancing and scraping on a thin floor a few inches above my head. Just below steam, iron, water, wood, mules, and soldiers making all the noise possible besides shaking my arm, pen, paper & stool.

Our command consists of about 300 enlisted men, 2~~50~~ officers and 30 colored servants.

Head Quarters 11th Mo. Infty. Vet. Vols.
Special Order No. 1

It is my order that Mrs. E. P. Hawley or Miss M.D.H. report without delay to these Head Quarters upon our arrival in St. Louis which I will communicate to you by telegraph. Duties: business & pleasure.

III. Whichever the exigencies of the Household Service will best spare for a few days. I will see to transportation, etc.

Hoping you are all well and doing well. I, in haste, send love unbounded, etc.

Yours affctly.,

T. S. Hawley

The veteran soldiers of the 11th Regiment Missouri Veteran Volunteer Infantry returned to duty on May 2, 1864, after extended furloughs. Thomas Hawley spent the night of May 5 sleeping under the stars without the benefit of a tent, but this did not perturb him. The members of the 11th Missouri Veteran Volunteer Infantry left Cairo, Illinois, and traveled on the riverboat, *Miami*, to Memphis, Tennessee. The regiment was waiting to be re-equipped as the new veteran regiment and there were about 300 soldiers present for duty. This was the lowest amount of soldiers needed to maintain regimental integrity and the regimental officers had communicated the desperate need to gain new recruits with the adjutants general in Missouri and Illinois. The regiment was at a decided disadvantage in regard to obtaining new recruits because most of the soldiers were from Illinois but the regiment served under a Missouri flag. Therefore, it was difficult to obtain recruits. Finally, the adjutant general in Illinois allowed the regiment to recruit in Illinois with the provision the regiment would be renamed an Illinois regiment; however, recruiting continued in Missouri and Illinois but the regiment never changed its name. It was an agreement between Colonel William Barnum of the 11th Missouri and Lieutenant Colonel Robert Buchanan of the Seventh Missouri Infantry which increased the number of effective soldiers for the regiment.

The "Irish" Seventh Missouri's term of service was also expiring but less than 200 men agreed to re-enlist and Barnum and Buchanan worked out an agreeable transfer of the men of the Seventh Missouri into the 11th Missouri Veteran Infantry which was to be accomplished by December 1864.

Thomas Hawley wrote on May 6 about the arrangement by which supplies were allowed to be transported within Union held territory in Tennessee and he alluded to the fact a wife of a Confederate general was allowed to transport supplies with the approval of the Union Army. Hawley also recorded the stillness of the evening which was punctuated with artillery fire, ever reminding the good doctor the war was present.

Camp 11th Mo. Infty. Vet. Vol.
On Hernando Road 2 Miles south
East of Memphis, Tenn. May 6th 1864
Dearest Parents,

I have just set up my field desk under the friendly foliage of a wide spread. Let's see what it is. Give it up, can't tell (after deliberating two minutes, eating a handful of these nice hazel nuts). Think it is a species of elm. We are in a very pleasant place, shade trees all around and we do so much enjoy them now.

We embarked on the steamer Miami, *a small craft Monday night with orders to report to the commander of the 17th Army Corps at Cairo, Ill. We arrived there about noon next day, removed to the fine new steamer,* W. R. Arthur, *with orders to report to Memphis, left next day, had a pleasant trip arrived the day after, yesterday about 11 o'clock immediately started for here. As yet have no tents but hope to get them this afternoon. We slept out last night. I lay awake sometime gazing at the beautiful firmament, the starry decked heavens but my thoughts were with the dear ones at home with whom I have just spent the most pleasant, the happiest month of my life. So blissfully happy but so exceedingly short. Then I thought of our divine protector, our heavenly father and I asked his blessing upon each one of the family. There has not been an hour in the day or days since I left, unless I was closely engaged, but that I thought of you. I have learned to enjoy to appreciate home more than ever before. My health is good for which I deserve to be thankful. This is the third letter I have written you since I left. I said in one I would send a R. R. ticket. I have since found it in my pocket book. I will sent it in this.*

But guess I will not mail this until tomorrow. I was over [to] the city today on business. Everyone hurrying, streets full of vehicles. The surgeon of 108 Ills. Infty. said one of his captains took up 50,000 dollars worth of permits on one road, the state line road. These permits are written permission for Mr. or Mrs. so & so to take through the lines, such an amount of sugar, sundries or dry goods. So you see, this is a fine Rebel Depot. A Rebel General's wife, Mrs. Tach, get passes through the lines for 30 days as often as she wants them and permission to purchase anything she wants in unlimited quantities. [S]he is quartermaster general of transportation. So she can nearly supply all the south. This corruption will almost be the ruin of our country.

Last night the Guerillas fired nearly all night on our pickets. So near we could see the flash of the guns. Once we got up and put on some of our clothes but soon layed down and slept well. We had for dinner, lettuce, eggs, butter, fresh meat, radishes, etc., onions. Some purchased at market. Trees nearly out in full foliage and some so at Cairo, plenty of fine flowers. Will try to send some. Mr. West & Lady and Krafft & Lady wish to be remembered to you ens all [you all]. So of Mr. Mrs. Miss Pruinss. By the way while I think of it, give my love and compliments to every body and some body in particular. The sun is going down and its rays lend too much heat & light to this page and me for comfort.

So adieu for a few hours.

Sunday 1 P.M. Just returned from the city and church had [with me] my old friend Dr. Grey whom I have written you about before, formerly of LaGrange, Tenn.

Thomas Hawley's letter of May 7, written on the riverboat *Sunny Smith*, related the expedition of the 11th Missouri Veteran Infantry, the Second Iowa Artillery, and a detachment of cavalry into Arkansas in search of Confederate troops. The expedition went as far as Madison, Arkansas, along the St. Francis River, but no enemy was found and the regiment returned to Memphis. While the 11th Missouri Veteran Infantry was marching in Arkansas, the non-veterans of the 11th Missouri Infantry were returning to Vicksburg after the disastrous Red River Campaign. Hawley speculated about where the regiment would be sent and he thought perhaps it would be sent to Grant in Virginia or Sherman in the Atlanta Campaign.

The health of the soldiers in the veteran regiment was concerning with as many as 10 percent to 15 percent of the men being sick. Major Eli Bowyer was reported to be in good health and Thomas Hawley wrote of his desire to be under the command of General Joseph Mower. Mower had attended Norwich University for two years beginning in 1843. He enlisted in the United States Army Engineers in 1847 and fought in the Mexican War until 1848. He was commissioned second lieutenant in the First United States Infantry in 1855 and served in the army in Texas until the beginning of the Civil War. Mower held the rank of captain at the beginning of the war and commanded artillery batteries in the siege of New Madrid, Missouri, until his promotion to the rank of major in the 11th Missouri Infantry in May 1862. Since joining the 11th Missouri he had successfully led the regiment in battles at Iuka, Corinth and Vicksburg and was rewarded with a promotion to the rank of brigadier general and divisional command. He was greatly respected by the regiment and the army.

Also included in the May 7 letter were allusions to conflict between Lieutenant Colonel William Barnum of the 11th Missouri Infantry and the officers of the regiment. The conflict with his commanding officer led Hawley to threaten to leave the regiment if he was not treated properly by Barnum. Regimental surgeon, Melancthon Fish, who had been absent, from the regiment since Thomas Hawley rejoined the 11th Missouri a year ago, was finally encountered by Hospital Steward Zeba French in Memphis. French related Doctor Fish expressed his sympathies for Hawley shouldering the entire responsibility for the medical care of the regiment but "not enough to join the regiment." Nevertheless, Thomas Hawley was happy with his duties.

On Steamer <u>Sunny Smith</u>
Below Memphis, Tenn.
May 7th 1864

Dear Parents,

We are now returning from a fruitless search for Rebels in Ark. We left Memphis 4 days ago on this ship with a section of the 2nd Iowa Batt., 13 cav. men and 250 of the 11th Mo. I. V. V. The rest not being supplied with guns. Genl. Washburn said we would perhaps be fired on several times by guerillas and that we should go to Madison in St. Francis County on the St. Francis River and then Col. Coon with 300 or 400 cavl. to be ferried over the river and scout between the two rivers, St. Francis & White. We went to Madison, but [no] molestation found, the place all quiet, remained all night then the cav. came across 40 miles west from Memphis. Set them across the river the next morning. After a short scout, they returned, reported no enemy near. Put them back and left again for Memphis not having seen any Rebels on the entire scout and have had so far a rather pleasant trip. The St. F. River is a small, torturous, deep stream up as far as we went. Low banks, rich soil on either side, not many farms but a quiet, a pleasant stream to navigate.

My health has improved since I left a few days ago. I now wish they would send us to St. Paul on another voyage of discovery for our health. They may send us to Genl. Grant or Sherman any day but all that is uncertain. Our command is at Vicksburg or was a few days ago. I guess we will come together soon—they to us and we to them. Several steamers have been fired into recently but so far as I have heard, fortunately not many injured. We have quite a number of sick or had 30 or 40 but none dangerously.

Dr. French was left at Memphis, in charge of sick in camp as we expected to be gone 8 or 10 days. I asked him to send word of his whereabouts.

I hope you all got to see that pride of the south, the Magnolia, but I guess if not spoiled, it must have been very much bruised. I wish you could see them as we have them here in all their pure white beauty and rich fragrance.

The weather has been rather pleasant because of fine rains in the last 4 in 6 days. Before it was rather dusty and warm, a good refreshing shower in this climate makes a vast difference in the temperature for at least 10 days. The evaporation is so great it cools the whole atmosphere.

Major Bowyer is well as usual and doing well and we all want to see Genl. Mower take command of our divis. or brigade. He has some accounts to settle with our present commanding officer. You know his name, which may settle a rather unpleasant relation. He is becoming exceedingly offensive to officers and some men. The regiment is badly cared for, poorly disciplined, do almost as they please. If the Lt. Col. does not treat me courteously about the time that all men & officers are to be mustered out next August, I am under no positive obligations to remain. You cannot guess what an unpleasant man he is when he happens to be out of humor. I may look around and do better or wait a short time but would rather continue in active service at least another year if necessary. But all this, I will mature as new rotation or movements are developed and trust in providence for the best. We will arrive at Memphis about 10 o'clock tonight if all goes well and I will finish the next page there and mail as soon as possible. The boat has proved rather a rough place to write upon, although I am writing upon the clerk's desk and upon his paper. We were ordered to take nothing with us on this last trip. Indeed it was not necessary but boarding at 50 cts. per meal is rather expensive, so the druggist and [I] bought a box of bread & meat but this soon gave out. So I eat breakfast and dinner at table and crackers & cheese in my state room for supper. So I came off with something left and feel all right. More soon.

May 8th Pleasant morning. Some rain last night. We arrived at Memphis last night about 12. Early this morning, started for our old camp, found all well, i.e., old friends, not many sick in hospital and just in time for breakfast. This afternoon I propose to send you this scroll. Dr. Fish is in the city, says he feels sorry for me but not enough to join the regt., said so to Dr. French. Thinks Dr. F., will soon be assigned a place.

Just heard that Genl. Mower was to be here every day. I am quite well and in good spirits. Much love to all the dear ones at home. I would give so much to see your smiling faces this pleasant fine morning.

That leave of absence was so exceedingly short and it just gave me a fond taste of the sweets of home, dear home. It takes a strong sense of duty to keep me in the army at all. I am a home chap all over. Love to all dear sisters, brother and parents and may the good Lord prosper and keep you in perfect health and happiness and may we soon be an unbroken family here below to be finally, after

lives of usefulness, encircled around the family altar above, not one missing. The sincere prayer of your most affectionate son & brother
Thos. S. Hawley

On May 13, Thomas Hawley wrote his next letter to his younger sister, Fannie Hawley, who was a teacher in Olney, Illinois. Most of this letter contained familial references, but Thomas Hawley gave an excellent description of Memphis in the spring in regard to architecture and vegetation. In regard to the war, he reported there were rumors the regiment would return to the Red River region of Louisiana to correct the losses which occurred during the recent campaign. He also stated there was a high likelihood the regiment would stay in Memphis throughout the summer, but he preferred Alabama or Georgia to his location at Memphis.

HdQtrs. Med. Dept 11th Mo. I .V.
Memphis, Tenn. May 13, 64
Dearest Sister Fannie,

Last evening I was so disappointed at the non-reception of a white winged messenger from some of the dear ones at home that I opened my valise to read some old letters and what should I find but two very interesting letters from my dear little sister whose kiss I would go a long ways for now if I dared. One was written while you was in the office dealing out letters every few moments (and pardon me for saying it) in my opinion is the most interesting of all. Well written in a fine lady's hand and well worded. I read it and one or two others. I concluded to answer immediately if I had not done so ably when on that ever to be remembered leave of absence. Oh what a good time. Now sister, I hope the instrument came to hand in good order and will please you. I have just now forgotten whether I wrote you when in St. Louis or not. If not, it was from the want of time. I rushed frantically over to the duch [Dutch] City of Belleville, did not see many friends. I hope you can readily learn to perform on the guitar but do not devote time to that which should be given to other studies, to perform well on any instrument is a fine accomplishment but my dear, by no means, the only prerequisite to a good English education. Besides many things must be learned which your teachers cannot well give you direct lessons in, but are limited to advice and wise counsel, perseverance, close application, patience, will do wonders.

Soon you can astonish your best friends by the rich stories of a well-trained mind. Treasures worth more to your real happiness in this world than all the gold of California. Please improve every precious moment for the next few years; but why do I always urge you to close study when I have every evidence to think [it] improves the time well? Because I love you so dearly and am exceedingly anxious for your future welfare.

Four. 1864 179

I wish you could visit this city and the suburbs this pleasant May afternoon. There is some palaces almost, finer residences all around the city for 2 or 3 three miles out from the business part. Almost every acre is taken up in arraigning beautiful parks and yards for dwellings. Houses mostly of the gothic or cottage style some with statuary fountains and endless variety of evergreens, magnolias, live oaks, American hollies, cedar, cypress, arbor vitae, etc. When you become interested in botany and want several varieties of plants for your herbarium, I'll try and send you some from the sunny south. When my old friends meet me now, they say I look well. My health must be good.

There is a rumor that we may visit the miasmatic region of the Red River. I hope not and think not. Our destiny to us is at present unknown. I have written Sis, Ma & Pa twice I think up [to] today, no letter from home but I look almost every hour.

It is rumored our regt. may stay here as Provost Guard. If so, we may stay all summer but I'd rather be in Georgia or Ala. for health. Dr. French is better today, and wants to be remembered kindly to all. Please give my compliments to your teacher, Miss J., then kiss her for me. But mind you must not say so, Sis. 40 kisses for Evie Bell Hawley, Ma, Pa & sisters. 14 to Bub for me and 26 for yourself. A river, yes an ocean, of love to all. Write soon, give all the news. I am and ever shall be your affct.,
Brother Thomas S. Hawley

The cacophony of camp life greeted Thomas Hawley on May 15 in Memphis as he read his newspaper and prepared for sick call. He tended to 25 sick soldiers and then went to church where the sermon was delivered by a Southern preacher. Hawley related the positive news from the war in Virginia as Grant had recently fought the Battle of the Wilderness to a tactical draw and was involved in the Battle of Spotsylvania. The speculation about further action on the Red River continued but all was quiet on that front. He also mentioned the health of Eli Bowyer and Zeba French, and he prescribed for Captain William Notestine, a railroader from Olney, Illinois. He was one of the original members of the 11th Missouri and had worked his way up through the ranks through the merit of his performance. Notestine was well liked in the regiment and was a personal friend of Doctor Thomas Hawley. Finally, he mentioned the desire for peace in his letter and he hoped the "angel of peace speedily conquers by the sword of never ending peace."

Memphis Sunday Morning Bright
and early May the 15, 1864
Most Esteemed and Loved Parents, brother and three dear little sisters,
   Seated at the old field desk, face turned toward the sun rising, birds and

drums, singing, men talking, news boys crying their papers, latest news from Virginia this morning, Bulletin, then goes a bugle talking to the artillery, cuss the wad, then I hear our drums give a few warning notes for the sick call. Yes, that's it. Come & get your pills. Come & get your pills. I can't give the notes or I would. It also says to me repair immediately to the hospital tent and dispense the balms of Gilead. I have the call now, sounded at 6½ o'clock, breakfast at 6 o['clock] about 25 sick to attend to.

    2 olc P.M. Said sick attended to, went to church, heard a young Southern, Mitchell by name, do not know where he is from or of what denomination. I had hope to hear my friend Dr. Grey but he had gone to LaGrange. The weather is fine and health good. I am better than I was most of the time at home. But I do assure you my enjoyment is nothing in comparison to what it was at the dear old home of my youth. I have not heard direct from home since I left it now three weeks and I was just thinking it had been four. There is no news here of importance. No enemy near. All good news comes from Gen. Grant. None from Red River. We have not yet been assigned permanently to any brigade or division. The impression is prevalent that we will wait for our old command now up Red River and we cannot get much news from them as they are almost cut off from us. Major Bowyer is well as usual today, had some symptoms of chill. Dr. French was quite unwell but is much better. Well but rather weak. Capt. Notestine asked for some prophylactic for chills. His father is here, been down over a week & did not know his sons were here. Dr. Fish is at Cairo, will forward my interest, I suppose after August, by not re-mustering.

    We of the army received the glorious news from Virginia with the greatest enthusiasm. It talks of grand & sweet things. A peace, yes a permanent peace, one founded on eternal truth. A union indeed of states, of objects, and of principles, the dulcet sounds, and rumors of home, dear home, and its dearer ones, an unalloyed unity of happiness, a union of hands, of hearts and of war broken families. May the good angel of peace speedily conquer by the sword never ending peace to the continent of North America, at least. But my dear friends, a letter I am looking for from day-to-day and still I keep sending. I said I would write to each member of the family unless I soon received a letter. I mailed one for sister Fannie Friday. I guess have sent 4 others, I think, since I left home; and I have no helper in the medical department either. But I know you are each very busy and have written several times ere this. I hope you each continue to enjoy excellent health. It is our greatest blessing. I try to thank the giver of every good & perfect gift for this daily blessing, and ask his Christest blessing to each of you.

    I will try to write brother or sister M. this week. I hear a boat, hope it is the bearer of pleasant news to me and all my cousins, Uncle Samuel's boys. Wm. Friese and all his family ordered down the river to Island 63. Genl. Osbourne has stopped the trade to some extent at this post. Washburn, I mean.

Much love to all. I may add more if have time. Write soon to this [address]. You affct. son

Thomas

On May 28, Thomas Hawley wrote his Sunday letter from Memphis, Tennessee, and although he was unaware his garrison duty was about to come to an end as his regiment would be called to enter the war continuously over the next seven months. He began his letter with references to the Great Mississippi Fair which was presumably the Mississippi Valley Sanitary Fair. This was an event sponsored by the U. S. Sanitary Commission to replenish their coffers which had been depleted during the struggles and combat of 1863. The fair opened on May 17 in St. Louis. When the fair started, there was $2,500 in financial reserves of the Sanitary Commission, but the event successfully raised $554,000 for use to aid the soldiers fighting the war.[2]

The Union forces in Memphis numbered about 20,000 under the command of Major General Andrew Jackson (A. J.) Smith, the irascible, but highly effective, general whose nickname later came to be known as "Whiskey" Smith. Despite the nickname, it would be difficult to find a more dedicated and effective general in the Union Army than A. J. Smith. Prophetically, Thomas Hawley wrote General Nathan B. Forrest was causing problems with Sherman's supply and communication routes.

Doctor Melancthon Fish was present with the regiment for the first time in a year and he revealed he had decided not to re-enlist. Hawley also recorded Doctor Zeba French had passed the examining board and was ready to find a position as assistant surgeon; and he also mentioned Charles Sheppard, his clerk. Charles Sheppard remained with Hawley until the fall when he was transferred to the United States Naval Academy in Annapolis.

Memphis, Tenn.
May 28th 64

Dear Parents,

I received quite a good, long letter a few days ago written on the 23 inst. This informed me of your good health and the prosperity of the school which I am truly glad to hear of. The letter was written by Pa & Sister Fannie, many thanks for it. Pa, I suppose some of you ens will visit the Great Mississippi Fair. If you cannot leave school that long after it is out and we remain at this point, pay the Gallant 11th Mo. I. V. V. a visit. They all, or most of them, remember your former visit. But since that time we have lost many good and true hearted fellows. At present, one would not know the regt. by her officers, only 2 or 3 with us now that came in as true officers. Some discharged, some resigned, others killed in battle. I hardly know what we will do, have only 400 men. They may consolidate with some other regt. and muster out half the officers of each. Col. Barnum told me all persons belonging to the old organization not having reenlisted would be mustered out of the service by next August, i. e., if they did not desire to continue longer. I rather think if I cannot be mustered as surgeon at that time, will seek some other place for practicing. Dr. Fish will not be re-mustered so I hear, and will aid me all he can to get the promotion as surgeon. During the last week [I] was not so well as before, owing to the change from a northern climate to a southern. Had no chill, but symptoms, am now better, sickness rather on the increase.

There is rumor that Genl. Smith's command will be ordered to join Genl. Grant instead of Sherman. There is nearly 20,000 troops at this post. I cannot see what they are keeping them for when Genl. Forrest, that Blackest of Rebs, is menacing Genl. Sherman's communications in east Tennessee, but the news is indeed most glorious from both our commanders. What do our Republican friends think of Maj. Gen. Dick Oglesby for governor of Ills.? I think he will do but Hansie will make a poor auditor. The Union majority should run up to 20,000 this fall for the glorious state of Illinois. All quiet at this post, no long trains of goods and cotton going and coming all day as it was two weeks ago. Genl. Washburn is well liked by most of the Army. I guess [he] is trying to do the fair thing by his government and the Union men and is hard on Mr. Rebs.

Dr. French is well and thinks some of getting a position as asst. surg. in some colored regt. and I think will as he has passed the examining board and has been recommended to Adjt. Thomas. I shall miss him very much as we have been together so long. Chas. Sheppard is with me as clerk from Lawrenceville. Step son of Maj. Grass. A very good boy.

If you need any funds, use mine there and you can make some arraignment during vacation. What does Amos contemplate doing? I hope he can find some good place soon. Please write soon and often. Maj. B. is well. Much love to each one and all. We are in good circumstances here. Weather rather pleasant.

Your affct. Son,

Thomas

On June 2, 1864, Thomas Hawley wrote a letter to his sister, Fannie, from Memphis, Tennessee. It was clear from the letter Thomas Hawley and Miss Carrie Joy were a topic of communication within the family. The exact nature of their relationship was not known from his letters, but the pair was close. From a historical point of view, the culmination of the relationship was unknown to Miss Carrie Joy and Thomas, but these two young people would be married in less than a year of this letter. Also, at the time of this letter the non-veteran 11th Missouri Infantry was serving with the 33rd Missouri Infantry and was preparing to engage in a particularly bloody fight near Lake

Village, Arkansas, in an attempt to stop the Confederates from vexing Union and civilian river traffic on the Mississippi River. The 11th Missouri Veteran Volunteer Infantry moved from Memphis into the Tennessee countryside and the regiment camped on the land of Judge James. The regiment was ordered to move off the land when the judge complained about the Union soldiers taking up residence on his property. Immediately after this complaint, Thomas Hawley was ordered to move his hospital back onto the James' property. Hawley was irritated at this because he felt Colonel Barnum did not initially select the proper site. Finally, there was some matchmaking occurring as Thomas Hawley wrote of Fannie Hawley's romantic interest in Doctor Zeba French.

Tent under the poplar
tree near Judge James
Not far from Memphis, Tenn.
June 2, 1864

Dearest Darling Sister,

According to [my] promise, but I guess you think rather dandily, I presume to address a few sentimental lines. Not that I love you less but that I love you more. Your good, kind, loving letters always give me, your elder brother, much comfort and pleasure. If I only knew how to add one moment of pleasure to your life, one more spark of happiness, I would take pleasure in doing it. It gives me much pleasure to see the energy and perseverance in which you, as it were, commence upon the duties of life rather independently but steadfastly.

Sister, I need not tell you who is the most frequent subject of my thoughts. You know and do not feel jealous either. You are indeed a good, good sister. Oh! I always knew that.

But now my pet, please retain perfect possession of that priceless treasure, your heart, until you know it is in safe keeping. For I think to be disappointed would kill one outright or kill at least all that makes this life desirable. This is a strange feeling that takes possession of one's whole soul—body and mind, yet I do assure you it is not unpleasant. I have been complaining a little this week but feel better today. Yesterday and last night had a refreshing rain. All nature animate & inanimate praise the giver of all good and perfect gifts this pleasant morn. The dust has been intolerable for 8 or 10 days but thanks to the little June rain, more dust has been put under our feet entirely subjugated for a few days at least. Yesterday we removed from the Hernando Road to the Pigeon Roost Road into Judge James' lot, moved in today. Maj. Genl. Washburn says leave that lot immediately because the family complained and 400 men to be comfortable would disturb a cow, a mule and old man and lady, but not materially injure their property. But Mr. Soldier boy, you must not rest your weary bones under the shade of my fine & big tree. Begone you Dog!

Well, just here the adjt. gave me the orders from the col. saying you will move the hospital this evening over near the Judge James' house. So Dr. French has just gone with ten men to pull up stakes, etc., and move just as we are nicely fixed up. All because the col. did not select camp in the right place at first. More rain. Not a good time to move the sick.

Yes, here it comes, harder & harder. Now it pours down through the big poplar tree paptering patterns on my canvas roof but cannot quite get through. Oh! I must tell you, but I spick [expect] you know. This big brother of yours was made the happy recipient of the prettiest little heart-keeper, the cherriest lips and most kissable cheeks, you or any other one ever saw. Well Sis, I gave your Darling Dock the best compliments and—all of which was duly received and freely appreciated and lots returned. Tis all O. K. So they say.

About the answer you give folks when asked if Miss Carrie will return to Olney. My Dear Sis that's right. I think only the truth. You folks are sharp to cheat the people of Olney. I am glad of it. Dr. French I am sure, or pretty sure, not engaged to anyone. I do not care if you like him. He is a dear, good fellow. Did I ask you to do too much in dismissing Harry? I feared I did. If your health is good and you preferred it, why teach during the collegiate vacation if you can get a good school? I am looking for your dear adjt. but I guess he will not come now for some days. They have gone up White River. Most of the troops left Memphis yesterday for Mississippi or some other part. I guess we will stay some time. Kiss my Dear Carrie often for me & give muchest love. Love to our dear parents, bro. and Fannie & E. Bell. Also love to Dora. Tell him remember these speeches. Please write soon to your dear brother,

Thomas

Good lines

The following letter was written but the date is unknown. It was written prior to July 1, because Thomas Hawley wrote of the anticipation of Mark Sappington's promotion which was acknowledged in the letter written on July 1. This letter began with Hawley extolling the joys of church and description of his walk to church. Although the roads were dusty, the vegetation was beautiful. The efforts of the Union armies to the east were explained. Also, Hawley was considering his future home in East St. Louis if the war ever ended, and he encouraged his father to look for a suitable location to build a house.

Subject—19 Psalm part of the 12. V.

Self knowledge an excellent sermon. The major thought the best he had heard for months. I excepted several I had heard in that time.

I do enjoy preaching so much. Yes, I do love and enjoy the privileges of the sanctuary. I think I can say truthfully more since my visit home than ever before. Indeed think I am a better man, know I have more to live for. Your loving kindness toward me is too much. Oh, how ungrateful I would be not to follow so far as in me lives your good counseling and righteous example. Almost every member of the family said they did and would pray for me and others will do the same. This is indeed cheering to us, to me. I know I must pray for myself. I do and try to pray for you each one.

We walked two miles to church and back. The roads quite dusty, the sun boiling hot. The dense shade occasionally, truly refreshing, fine flowers in abundance. Dr. French and I propose to send some to Olney, hoping they may retain a portion of their original freshness and sweetness.

Lieut. Mark Sappington today looks rather well and is expecting a commission as Captain Quartermaster, rather a nice position, recommended by the President and confirmed by the senate. There is no news of importance except that we hear from Northern papers. We all wish and pray that the Army in Virginia may be abundantly successful, also so of Genl. Sherman's Grand Army but think it will not need the prayers so much as the first. I had no time to see about money while in St. Louis. Pa, do as you think best with it, but if you attend the fair in St. Louis and wish, I would like for you to look around and if you find some good property lots or lot near the city of East St. Louis worth 500 or $1,000, and can get them on time, go on and make the purchase. I think there is no danger and property must come up in that neighborhood I think, but if you have time please look around and let me know if you can. I fear though, it is asking too much. Or a good bargain in Olney make a strike, but I will not practice there I think.

Dr. French is quite unwell again today from chills and medicine he took but think he will be up tomorrow. Not much sickness in the regiment. Please get Mr. Wilson to take another doz. pictures for me and I want Ma and Pa to get some taken. Please pay for all out of my funds. I do hope Brother Amos is getting along well as to health and business. I think he can get a good place soon in Olney by trying. Let us all hope for the best and persevere. Bro. Amos, I will write you this week if I have time.

One and all, please write to me as soon as convenient. Evie Bell, I love you. Oh! so much. So I send a kiss. Fannie, I hope you will like your instrument. Mr. Peters said it was among the best they had. I feel confident you will learn soon and rapidly. Sister Myra if you love me, say so. I know you do. I love you more'n ever.

But it is no use for me to try to tell half my dearest love for you all.

You can direct to our regiment at Memphis for the present.

Everlasting love to each and all

from Thomas

Like the previous letter, the following letter was written without a date. It was a letter written to Thomas Hawley's youngest sister and contains information of a familial nature. Thomas referred to his youngest sister's dog, Fido, and offered his best to his cousin Theodore.

[Unknown date]
So my Canvas House under
the shade of a fine forest
trees, I write you my
Dear Little Sister Evie Bell,

I would love to steal a kiss but then I did steal lots when at home. Didn't we have a good time. Oh golly. I was so glad to hear you read and it was done so well and quite a hard lesson too. I saw plenty of little boys & girls at the picki nick or picnic a few days ago. It was warm & nice, soft, grass to romp on plenty of nice sweet flowers. All enjoyed themselves very much. I thought of Evie Bell, my dear little pet, and her pet, Fido. I'd like to shake his friendly paw this afternoon. I know he'd jump and skip to see his "Brother Tommy," ask him now, wouldn't you Fido? I found Dan and Miney all right in St. Louis. Give Dora my love. He is studying hard I expect by this time as he used to. Tell him not to box Frank over the ears so much.

Are your little chicks all well? I fear their toes got cold during the snow storm. Why not make socks for them. Their feet look so red and cold. Tell Fannie I cannot send her any kisses just now. But you may kiss her four times for me, and Adda twice. Now study real hard if it is not too warm, then play for plenty of fun, then help Ma and sisters all you can and write to me just as soon as you have time and remember who loves you this world full. Your

Brother,
Tommy

On June 12, Thomas Hawley's weekly letter to his family revealed the first rumors of the Battle at Brice's Crossroad in which Major General Nathan Bedford Forrest defeated Brigadier General Samuel Sturgis. Hawley also noted the non-veterans of the 11th Missouri Infantry re-joined the regiment after their recent march as part of the 33rd Missouri Infantry on the disastrous Red River Expedition. Rumors circulated around the post that the regiment was to be part of a new expedition up the Red River.

Camp 11th Mo IVV
In Judge James' Park Memphis
Tennessee June 12, 1864
Dearest Parents
Another week has rolled round and today finds us in a very pleasant camp.

Indeed all officers in the regt say it's the most beautiful camping ground the old 11th ever occupied. The health is good, only 25 or 30 sick, 9 in hospital all able to sit up. But I regret to say the best interest of the service will not permit us to remain here long. We have recently received orders to be ready or at least, I got verbal orders from the medical director to be ready that the Army must again proceed up Red River that we would start in 8 or ten days but I guess from what I hear the expedition was to be sent after the Rebs who are trying to blocade the Mississippi and would not go far up any of the rivers. But quite recent rumors or disasters of our armies in this state at Ripley 50 miles east or south of this place, will send us in that direction. Rumor says 13 regts. of infty, 12 or 15 pieces of artillery, 200 wagons and numerous other munitions of war fell into the hands of the enemy. The men say all through mismanagement. Brig. Genl Sturgess was in command. We are ordered to be ready to march at a moment's warning and I guess it will be there instead of up or down the Miss. The non-veterans of our regt. joined us today. All say half the Red River disaster has not been told and cannot say enough against Banks, nor praise and extoll Genls. Mower & Smith high enough. The weather is quite cool, have had rain and rather warm, sultry weather for ten days, but since it has turned cool, it will not rain for 8 or 10 days. Dr. French and I called this evening to see Judge James, his lady and sister-in-law, had a pleasant chat which they enjoyed well enough to cordially invite us to come often, gave us each a fine magnolia and sent the maj. and I a bowl of fine ripe raspberries & cream. I tell you they were fine. I saw Jas. Krafft yesterday, looks well but tired just returned from the Red River expedition says all at home are well. I must call to see him this week, also the adjt. of the 49 Ills. near us. I saw Dr. Messer is unwell and in the Officer's Hospital, better now. Called to see Maj. Campbell at same place but he had left for Olney same day, case critical.

My health is good. Dr. F[rench] and Maj. B. well. Indeed all doing well. Maj. B and I heard Dr. Grey preach a good sermon today on Romans, Chap. 14 and 17. Last evening Bro. Allen of the Christian Comm. gave the boys a good talk, had prayers in our tent and remained all night with us, left this morning after breakfast for other fields of labor. There is a probability of our regt and the 7th Mo being consolidated, at the least Lt. Col. Barnum is working for it with all his might. They have near 200 men. Mr. Notestine called to see us today, is well. I am glad to hear often that you are all well and hope & pray it may continue. Much of the best, a strongest love to each one and all. 40 kisses to E. Bell. I'll send some to Fannie in letter and Sister Myra tell Bub to please answer my letter. Love to Dode and Misses Dode, etc. Fannie mucher love to dear parents from your affct. Son,

Thomas

From June 16 through June 27, the 11th Missouri Veteran Infantry was detailed to protect the work crews repairing the railroads between Memphis and LaGrange, Tennessee. Thomas Hawley accompanied the regiment and wrote a letter on June 19 to his mother. He began this letter lamenting the ravages of war as he ended his first three years of the conflict and although the Union had the upper hand, the war was far from over as Hawley would learn during the last six months of 1864. He wrote the veteran soldiers were improving daily, and Hawley commented on the value of the veterans and remarked on the uninitiated recruits.

The Battle of Brice's Crossroad was fought on June 10, 1864, which is also referred to the Battle at Guntown, the designation Thomas Hawley used in his letter. General William Sherman was concerned Confederate General Nathan Bedford Forrest would damage his communication and supply lines while he advanced on Atlanta. He sent Brigadier General Samuel Sturgis with over 8,000 Union troops to threaten northern Mississippi in hopes of pulling Forrest from Sherman's supply lines and this maneuver worked. The two forces battled on June 10 and resulted in a decisive Confederate victory as the Union lost 2600 men compared to less than 500 casualties for the Confederates. Thomas Hawley wrote in his letter the stragglers made it to the Union lines near Memphis having retreated over 80 miles from the battle. The condition of these stragglers was severe and Hawley recorded conversations he had with these men and described their condition in detail. Also, Thomas Hawley recorded the United States Colored Troops of Colonel Edward Bouton's Brigade provided actions which allowed most of Sturgis's force to evade capture. These soldiers fought bravely and about half of the Union soldiers listed as killed-in-action were from the 55th and 59th USCT. The defeat at Brice's Crossroads prepared the way for actions in July that would involve Thomas Hawley and his regiment.

Camp in the woods
on Memphis and Charleston RR each
of the former 30 miles Hd. Qutrs. Med.
Dept 11th Mo. I. V. V. June 19th 1864

A Bright Sunday Morning

I greet you, Dear Mother, with a kiss, in thought if not in deed, and in thought am often with you, my head on your lap resting. Oh so pleasantly, or as in informer days, seated on your lap having a nice chat but here I am in reality hundreds of miles away seated on the hospital knapsack with a prescription book for a desk and sick and wounded men around, bring[s] my thoughts to this horrid war with all its terrible results, blood, rapine, murder and carnage and every day scenes in this our once happy, peaceful, moral nation but where are we hastening to now with the speed of the wind? To utter destruction, morally, civilly and financially. Yet with the divine aid of an almighty army, good, great good, can be brought out of all this wickedness and I have faith to believe such will be the case but God will and does require all the profusely righteous people of the land to labor most arduously for this beneficent end. Will they, are they doing it? They are doing more than any other nation [has] ever done or conceived of before. Still they are not doing all they can do. However, they are doing more & more every day. Our old veteran soldiers are getting to be better men every day, more moral [than] the new recruits on the worst day. Here I was interrupted by a soldier that wanted a wound dressed.

I wrote you or Sister a few items in regard to this conflict between our forces under Genl. Sturgess and Confeds. under command of Forrest. F. attacked our men near Guntown, took them by surprise, demoralized them. Indeed many of them were panic-stricken, threw away their guns, cartridges, coats & shoes made straight coat tails for Memphis. Stragglers have been coming into our lines every day and night since. Some poor fellows literally walked their feet off or rather run them off. They run & walked and jumped logs & brush a distance of over 80 miles in 30 hours. Feet & legs swollen black as a hat, even sloughing, poor fellows. I have seen many poor Negroes. They escaped better than the white troops, understand slipping through the woods and keeping the right direction. All say they fought well. All say they didn't "treat" until the officers ordered them to, said they "loves to pop Mr. Secesh." One said they often heard the bloodhounds after them. They "coch" [caught] lots poor fellows. Could hear the secesh say, halt! Then shoot "specks." Many a one was killed in the thickets. Most of them had nothing to eat for five or 6 days, but all cheerful and gloriously glad to enter the Union lines, said they'd soon be ready for secesh again. I asked some if they had not rather be with their old masters instead of this hard fighting. Quickly they answered firmly. "No, sir. I had rather fight all my life than go back to him." Many of the officers say if it had not been for the Colored troops all the white soldiers [would] had been captured.

Men now repairing the road to LaGrange, have rebuilt 3 bridges and several more to finish a large one at Wolfe River. Then I understand Genl. A. J. Smith will make LaGrange a base for an expedition south. I cannot say when we will be ordered to operate. Some talk for our returning to Memphis soon. My health is very good for which I am thankful. Maj. B[lowyer], Dr. F[rench] and Capt. Notestine are well. Dr. Fish in Mo. with the sick. The weather is pleasant. All our tents, wagons, cots, etc., still in Memphis, ordered to take nothing with us, i. e., in the baggage line. Have some blackberries, fresh beef & new potatoes occasionally. Many thanks for numerous papers recently received from Division Post Office. Some had been on the Red River expedition. I brought several out here. The boys have no word or daily papers, and read these with avidity. Indeed they always do, at least, many of them. I suppose the school is broken up for the summer, hope you [are] all well, try to enjoy vacation and are, and will be, well. The Lord Blesses me even in camp sometimes in answer to your & my prayers.

Much love to each member of the family. All write often. Remember as ever your affct. son,

Thomas

I have no difficulty in reading your good letters when they come.

Two days later Thomas Hawley wrote a letter to a group of unknown recipients, but presumably this letter was written to his family as he signed the letter son and brother. He was still with the regiment assigned to protect the repair of the railroad forty miles east of Memphis. The soldiers of the regiment were repairing a bridge which had been destroyed by Confederate raiders. There is little news reported in this letter and Hawley wrote of the general good health of the soldiers and mentioned a few names specifically. He described his makeshift bed which included sleeping on fence rails covered with vegetation and a blanket.

Tuesday Morn. 40 miles
east of Memphis June 21, 1864

Dearest Friends,

Still all well, yesterday moved camp to another railroad bridge. We guard the hands while they repair the road. We only marched ten miles. We draw fresh potatoes by the tops and pork and fresh meat are detained by our unerring rifles.

This is nearly all the paper I have here and may [have] wrapped the scrap up in it yesterday by mistake. We will soon change [locations] again, are within 16 miles of LaGrange now. The weather is fine and climate salubrious. Our health good but few sick in camp. I hardly think we will be on the Mississippi River this summer which we all feared, you know. Will you visit our friends in Crawford this summer or in Mt. Carmel? Had better. It will do you good. Sister will have rather a hard time I fear teaching all summer. Hope she will be all right. The war news is good so far. Maj. B. is well. Dr. French still in Mo., is all OK. Lt. Sappington is with us & well. No baggage here yet. Valise & trunks & cots all in old camp at Memphis. Also tents. We have a tent fly. Sleep on fence rails, placed side by side, on cross pieces, fine brush & twigs thrown on next, then a thin layer of wheat straw, then a large oil cloth, a few blankets. My shawl and quilt for cover, coats & pants for pillows. This you see constitutes our luxurious couch on which I sleep soundly, last night with Maj. Bowyer. Well it's nearly train time, so I must close with much of the deepest love for each one and all. I remain as ever true friend.

You affct. son and brother

Affectly.,

T. S. Hawley

On June 26, Thomas Hawley began his letter from Memphis where he was obtaining supplies for the regiment, and he was ordered to join the regiment still on guard duty near Moscow, Tennessee. He concluded the letter with an entry on June 27 from LaGrange, Tennessee, as he moved to join the 11th Missouri Veteran Infantry and all speculation pointed to an expedition against the Confederates was soon to begin. Hawley wanted an opportunity to regain the pride of the Union Army against Confederate General Nathan B. Forrest after his recent decisive victory at Brice's Crossroads. The confidence in the division and corps commanders, General Joseph Mower and General A. J. Smith, was evident in the letter. These were good commanders capable to facing Forrest who had the reputation of never being defeated. Doctor Zeba French, Hospital Steward, was ordered to remain in camp to care for the wounded and the sick.

Thomas Hawley had just sent money home for the family and wrote communication would be difficult because he was planning to begin the march. He wrote he had returned to LaGrange and despite the regiment's absence from this location, the town was in good condition. He mentioned an acquaintance, Mr. Rosena, who was a Union supporter and the difficulty he had living in a pro–Southern community. Finally, the general health of the regiment was good, but the weather was hot. For soldiers marching in the Mississippi or Tennessee sun in woolen uniforms, it was a trying time.

Memphis, Tenn.
Hd Qts Convalescent Camp
11th Mo. I. V. June 26, 1864

Dearest Parents,

Today I am compelled to return to our regt. at Moscow, Tenn. and I guess by tomorrow will all move to LaGrange from there onward. Genl. Mower and A. J. Smiths's Division are on Wolf River near Moscow. There was a long bridge over it which the rebels under Genl. Forrest destroyed as they did almost every other on the road. I came in the city day before yesterday to procure supplies. Dr. French will remain here and attend sick in camp and hospital. All anticipate rather a hard march some distance south but cannot find out exactly where we will strike. Cannot tell how long we will be gone perhaps a month, maybe longer, though I think not. We will have quite a force and should we meet Forrest under the able generalship of Genl. Jos. A. Mower, will return our lost fortunes.

Please write as often as you can but should you not hear as often as usual, you will know what to attribute it to, for our transportation will be rather light and we may not be able to write or send them after written. I was paid yesterday and sent home per Adams Express one hundred and thirty dollars. Express fare paid $1.25. If you need any of it, send it up to any purpose you may see fit. I mean use it at your pleasure.

LaGrange, Tenn. June 27th. Just arrived at this post found all quiet. I was among the first of the infantry officers who came here though there had been cavalry here some time, 24 hours, and did not find many calv. secesh for their furloughs expired rather suddenly and they left for a more genial clime. All is quiet so far, nothing destroyed by the Rebs at this post although they set fire to the two bridges several times and the citizens put it out. Depot and other buildings all right, they rebuilt fences and have gone to cultivating vegetables, etc. from a necessity to live on because they could not purchase other necessaries of life. Mr. Rosena, a Union Dutchman, said he had seen many men working in their patches like slaves who never could work before. They said the Yankees would never come here again. So worked with the full confidence of raising a good crop. Thus have they been deluded to raise vegetables for Union soldiers. We would otherwise suffer from scarcity of such food this time of year but blackberries, plums or a species of plums, cherries and a few apples and ripe peaches will soon be in abundance and if we make a raid into Mississippi such things will be in abundance for the use of the entire army.

We moved into an old fort constructed in the middle of town last winter by our men and under the immediate supervision of Genl. Mower. This is still standing despite the ravages of Mr. Rebs and time's ruthless hand. Numerous vacant houses inhabited by spiders, rats and wild birds, mark the demon's war path. I told them said Mr. Rosena, "War was not child's play, your churches and colleges will be used as hospitals, houses ransacked and robbed and some burned, fences destroyed. You will want for the common necessities of life, for the comforts of home, you will suffer. The north, I tell you, will fight and you will finally be whipped. They told him he lied, was a d____ Lincolnite. They would hang him, etc." Most of the citizens will attest the truthfulness of these bold assertions by the staunch old Union Dutchman.

It is extremely hot, intensely hot, intolerably sunny is the continued sunny south. The general health of this command is good. The cars just came, this from east, the first day in 3 or 4 months. We join the brigade soon and I understand they are in the hot sun. The major is well. No further developments in regard to this movement. So far as I have heard, Maj. Thurston paymaster USA paid our regiment today. He came out with Col. B. & myself. I cannot say how long we *will remain at this post. Perhaps I cannot write for some time but be assured I will write at least once per week if possible. My health is good and I always improve on the march. I have not heard from home for over two weeks. I could not finish this in the city of Memphis. So finish it now & send immediately if possible. Give my compliments to Mr. Gunn & lady. Love and kisses to the girls, great & small. Much love to my dear ones at home. All of whom I love so dearly. Please write often. I have not heard of the Great Exhibition. Yours, in much love and haste, and always your dear affct. son & bro.,*

Thomas

On the verge of an expedition against Confederates in Mississippi, Thomas Hawley wrote his weekly letter and this week he was still at LaGrange, Tennessee. He began this letter with the fire of patriotism and love of family. He also mentioned Lieutenant John Cowperthwait had opened a variety store in Olney, Illinois, after resigning from the regiment. Lieutenant Cowperthwait was a native Missourian and he moved to Olney after leaving the 11th Missouri Infantry.

Thomas Hawley revealed in his letter the plan for the impending expedition into Mississippi. As Sherman continued his march through Georgia toward Atlanta in the summer of 1864, it was important for the Union Army that Major General Nathan Forrest be prevented from attacking their supply lines and from causing other damage for which he was particularly adept. Sherman wanted to keep Forrest busy in Mississippi to prevent his interference in the Union campaign in Georgia. Sherman sent a message to Major General George Thomas, commander of the Army of the Cumberland, on July 2 stating, "I see Forrest is at Tupelo; that the enemy has detected the fact that a heavy force, under A. J. Smith, is moving out of Memphis, as they suppose, to re-enforce us."[3] The expedition by General Andrew J. Smith was designed to draw the Confederate forces under Forrest into a conflict in the state of Mississippi and away from Sherman's rear in Georgia. Sherman had no other plan for Smith than to hold Forrest in place and perhaps to destroy his force. Smith's expedition would be the third attempt to control the Confederate cavalry that had been causing so much trouble. Brigadier General W. Sooy Smith was given this task during Sherman's Meridian Campaign early in 1864 and Smith was defeated at the Battle of Okolona, Mississippi, on February 22, 1864. The second attempt was made by Brigadier General Samuel Sturgis who was defeated at the Battle of Brice's Crossroads on June 10, 1864. A. J. Smith was a wily, experienced general with excellent, well-trained troops under his command and Smith was determined to show Forrest that he was indeed a different general than was Samuel Sturgis and Sooy Smith.

During this expedition, Sherman told Smith "to punish Forrest and the people now or risk compromising the effect of past victories."[4] Confederate General Joe Johnston needed Forrest out of Mississippi and he wanted Forrest to concentrate on Sherman's supplies and communications, but Confederate President Jefferson Davis decided to overrule Johnston and keep him in Mississippi. So, the stage was set as General Smith's divisions of the XVI Corp started their march toward Tupelo, Mississippi, and Major General Nathan Forrest and Lieutenant General Stephen Dill Lee were there waiting for him.

Thomas Hawley wrote of his future plans in the army as his term of service was set to expire within 30 days and he had concluded he would not re-enlist without being offered the position of regimental surgeon. Clearly, Hawley was already serving as the chief surgeon for the regiment and Doctor Melancthon Fish only occasionally was present with the regiment. It was noted in this letter Doctor Zeba French planned to resign at the end of his service in August 1864. Thomas Hawley also lamented the death of the regimental apothecary, William Lymans.

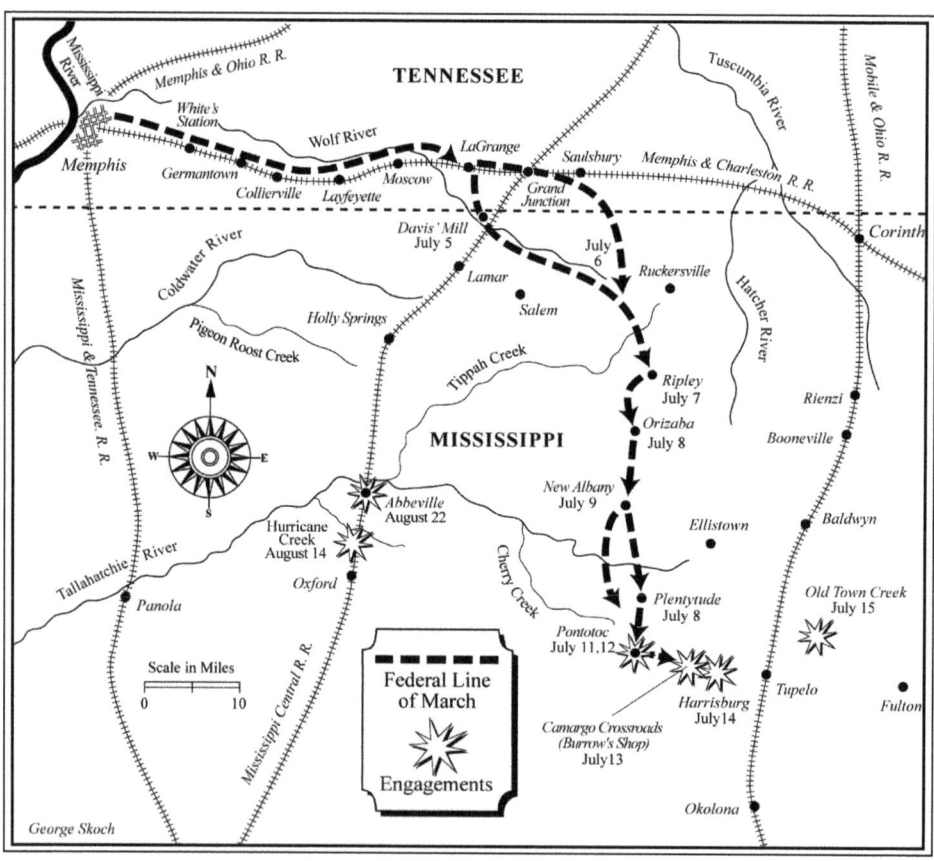

LaGrange, Tenn.
July 1st 1864

Dearest and Most Beloved Parents, Bro., and Sister,

A good letter from sister Myra came to hand yesterday bearing the date of June 22nd informing me of your good health and the anticipated enjoyment of the few weeks of vacation. I could not bring anything out here so I have forgotten to whom I am indebted for letters but as usual will write the weekly message to the dear readers seated around the family circle of which one chick is just now in the United States service and all others are as I am, strongly devoted to the best government. This gives me great pleasure not one drop of tainted, traitorous blood flows in our veins. All are boiling over with pure patriotism. Maj. B. received a [letter] from home June 27 saying all was well at home. She almost always speaks of the family. I am glad to have this source to hear from you as I am deprived from quite recently. I see by the <u>Olney Journal</u> Lt. Cowperthwait, formerly of our regiment, has established a variety store in Olney. He is a good, loyal, devoted soldier and kept on duty entirely to caring for the constitution. I fear he never will recover from the poisonous influences of this climate. If you can form his acquaintance and wife, such folks should be encouraged instead of Livingston, Bryres, etc.

Confidentially, for this is contraband news and straight from general headquarters, this command marches in a few days. Tomorrow, I guess for the south & south east perhaps for Columbus, Mississippi, and destroy the Ohio and Columbus Railroad at or near Tupelo. If successful will only be gone 4 or 5 weeks but during this time may be cut off from communication with our home friends and for a time with the United States of America. We hope to do some good at least in seeking the close of this wicked and unholy Rebellion. The Rebels are at the present running the Ohio & M[obile] RR up to Corinth, Miss. By this means, they defeated Genl. Sturgiss so readily, and by his intrigue and connivance in or with Genl. Forrest, a large amount of property was turned over to the Confederate forces.

Dr. French is well and doing the same. Capt. Notestine is well. We will march early, generally starting about 3 o'clock and continuing on the road until 8 or 9 o'clock P.M. The weather has been unusually warm and troops cannot march much or fast without losing more men from the effects of heat than from bullets of the enemy. The war news from this department is meager. A citizen came up a few days ago from Tuscaloosa, Ala. Says the citizens almost destitute. Adult white males all gone to the army. Females who a few years ago hardly knew how to prepare a meal, & tots are now working in the fields, sometimes with the darkies. The land looks destitute & forsaken. Lt. Mark. T. Sappington has been promoted to Capt. A. QM., i. e., Capt & Asst. Quartermaster U. S.

V., a fine berth and one that is eagerly sought for by most quartermasters. I do not know whether he will remain with this division or be ordered to some post at another station. He has numerous army friends but drinks too much sometimes.

Mr. Jno. Baird formerly Sergt. Co. E our regt. will go with him. Mr. B. said today he was going to Olney in a few days and would take messages for many & so I will send this if possible. There is a pleasant breeze here most of the time so the intense heat of the sun is partially neutralized. Quite a number of our old Spartan band will leave us in August next. Those not reenlisting will be mustered out. I have thought I would not remuster under Lt. Col. Wm. L. Barnum for any position except surgeon, neither will I. If I cannot get that immediately and without much trouble, there is a strong probability of my becoming a free American citizen. This must not be known about at present, should we change commanding officers. I will not stay, I mean say what I will do.

My health at present is good for this time of year. Indeed I guess better than it has been at this time of year for two years and if the weather is not too inclement I am always much better in the field on active marches than at stations or camps.

I heard Col. Black was wounded and Henry Mann killed. Is this true? How are all the friends in Crawford Co.? I have not heard for a long time. I hear Dode has started home. I will answer his letter then when I have time. I am pleased to hear Fannie speak so determined in regard to studying hard in order to obtain a good education. Sister Myra must not have too many irons in the fire at one time and become nervous and excitable. I hope, and know, you do enjoy pleasant seasons, may they ever continue and give more payment. I had thought if we remained in Memphis, it would be pleasant to receive a visit from some of the dear ones at home and perhaps pleasant to them.

You know I have spent some time of these three war years in this place and have a few pleasant acquaintances. Maj. Last of the 10 Mo. Calv. is sick and sent for me to treat him, wants me to come often at a pleasant family's. I almost even have a treat of tolerable music, good for us in camp at least. This is a pleasure. We may march to Holly Springs, then you know I will have the pleasure of seeing my southern Bell, Miss Annie, if she has not gone up or south to Ricon, Ga. We lost one of the best men in the Medical Department, the apothecary. I had him detailed last June at Young's Point, La. from Co. D, was a model young man. Never drank, seldom swore, always quiet and good. He lived in or near Louisville, Clay Co., was a staunch friend of mine, died at Overton Hospital, Memphis of inflammation of the bowels the first of the week. I should have recommended him as asst. hospital steward when Dr. French was promoted or mustered out as he will be I guess in August. What has Bro. A. done with the store and what is the business prospect in Olney?

Much love to all to each and every one. Thanks for the newspapers which *still come to hand often with a few short words saying all are well. Much love to dear little Bell, Sisters Fannie, Myra and her feller, please write often. I like the pieces selected for the program or exhibition. Most excellent. Compliments to all inquiring friends. Mrs. Bowyer spoke of Bro. Balhts death of lung fever. He was a good man and I hope is happy in Paradise. May we all be always ready, may the good Lord bless you, one and all, and ever keep you as under the hollow of his hand. Remember I shall ever try to pray for you.*

You affct. son & bro.,

Thos. S. Hawley

Thomas Hawley's next letter held a detailed account of the expedition of the XVI Army Corps under the command of Major General A. J. Smith to Tupelo, Mississippi, which took place from July 5 until July 21, 1864. The culmination of the expedition happened on July 14 and 15 when the Battle of Tupelo was fought which resulted in a Union victory over Lieutenant General Stephen Dill Lee and Major General Nathan Bedford Forrest. Not only was Forrest defeated which was a rare event, he was also wounded in the battle. The expedition was undertaken under extreme weather conditions and on July 2 the 11th Missouri's Sergeant Charles Treadway recorded that he anticipated no movement of the regiment until "the weather gets a little cooler. It is so hot here that it appears as though the earth will burn."[5]

As Smith moved toward Forrest and Lee, the XVI Corps reached Davis' Mill just inside the state of Mississippi on July 5, Ripley on July 7, New Albany on July 9 and was within five miles of Ponotoc on July 10 as the march continued in a general southward direction. As Smith's column moved southward skirmishing intensified as Forrest tried to lure the Union column toward Okolona where Forrest intended to fight him on his chosen terrain. Confederate generals Stephen Lee and Nathan Forrest decided a battle with Smith could be successful based on past victories over Sooy Smith and Samuel Sturgis, and so "decided to fight Smith where he showed an inclination to fight or attack at the first sign of retreat."[6] Doctor Thomas Hawley provided a gruesome description of the march through this part of Mississippi in his July 21 letter.

Lee and Forrest caught up to the Union march on Tupelo on July 13 and two skirmishes occurred from Pontotoc to Harrisburg, just west of Tupelo. The skirmishes were easily swept aside by the Union troops and the Union corps camped overnight at Harrisburg. The next morning the Confederate troops of Lee and Forrest attacked the Union soldiers who were behind light defenses and the Southern attacks were repulsed. The Confederates suffered losses of about 1300 killed, wounded and captured compared to less than 650 for the Union Army. On July 15, General Smith awoke to find his food spoiled and then fought his way through the Confederate lines to return to LaGrange.

Once the Confederates realized the Union forces were withdrawing they hurried to find a way to inflict what harm they could. Smith's corps found it necessary to fight their way out of the ring of Confederates and accomplished this before the concentration of Stephen D. Lee's troops arrived. Most of this action occurred near Old Town Creek where the Confederates attacked the rear of Smith's column. Mower's First Division skirmished with the dismounted Confederate cavalry as the Union began their march and as Mower's division crossed a creek bottom, the 11th Missouri came under artillery fire. The regiment recorded five casualties which occurred during the skirmish and artillery fire. Smith ordered reinforcements to meet this threat and the Confederates withdrew from the action. It was at this time that General Forrest was wounded in his right foot. This action ended the second day's fighting near Tupelo.

LaGrange, Tenn. July 21st
Back again to the United States
Dearest Parents, Brother and Sisters,

We arrived in this place safe and without the loss of a man this morning bright and early having started from Davis Mills six miles south east of here at 3 o'clock this morning. I suppose some of the papers have contained accounts of our march or battles and perhaps exaggerated rumors for I guess they got nothing but rumors, and that as always <u>reliable news</u>. I think I mailed you a letter the day the 11th left July 5. Since then have heard from no one of my friends either by letter or paper or indeed from any part of the U. S. except through the secesh Grape Vine Telegraph not the most authentic source you know. We marched about 8 or 12 miles per day up to July 13th when we arrived at Ponotoc, Miss., 20 miles from the Mobile and Ohio Rail Road about 80 miles without anything of special interest transpiring.

The first few days many cases of sunstroke. I only had one and three days after he was marching. Some taken sick, ride a day or two in the ambulance and go to marching getting stronger each day. The men would go many round-about ways to get a few green apples or peaches and numerous potato patches were dug early and speedily. All kinds of fruits the soldiers enjoy eating heartily, almost voraciously of them and strange as it may seem to you, I think it did them good, that is, with the exercise they had and the diet. They had been accustomed to salt meat and no green succulent vegetables. The system craves something of the kind and there is ever a feeling of hunger unless this demand of nature is at least partially supplied. Fresh meat we all had in abundance, lamb, veal, chicken, pork, beef old & young.

In short we march, Rebel property suffers and we passed over part of the same ground crossed as part of General Sturgis' forces. Could often see the wreck of a wagon, the skeleton of a mule or horse, a few muddy army blue rags. Looking closer in the bushes and gullies, we often saw bones of the human skeleton. A skull or other bones well distinguished. Some never buried at all, others in narrow, shallow pits that the hogs routed out and devoured the flesh. Then to hear the tales of many of the men who had run the gauntlet of death was truly distressing and exasperating. We could see houses burn without any compunction of conscience. Nearly all the household property was destroyed or captured. Gardens, orchards, fields near the road stripped. The harvesting done up in the shortest possible style and without any positive orders against it. After the first three days only ⅔ rations issued, for 6 days then ¼ and the last two days almost nothing but not many of the men really suffered from hunger—bread or as we call it, hardtack, was above par.

At Ponotoc we remained one day then marched for Tupelo, Miss. & RR. The rebels after us. They attacked us on the right flank and rear at [the] same time but did not drive us far. No, not [at] all, but got badly repulsed and severely punished. The attack on the flank of the moving column was directly on the rear of our regt. As it was turning an angle in the road the Rebel cavalry rushed up and fired most of the balls whistling over our heads killing a man just in front. I was riding with the major just behind the men and in front of ambulances. No one of our regt. hurt, in afternoon had another fight. Next day they attacked us in force but Genl. Smith & Mower had chosen a fine position and we thrashed them finely losing in all less than 300 and they nearly 1500. I had to work hard for a time but am all right. Just then the tent poles came down but no one hurt. So I am still all right, well and doing well, and oh so anxiously looking for letters from the dear ones at home for it seems almost an age since I heard from you. It is almost meal time. With a boundless ocean of love for each dear heart at home, I wait the coming of the mail for this regt. and I will know some kind loving message will be with it from home. Please all write soon. I will write tomorrow or next day and give some details. We go to Memphis soon. All our things are still there. Much love to all from your affectionate son,

Thomas

I write this hasty note on time after our arrival within the lines hoping it may arrive soon enough to relieve some of the anxiety I know you feel.

The 11th Missouri Infantry moved to Memphis in preparation of the non-veteran members of the regiment mustering out at the end of their term of service. A little surprisingly, Colonel William Barnum decided to resign along with several officers. Thomas Hawley mentioned Lieutenant George Pickrell, Lieutenant John Finley, Captain Menomen O'Donnell, Captain Jesse Lloyd, Lieutenant James Wilson and Captain Charles Osgood. These were men would had served through three long years of war. On a positive note

Major Eli Bowyer, Thomas Hawley's close friend, was given command of the regiment and a rank of lieutenant colonel. Thomas Hawley was being enticed to remain with the regiment and Doctor Melancthon Fish was again absent and reported to be in Georgia. Thomas Hawley could not be promoted to the rank of regimental surgeon as long as Fish held the position of surgeon. To keep Hawley connected with the regiment, he was offered a contract to perform medical services rather than a promotion. Thomas Hawley wrote if he accepted the contract he would stay no longer than the following spring, and this was disturbing to him because of his obligations at home. Doctor Zeba French resigned from the regiment but had taken a short term contract for a couple of months.

Thomas Hawley referred to a possible expedition to begin in 8 to 10 days. He was correct about the expedition, but the march started the next day lasted the entire month of August. This expedition included two skirmishes and the destination was Oxford, Mississippi.

Memphis, Tenn. July 31st 64
Dear Father,

Your welcome letter of the 25 inst. came to hand on the 27 inst. This is doing very well. Most of our mail comes to hand 8 or 10 days after leaving the north except the daily newspapers. They come here in about 2 and 3 days. The river is quite low and navigation is impeded by it. The health of this command is as usual, about 30, only 3 or 4 sick in hospital. We will lose some good men and officers on the 5th of August, about 100 men and 6 or 8 officers. Col. Barnum, Quartermaster Geo. Pickrell, Adjt. Finley, Capt. O'Donnell, Capt. Lloyd, Lt. Wilson, Lt. Blew, and Capt. Osgood talk of mustering out. The 7th Mo. I. are ordered to consolidate with this regt. They will bring in about 200 enlisted men and no officers. So we hear Maj. Bowyer will be thrown in command immediately and will I guess soon after be mustered out as major and recommended as Lt. Col. to which office the men and officers elected him last winter. He seems very desirous that I should remain with him, thinks my prospects fair for promotion, will do all in his power for me. Yet does not wish to exercise an undue influence. I have thought over the muster seriously, and prayerfully, and about come to the conclusion to muster out as asst. surgeon and wait a short time for the promotion if Dr. Fish is mustered out, if not, I cannot stay. The divis. surgeon is anxious for me to stay and offers me a contract with the 11th until the chances are developed. Dr. Fish has gone to Atlanta, Ga., cannot say how long he will stay, 3 or 4 weeks probably. The contract will not last longer than three months with the same pay, etc., as asst. surgeon. I need the advice of you & Ma. Wish I could see you and talk the matter all over but three months are not long and medical officers are scarce. Not enough to attend the sick hardly. In this divi-

sion of 16 or 18 regiments & 3 or 4 detachments, there is only one surg. to each regt., when the genl. allows, three to full and 2 to half regts. Dr. F[rench] will take a contract for two or three months, I guess. I want him with me. We all want him as asst. surg. if he can get a commission. The health of all is good. We will probably start another expedition soon since of our division has gone out on the railroad already. I hear they are building the road to Holly Springs, Miss., will make that a base to operate against Forrest and perhaps Columbus, Miss. I hear the expedition will start in 8 or 10 days. Our brigade perhaps sooner. Maj. B. wants to know how you'd like to spend a time with us if you do not teach this winter. It might agree with your health in the south if you have no definite plans for the time. But we must all be governed by circumstances.

I will let you know my plans soon. Soon as prospects are developed here. By the last of the week I shall know more. I have written you almost twice a week since our return, i.e., to some one of the family. I think you did well with the books & stationary, better than I first supposed. I hope you took enough to pay well for the trouble and anxiety. I am well rewarded if Bro. Amos gained a few extra dollars for the time lost. At the end of 2 or three months if I am not commissioned surgeon, will come home and providence willing, will not stay away longer than next spring. I am under obligations to one & all to return then. Indeed, only stay now from earnest solicitation & because surgeons are needed and our braves may need my aid. I hope all are entirely well by this time. Ma's kind letter came to hand today written 27 inst., good time, will answer it soon. Tell Sister Myra not to be too hasty and wait a time for my suckers. Much love to each & all.

Your affect. son,

Thomas

You did well with the lot purchase. I am glad [you] have settled the other business.

In August 1864, the 11th Missouri left La Grange, Tennessee, and marched to Oxford, Mississippi, in an attempt to prevent the concentration and attack of the Rebel cavalry under command of Major General Nathan Bedford Forrest. General A. J. Smith's XVI Corps moved from Memphis to LaGrange and marched toward Oxford, Mississippi. Thomas Hawley's letter of August 1 was his shortest letter of the war as he scribbled a few lines to tell his family he was ordered to begin the expedition against Forrest and the family was experienced enough to realize his communications would be restricted.

[August 1, 1864]

We are ordered to leave tomorrow Aug. 2. I guess to Holly Springs, same style as the last trip. I will try to write again or I may stay back a few days.

Thomas

The next letter was sent from Abbeyville, Mississippi, on August 15. The letter revealed Thomas Hawley did not depart with the regiment due to his expiration of service which occurred on August 6, 1864. The letter recorded Hawley's efforts to re-join his regiment and although the assistant surgeon did not carry a musket, the letter showed the dedication he had for the regiment. He realized the regiment was advancing against the enemy, but had no surgeon and he felt obligated to reach the men to provide the medical attention they needed. He traveled with Acting Quartermaster Lieutenant James Lott and reached the regiment to find the men in good condition with Eli Bowyer firmly in command.

On August 14 Colonel Lucius Hubbard's Second Brigade was involved in a skirmish at Abbeyville, Mississippi. Little is recorded about the skirmish at Hurricane Creek and the 11th Missouri regimental records chronicled, "Skirmishing with the enemy driving them across Hurricane Creek and then returned to camp."[7] Doctor Thomas Hawley recorded on August 14, 1864 the regiment "was marching towards Oxford after Mr. Rebels, found them in considerable force, drove them 7 miles after considerable artillery firing and heavy skirmishing.... No one hurt." The skirmish lasted from 45 minutes to two hours based on various accounts and the skirmish was fought through intermittent rainfall. During the skirmish, both sides shelled each other with artillery, and it wasn't until the Union cavalry flanked the Confederates that the skirmish came to an end.

While Smith's corps was seeking Confederate forces, they marched on Oxford, Mississippi, where the wrath of the Union Army was felt and many of the houses around the courthouse square were burned.

Thomas Hawley also wrote in this letter the final break with Colonel William Barnum. Barnum had struggled to gain the respect of the officers and men of the regiment and Hawley wrote, "The Colonel, we cannot always trust." This reference related to the conversations Hawley had with him regarding his position and possible resignation. Finally after successfully establishing the veteran regiment of the 11th Missouri Infantry, Colonel William Barnum mustered out at the end of his term of service.

Hd. Qtrs. Med. Dept. 11th Mo. I. V.
Near Abbeyville, Miss.
August 15th 1864
Dear Parents,

You will see by the address of this my whereabouts. I arrived here yesterday about 3 o'clock having left Memphis with the Act. Quartermaster Lieut. Lott on the 12th inst; but on account of heavy rains, the track was damaged, delaying our train several days. Ours running off in advance of us, another stopped by sand washed over the rails and the engine of our train thrown clear off the rails and track by heavy banks of sand washing down the sides of a deep cut concealing the iron rails. Fortunately no one was hurt and we had to go back to Holly Springs four miles and wait until [the] next day. The R. Q. M. and I went to my old boarding house where Van Dorn came to see me almost two years ago, Dr. Bonner's. The Dr. was apparently glad to see me. So we made it our home for the night, had a good domestic breakfast. The first I think since I left home. At nine started on another train for the river, called Tallahatchie. The present terminus of the railroad and four miles from our camp, an ambulance was in waiting for us. We found the regt. in tolerable good health. Maj. B. in command. He is suffering some earache but is better this afternoon. They had just returned from a trip to near Oxford after Mr. Rebels, found them in considerable force, drove them 7 miles after considerable artillery firing and heavy skirmishing.

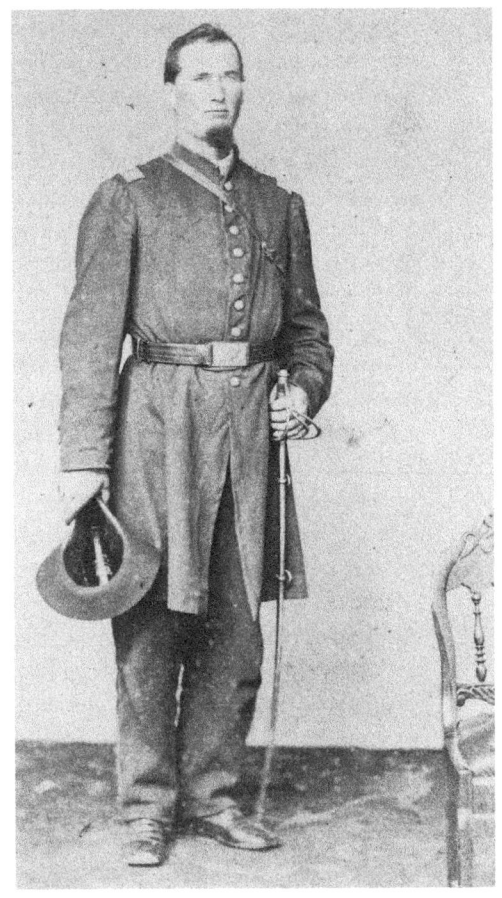

Colonel William Barnum (editor's collection).

Returned the same day after dark. No one hurt. Dr. French has, ere this will reach you and I doubt not, communicated all the news and perhaps my relation to the regiment.

I remained in Memphis from the 5th until the 12th inst. awaiting Genl. Washburn's decision in regard to the officers to be mustered out of the regt. The day before I left, his adjt. general informed Col. Barnum that he would issue an order or authorizing them to go home and await the final settlement of their accounts with the government when they would be formally mustered out of the United States service. The colonel, we cannot always trust but he said he would do all he could to have me mustered out as I wished it but he feared I could not get out as readily as medical officers are so scarce in this army. But they will not retain medical officers after their term of service against their will, at least, not after this campaign is over. I feared the regt. would get so far away that I could [not] join them, as they had no surgeon and my horse was with them and other property and the medical property had not been transferred to another medical officer. The regt. wanted me and might want me as surgeon, and officers said I could just as well be mustered out after this campaign was over and I had dear friends here. Also felt it my duty to remain with them until this affair was over. It may detain me from getting home so soon, and it may not, for I was not sure I could be mustered out. Besides Col. B. said he would send the order if received to me by special courier. I think for present indications we will [be] cut off from the railroad for a few days and advance into the interior of the state but I cannot think we will go far, for as yet, we have found no large force in front sufficient to cope with ours. We rather think it a ruse to keep some, at least, from reinforcing Mobile or the Atlanta army. And if Mobile is taken and Atlanta, this portion of the so-called southern Confederacy will be only a name for a thing, a monster that was but now extinct. I think the popular heart north has great reason to rejoice at the pleasant prospect of a speedy closing out of this rebellion. Called to see the 117th, saw Jas. Krafft, found all well and after a very pleasant chat, left. Also saw Adjt. Hay from Belleville doing well & Col. Moore.

 Morn. of the 16th. All well and doing well. Be not surprised if our lines of communication should be cut off and no letters come to hand for two or three weeks. I hope this will not be the case, but it may be. My health is good.

 Maj. is much better, indeed I may say well.

 Capt. Notestine is well. How is Br. Amos? I hope he will write soon. I have not heard for a long time. How is he doing?

 The weather is pleasant. Well, here is the sick and it is nearly mail time. So with much love to each one and all, and wishing you all health and happiness, I close this letter.

 Many kisses for the little ones.

Most affctly. your

obt. son & bro.,

Thos. S. Hawley

  Thomas Hawley's next letter was written after the second skirmish of the expedition to Oxford and this clash with the Confederate cavalry occurred at Hurricane Creek, Mississippi. As the brigade marched from Oxford on August 22, moving northward, the rear guard was attacked by Confederate cavalry. The attack was made by Brigadier General James Chalmers who intended to strike the rear of the Union column which he felt was vulnerable as it crossed a bridge over the Tallahatchie River. Unknown to Chalmers the bridge partially collapsed delaying a large portion of the Union force. The

Confederate cavalry charged into what they thought was a small group of soldiers but instead rode into a camp of infantry which quickly repulsed the attack. It was recorded the Confederate Cavalry lost ten troopers killed and nine wounded. The Federal loss was none killed and ten wounded. The Seventh Kansas Cavalry pursued the retreating enemy and during the chase lost one man who was killed. The 11th Missouri recorded one man wounded, Sergeant John M. Clements, who was severely wounded in his left arm with a musket ball.

Maybe one of the most ironic events of the Oxford expedition was while seeking to neutralize General Nathan Bedford Forrest, it was reported to General A. J. Smith Forrest had been spotted near Memphis, the original location of the Union force seeking him at Oxford. Thomas Hawley included an interesting conversation he had with some captured Confederate soldiers and he referred to them as "poor deluded fellows" because of their demand for their rights.

Thomas Hawley continued his letter with an addition written on August 27 and at that time he was located at Holly Springs, Mississippi. He reported the railroad was again destroyed in various locations, and also reported rumors the regiment would be moved to the Georgia campaign. He finally concluded his letter with a section written on August 30 from Memphis.

Hd. Qtr. Dept. 11th Mo. I. V.
Near Abbeyville, Miss. Aug 24th 64
Dear Father, Mother, Bro., and Sisters,

Once again I have this delightful privilege of writing to the dear friends at home which has been denied me for a week or two, but if this be pleasant, infinitely greater must be the pleasure of holding conversation, face-to-face when the time is unlimited and all can hold sweet communions by actions, words and thoughts. Not having heard from you for some time I am naturally growing exceedingly anxious and will look for letters the moment our lines are open which we expect will be in three or four days. You will hear the news of our armies and the movements of the enemy before this can reach you and much more definitely than I can give them. I think I wrote you as soon as I arrived at this camp which was the 14th inst. The day previous the brigade had quite a skirmish 7 miles south of here on Harry Carn [Hurricane] Creek driving the Rebs off. Luther Zimmerman of Co. H has not been heard from since. No one knows whether he was killed or not, has been captured several times before. His father lives on Jos. Rieley's old place. The present health of the regt. is quite good. Maj. Bowyer and Capt Notestine are well, also, your most obedient, for which I am thankful. We are within a few miles of the Tallahatchie River, between it and Abbeyville in the south. The weather has been pleasant for the last week.

On the 21st inst. started for Oxford, Miss. 12 miles south of this [place], march[ed] in without much opposition on the 22nd inst., found quite a fine little town once inhabited with 2000 souls, now by perhaps 1200 old men, women & children, had not felt the devastating effects of war much, although Genl. Grant once occupied the place. Soon after our arrival there, the comdg. General A. J. Smith received a dispatch to the effect that Genl. Forrest was or had been in Memphis and had done considerable damage, after mature consideration, they concluded to return to this camp and await results, as the object of our expedition would be accomplished as well in this way as any other, and there being no enemy in force in front. Besides our supplies were growing short by our long detention on acct. of rains. Yesterday about 12 [noon], arrived in camp, had not been here half an hour when the enemy came upon us evidently thinking we were still crossing the river. Our boys were soon in line and heavy skirmishing commenced, lasting all together half or ¾ of an hour when Mr. Rebs beat a hasty retreat, leaving about 12 killed and as many wounded in our hands. Also 8 or 10 prisoners, one Captain Turner of the 5th Miss. Our loss was 12 or 13 in all. The Rebs carried off more than they left. I hear they got one of our wagons and ambulances. I had a chat with the prisoners. Rather intelligent, healthy men and say they are most agreeably disappointed in regard to our treatment of prisoners of war but are determined in their resistance to the old government but wish the war closed but upon their own terms. They want their <u>RIGHTS</u> as usual and are conscripted for during [duration of] the war, health permitting, "poor deluded fellows."

I hear the army will remain here some time. The railroad again to be opened and supplies forwarded. The road was abandoned from Grand Junction to this point on the 18th inst., I think. I cannot say how soon it will be repaired nor how soon I can send this and those I look for in return will come. The officers with me asking to be mustered out have had their request granted but as yet we have no official return. So I do not know exactly my standing or relation to the army, will hear soon, I hope, and inform you. We do not know whether Forrest destroyed our camp and property in Memphis or not. I left my trunk at a private house, Judge James,' rather think they are all safe, shall hope so until I hear different. We all think and hope Forrest did not do much damage in Memphis. With your permission, or not, I must wait for news and particulars.

Holly Springs, Miss. Aug 27, 1864

All well. Arrived at this place yesterday without any trouble, middle of the day, very warm. All quiet and seem in no haste to leave. I think we will start for Memphis in a few days but know nothing positively of it. It is only 45 miles across the country in a direct road. The railroad has been destroyed between this point and Grand Junction. So our communications are not yet opened. We hope to send letters in a few days.

I am strongly thinking of home every day but am uncertain what was done with my van. Shall write you positively when we get to Memphis. I only write a few thoughts in this as time permits, desiring to send it by the first mail. I heard from one of Genl. Mower's staff that this army of Genl. Smith's was ordered by Genl. Sherman to Atlanta immediately. Can't say which way they'll go.

Memphis, Tenn. Tent neath the poplar tree Aug 30th 1864

Regt. arrived at this place 3 P.M. safe and sound. Health generally good. We started from Holly Springs last Sunday, marched 20 miles next day to LaGrange, Tenn., ordered to embark but by some delay, train did not start until today. Nothing transpired in this march worthy of note except that already written. There is a rumor that this army is to go to Genl. Sherman in Ga. soon. But I guess orders will not go. The hundred day troops will soon be mustered out, then they must keep some old troops here or Genl. Forrest will call in and hold permanent possession. He's done no damage worth mentioning while here [but] lost almost as many men as he took prisoner. Nothing burned and not much stolen. They only remained in town ¾ of an hour.

Sister Myra's letter of the 25 inst. I found here and a composed one from Pa, Ma & Fannie written before the 20th. Glad to hear all well, feared you would suffer from the prevailing epidemic. I would be pleased to hear from Bro. Amos directly and all about his business. Maj. Bowyer is well. Dr. Fish is here & wishes to be mustered out or so I hear. Maj. B[owyer] is now the cmdg. officer, is well liked by men & officers and Genl. Mower. We have a small but good regt. of men. We had plenty of vegetables to eat on the last expedition. Several houses destroyed by fire on the road [and] the court house in Holly Springs. My property here is all right. I hope we will be paid soon. Pa, I am much obliged to you for paying the order. Ma did that small sum come to hand? Oh, so much love to each, one and all, the dear old folks and the dear young folks. I'll try and answer your kind letters. Your affectionate son & bro.,

Thos. S. Hawley

There was little rest for the 11th Missouri Veteran infantry after their expedition to Oxford in August. The soldiers returned to Memphis on August 30 and remained in camp only three days and were soon marching into Arkansas on an expedition to neutralize the Confederate forces on the western side of the Mississippi River. Thomas Hawley's letter of September 5 provided an excellent description of the movements of the regiment as it began this march. He wrote about the concern of Arkansas troops concentrating with the intent of invading Missouri, and the objective of the expedition was to neutralize this threat. The expedition was under the command of newly promoted Major General Joseph Mower and Hawley recorded in addition to the infantry, Mower had 11 steamers and two gunboats as part of the expedition. Thomas Hawley described his assistant, Daniel Johnson, who had worked for the doctor for more than a year. Johnson was a freed slave who found a livelihood with the medical department of the 11th Missouri Infantry. The war continued in other theatres and the success of Sherman at the Battle of Jonesboro, Georgia, resulted in the fall of Atlanta on September 2.

Saint Charles, Ark.
80 Miles from Mouth of
White River Sept. 5, 1864
Dearest Parents,

Only remained in Memphis three days then our division, the first, was ordered to prepare for embarking on steamers, Sept 2nd. Camps and convalescents to stay back as usual, by great haste had time to get our clothes washed and some food prepared. We embarked on the little steamer Jas Watson *and left the city on 3rd inst. The second day was the hottest of the year and the troops had to lay almost all day on the levy [levee]. Several cases of sun stroke, had a pleasant but warm trip to this place. We may possibly stay here several days. Health of troops generally good. My health, I am thankful, is quite good, hope this will find all the dear ones at home quite well.*

I was so much hurried the short time we was in Memphis, have now forgotten whether I wrote you or not. Know I thought of it. Aug. 30 was the first chance I had had to write for 15 or 16 days and I feared your loving anxiety which I would not for the world unnecessarily increase for I bear you each and all too much love and may I ever prove myself worthy of it. Maj. Bowyer is well. This is a pleasant place and well-fortified, no town as I can see tonight. DeValls Bluff is 40 miles by land from here. This you know is on White River also as I think I wrote you. It was reported Marmaduke was trying to use this stream and invade Missouri. I guess the Illinois Copperheads had planned to support him in the event of a successful trip in the heart of that desolate state. Guess he is checked, even here. The new Maj. Genl., Jos. A. Mower, is a haste within himself and has command of this expedition with their flotilla of 11 steamers and two gunboats, quite a snug little army and under his guidance will do some work. I heard from you by letter when in Memphis as late as the 25 ultimo. Sis had just returned from the land of the Nelsonites in company with one of— (let's see) her friends and found all doing well. My dear father would perhaps go into the itinerancy again. Well, we must trust to the good Lord. It is all for the best and I know this is well counseled in all these doings. We hear one of the steamers will start out by daylight in the morning and [I] pen these few lines in haste by the dim light of a friendly lantern seated on the medicine case under a tent fly. My couch had been prepared by Daniel Johnson of African extraction—a good, pious, moral, faithful servant of whom you have heard me speak more than one year ago. And yet, he wishes to remain and I hope to take him home with me and perhaps sometime he can saddle my horse on dark nights when I have professional calls. Castles in the air you say. I hear Mr. & Mrs. Fish wiggle thin, filmy caudal appendages in the atmosphere of the Olney Male & Female College? Poor institution resuscitated only to be sunk deeper into oblivion. Good bye, my dear old Alma mater.

I confess I owe you ens lots of letters, shall pay up so, soon as lines are open to communication. Do not feel the least anxiety if you do not hear from me soon again. I write often when I can. Oh, so much love to each dear one of the home family circle of which I am an unworthy link. I remain as ever your affectionate son & bro,.

Thos. S. Hawley

On September 6, Thomas Hawley wrote a letter to his family from Brownsville, Arkansas as the expedition proceeded to DuValls Bluff, Arkansas. Prior to the Civil War, the town was simply a settlement located on the White River and its greatest asset was the store and boat landing. During the war, its importance was a result of its strategic location as a route to Little Rock, Pine Bluff and also Helena. It was also used as a port when the Arkansas River was too low to navigate. Because of these traits the Union Army fortified the town and stationed troops there to protect it from the Confederate Army in Arkansas.

Thomas Hawley's letter described the town as primarily a Union supply depot. The regiment marched eighteen miles in the hot Arkansas sun and the soldiers suffered the affects of the heat. He described the countryside and the lack of foraging opportunities. The political situation in the state was also commented upon in regard to the futile effort of trying to establish a Union government in this strong Southern-supporting state. Hawley wrote, "Genl. Price is somewhere in the state," and General Sterling Price was about to reveal his intent to the Union Army. Hawley also erroneously reported General A. J. Smith and the XVI Corps had moved to Georgia.

Hawley commented on his assistant Daniel Johnson and also his horse, Billey, and he described the clothes he had on the expedition, including, a "holey hat." He mentioned his staff of Edward King, Charles Sheppard, William Anderson, Daniel Johnson and a servant, Hesler. Regimental records contain information for Edward King, Charles Sheppard and William Anderson. Edward King, druggist, was a twenty-six-year-old, Connecticut native from Jacksonville, Illinois. William Anderson was a twenty-one-year-old cook from Palestine, Illinois, and Charles Sheppard was a twenty-one-year-old soldier from Lawrenceville, Illinois, who was soon to be transferred to the United States Naval Academy.

Thomas Hawley mentioned the political situation and his concern the nation would shift to a "peace-at-any-price" administration. Politically, 1864 had great significance because it was a presidential reelection year for Abraham Lincoln who was not optimistic about his chances to be reelected. Not only had Sherman been stymied at Atlanta, Grant was stalemated at Richmond and Petersburg. Many Americans were pushing for an end to the war that had gone on for too long, and too many families had been touched by the casualties of the increasingly unpopular war. Fortunately the recent fall of Atlanta aided in the will of the country to decide to see the war to a necessary conclusion.

[September 6, 1864]
11th Mo. I. V.
Brownsville, Arks.
Dearest Parents Bro. and Sisters,

Think it was at St. Charles on White River I mailed you the last letter. Next day we embarked at daylight, the morning after the fleet started for DeValls Bluff 90 miles up the river. About 10 that night, landed at the almost deserted Bluffs, next day marched out to the edge of a large farm, encamped until 2 o'clock next day. Then started for this station 25 miles west by railroad from DeValls Bluff. Brownsmith is 1½ miles from the station in an between. Col. A. B. Morrison is there in command of the post. The 61st Ills. Infty. is also stationed there. I hardly know what we expected to do in this department. Genl. Price is somewhere in the state I suppose and ere long we must thrash him.

DeValls bluff is a small village composed mostly at present of army store houses, depot, sutler, shops, hospital and Negro quarters with a few poor houses of residents. Not one fine residence in the [town] that I saw. Indeed it is quite a frontier place. The present terminus of the Memphis and Little Rock Railroad, one mile from the village is the border of a wide prairie 25 miles to this place with poor water. We marched at 2 P.M. Saturday until 11 at night about 18 miles, sun hot, not much shade. Our men suffered, started next morning at 8 A.M. arrived here early and expect to remain a few days at least. I did not see one farm in this rich fertile prairie but one house occupied. The ruins of two or three others. Consequently, no forage, our nice vegetables of southern production, at an end in this state. Even if the land flowed with milk and honey, the soldiers could get none. The poor state had gone through the miserable farce of electing Union representatives. A dozen men elected by as many voters to each. All of questionable loyalty, politicks. All the bitter, disloyal horde from the just subsistence of the soldier. The Union soldier suffers from scurvy, cannot get vegetables, has no money, citizens will not give one jobs. He cannot use force while the Reb citizen gives and almost subsists the Reb Army in passing through. Indeed they have subsisted and cared for a army of bushwackers all summer. All this is the old milk and water policy which is a lasting disgrace to any nation fighting for its life and especially upon this one which hangs the interests of the world.

Some of our men are getting sick. Maj. Bowyer, Capt. Notestine in good health. I am thankful my health is still good. We do not know how long this division is expected to remain in this trans-Mississippi Department, hope not long. We think with the proper rigorous policy this part of the so-called southern Confederacy might have been cleared of all large bodies of armed Rebs. But with our loved kindred at home, for once in almost four years of bloody battle now rests the great and responsible duty of protecting all that we have accomplished and of perpetuating this Republican form of government upon them depends our safety. They must say whether the legions of glorious dead have died in vain. Change this too lenient administration for a radical peace-at-any-price one and you prolong the war 20 years, lose much that has been gained and all think is now almost within our grasp. My dear ones, I had hoped to be with you once again this fall, at least for a short time, but for the present it appears to be indefinitely postponed. I must abide the decision if it is fully decided, with patience, think it would be dishonorable to persist in leaving just now when one's services are so much needed.

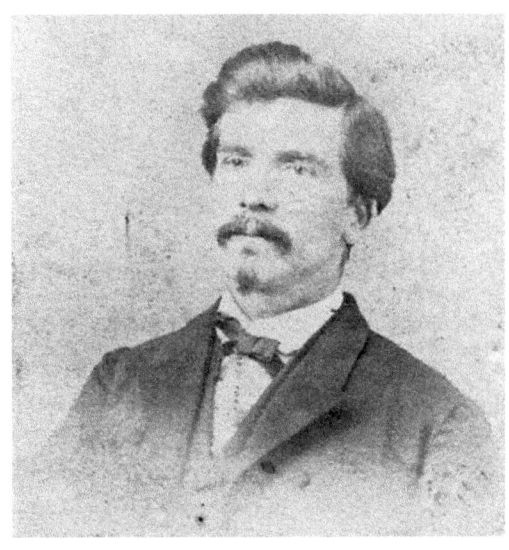

Edward King, Hospital Steward (editor's collection).

It is reported we have had warmer weather this month than at any time during the summer, had two cases of sun stroke crossing the prairie. Have you a remote idea where Pa will be, or rather all of you sent if he enters the service of the church in the Southern Ills. Conference. I cannot imagine without it would be as Elder of the Mt. Carmel district Headquarters at Olney. This I think would not be so objectionable provided he did not do himself, his friends and the church injustice by laboring too hard for his constitution.

Hope all will be for the best.

My Boy Dan and horse Billey are doing well, wish you could see them. Dan makes Billey come to him almost as far as he can call. Dan wants to go home with me. I have promised he might, is quiet, sober, never swears and is rather too *conscientious upon the important topic of confiscation. Never knew him to capture a chicken or shirt a porker. He has preached sometimes and discusses biblical subjects amusingly, is rather timid, only talks thus to darkies when I have overheard him sometimes.*

All our camp and garrison equipage, valises, etc., remain in our old camp at Memphis. My present wardrobe consists of two woolen shirts, 2 pr. pants, boots, 2 hdkcfs., holey hat, ½ doz. paper collars, old woolen blouse, etc. Tis enough & no more. As to fare, tis good enough for dinner, light bread purchased at Du V. Bluffs, pork, salt, tea, condensed milk, sugar, potatoes, pickles, etc. Have a good cook, William Anderson, from near Palestine, Chas. Sheppard of Lawrenceville, druggist of my teaching, Ed King of Jacksonville, clerk of my training, Dan Johnson, private servant, hostler, etc., makes up our mess or family circle, quite pleasant one.

Another article missed of our fare was from friends of the Sanitary Com., dried apples. Wm. procured ½ bushel of dried peaches by confiscation in Miss. We have not been paid for 4 months, rather nearly five months pay due us. Consequently, funds rather low but in this wild wilderness cannot suffer much from this cause. Officers can purchase of the division commissary, sugar 25, ham 25, coffee 60, pickles 50 per gallon, everything has doubled while officers' pay is less than it was 2 years ago, and that of all enlisted men has been increased. Do not understand. I am grumbling. If all would go at the war with hearty good will, determined to crush it out immediately at all hazards, I would willingly labor another 3 years for food & raiment and this Noble Army has many would do likewise & far better, health permitting.

Chas., I and Capt. Kendall are going to the depot for commissaries and will see Col. Morrison's camp, near, then I will write you of him. We hear Genl. A. J. Smith with the 3rd Divis. 16 AC have all gone to Ga. We have been with them for some time and rather hoped to be on the same journey. Please pardon if letters do not come to hand as often as usual while on this campaign. I will write as often as possible. I cannot answer the questions in the few last for they are at home, or rather old camp. Oh, so much of the best love to all at home. Kind regards to the Gunns, Fannie, Ada, etc. Lots of kisses to Fannie, Myra, Eva Bell, Mary & all. Please direct as usual. They will be sent from the DPO.

Most affectionately, your obt. son,
Thos. S. Hawley, MD

The 1864 odyssey of Thomas Hawley continued and was described in detail in his October 7 letter which was written from Cape Girardeau, Missouri. The sense of history was not lost on Doctor Hawley as he returned to the first garrison of the 11th Missouri Infantry over three years ago. He noted some of his old friends stated he looked better than he did three years ago. So, army life must have been agreeable to him. The letter provided a detailed account of the march from Brownsville, Arkansas, to Cape Girardeau, Missouri. He described the rugged march through creeks and sleeping on stony ground until they reached St. Genevieve, Missouri, where they boarded a steamer. As mentioned in the last letter written by Thomas Hawley, there was concern in the Union Army of a concentration of Confederate troops under command of Sterling Price and the fear these troops would invade Missouri. That is exactly what happened which resulted in the pursuit the regiment was currently involved.

Price's plan was to raid into Missouri and attempt to win back Confederate supporters. The raid also attempted to assist in the Georgia campaign by diverting Union resources to Missouri and possibly allowing additional Confederate troops to move through Federal occupied territory in the other southern states. Price's plan included moving through a large arc which included attacking St. Louis, Jefferson City, sweeping across Missouri into Kansas and returning through the Indian Territory disrupting Union positions as he swept all before him in a massive cavalry raid.

Price's cavalry force of 12,000 horsemen entered Missouri on September 19, 1864 through southeastern Missouri. On September 27, Price unsuccessfully attacked a Union force at Fort Davidson, near Pilot Knob, Missouri, and guerrillas attacked Centralia, Missouri, in central Missouri. These actions caused the XVI Army Corps under command of Major General A. J. Smith to move in pursuit of Price; and thus began one of the 11th Missouri's longest, uneventful treks of the war. Price's force continued its east-west arc — striking Cuba, Missouri, on September 29, occupying Washington on October 2, skirmishing at Herman on October 3, and reaching the state capital on October 8. Then, Price continued his raid through October, striking Boonville, Glasgow, Sedalia, Lexington, and Independence. It wasn't until the Battle of Westport on October 23, that the momentum shifted and instead of being on the offensive, Price began retreating back toward Arkansas which he finally reached on December 2, 1864.

As the 11th Missouri Infantry joined in the pursuit of Price, the effects of four months of almost non-stop campaigning was starting to take a toll on the men. The temperature extremes were noticeable and the result was sickness of the men who suffered from "hard shakes, colds, coughs, neuralgia." Despite the hardships, Thomas Hawley wrote his place in the regiment was improved over the situation under the command of Colonel William Barnum. Hawley concluded his letter stating, "We all hope the present campaign in the north will finally settle the war."

Cape Girardeau, Mo.
Oct. 7th 1864

Dear Parents, Bro. and Sisters,

Little did I think my next epistle to you would bear the above address when I last wrote over 300 miles away by the nearest road, but here we are among old friends and acquaintances who gave us a hearty welcome after three years absence. We, that is the 1st Divs. 16th AC [Army Corps], have been over 20 days in the wildness. Our history would give a similar record to that of the children of Israel only not quite so long. The last letter received from home was dated, I think, Aug. 30 and I guess by this time our anxiety is about equal to hear from each other. So I embrace this first opportunity to send the wanted word. The above lines penned this morning. Orders came to march to the river and embark for St. Louis, marched to town, remained a few moments, right about, came back to our old camp, no steamers there. I guess we will start for St. Louis or Jefferson City tonight or tomorrow. This as usual places us much farther north during the winter months than in the summer. Maj. B. was talking to me so I made the mistake. He is well. So am I for which I desire to be thankful. Some of my friends say I look better than three years ago. Indeed I am quite fleshy. If we could stop at St. L., I will try to see you if possible but I guess we will march on, travel directly through to Jeff. City.

I wrote you just before we left Brownsville, Ark. about the 16th ult. Genl. Jos. Mower in comdg. with two divs. of calv. under Col. Winslow and 4 brigades of 1st Div. 16th A C. Wagon train of nearly three hundred wagons left Brownsville, 25 miles from Little Rock. March directly north 7 miles and encamped on the 17th ult., next day march about 15 miles, 3rd day out we passed through Sissa and crossed the Little Red River which is navigable to this point, 50 miles from White River, 6 months in the year. Villages all rather new but desolate country, sparsely settled, log cabins. Austin is a small place 15 miles from Brownsville, a brigade of calv. had been here most of the time, face of country to Red River broken with some prairie. All the men waded the river which is knee deep. Bottom filled with stones, encamped on the bank. The men found enough pork, poultry and garden vegetables with some corn to make quite a variety of food and began to improve. We started with 30 sick, had to haul ten in ambulance all the way, but they continued to improve on the march, only average four or 5 sick between Red River and White. The country is rocky, uneven, almost mountainous. Only the valleys cultivated. March some days twenty miles over hills covered with stones and huge ledges jutting out of the hill tops. Many of the men without shoes or boots. These sharp stones lacerated their feet. Still they must plod on. At night, we must scrape the stones away to sleep, rations issued, rather scarce and the hard tack full of bugs and worms. Often when eating, I have pulled out worms from half an inch to an inch long but even this did not nauseate the stomach or disturb our voracious appetites.

Most every day on the march, reveille sounded at 3 o'clock, march half past four or at the first break of day and oftener leave before. After several days, long weary marches of rocks and hills, through brush and brake. The loss of several horses, mules and wagons. We landed on the banks of the White River encamped in a fine, rich valley. This was the first appearance of rich, well cultivated land. At this point is a pretty stream and was crossed about sunrise affording a beautiful interesting spectacle.

On steamer, <u>Minnehaha</u>, Sunday Morning near St. Genevieve. I heard the mail would not leave the Cape before Saturday though we would leave that soon if not before. So did not send this epistle, fear you will think I am tardy in writing. I hope you will get this before we leave St. Louis. Our progress has been slow owing to the low water. Our steamer is the largest in the fleet, consequently is behind all. Tis said we will necessarily change boats in St. L. as this cannot pass up the Missouri River. We are all suffering from cold. When we left Memphis it was extremely hot, mercury standing near 120° in sun, left our coats, etc., coming as we thought for ten days march, will get our own camp and garrison equippage soon. I hope for we cannot purchase anything as Uncle Sam has not paid us for 5 almost 6 months. I must have some things in St. L. or I will not go if I can help it. Men suffering from hard shakes, colds, coughs, neuralgia, etc. All from the cold, chills and without sufficient clothing. Some have no blankets, coats or shoes and many here among friends and supplies abundant. We all hope to be able to vote this presidential election, it and us, so near. Why not?

Our mail is, no one here knows where, nor how soon we will receive any. It would do my heart so much good to hear from you directly but so much more to see your smiling faces and hear your loving voices. I had hoped to hear from you soon but fear I cannot. I did still more hope to see you this fall. I shall still try to get out of the service next spring at least if not before. My place here has not been so tedious or unpleasant but quite pleasant since Col. Barnum left and Maj. B. was thrown in command. He so far sustains all my actions and knows the difficulties surgeons labor under among men and officers who cannot understand his or their official relations. We all hope the present campaign in the north will finally settle the war on the firm basis of Liberty, Freedom and Peace and crush the last link of hope the poor deluded Rebels have clung to so long, no help from northern traitors. We know they have the will but hope not [illegible]. My strongest purest love to each of the dear family circle of which I would be filled with unbounded joy to be a member at home this morning and with you attend the best of heaven's privileges, the sanctuary of God. The more I am deprived of the blessing, the greater I feel its divine origin and its necessity to the welfare of God's children. Much love to all the friends. Compliments to Mrs. Bowyer &

children, Jno. H. Gunn & Family also to Mr. Reed. All write soon to me, 2ⁿᵈ Brig. 1ˢᵗ Divs. 16ᵗʰ AC, St. Louis. I think this is best. I am ever you affct.

Bro. & son,

Thos. S. Hawley

On October 11, the pursuit of Price proceeded and the regiment was faced with chasing hard-riding cavalry by whatever form of transportation they could find. Thomas Hawley scribbled a few lines to his family as he passed through St. Louis on his way to Jefferson City, Missouri. He had enough time to express some money home and congratulate his father on his new position as Elder in the Mt. Carmel District.

St. Louis, Mo. Oct. 11, 1864

Dearest Parents,

Our stay in the city has been so short I could hardly realize that we are so near home. Only a few hours ride and then we have had so much to do. Maj. B. and I were paid yesterday for four months. We had to lend some to the officers. I expressed home today $200 in $20 new issue. Do as you see best with, guess I cannot come home until next spring. I just heard through Wm. Ridgeway that Pa was Elder of the Mt. Carmel Dist. I do hope his health, and that of all, will be good. Do urge Pa not to labor above that he is able to bear. Much love to all unseen. Yours affectly.,

Thos. S. Hawley

The veteran regiment of the 11th Missouri Infantry continued their relentless pursuit of the Confederate Army as the year came to an end. The 11th Missouri marched to Independence and then into Kansas, only to return to Pleasant Hill, Missouri. Finally, the brigade marched eastward towards Warrensburg and embarked by rail east and south. The 11th Missouri recorded this marathon pursuit of Price resulted in an aggregate of 1320 miles by rail, steamboat and foot. There are no records the regiment participated in any direct combat during the odyssey.

Sergeant Charles Treadway described the regiment's pursuit of Price, "marched to Brownsville Ark. We lay here for 4 days until all the wagons ware loaded then we took an Northeast direction and came out at Cape Girardeau Mo. got on some boats came up the River to St. Louis landed a few moments and then went ahead to Jefferson City took the cars and went to Salene Bridge which the Rebs had destroyed. Disembarked and marched to Sedalia thence to Lexington thence to Independence thence to Kansas City thence to Harrisonville thence to Warrensburg thence to Sedalia thence to Jefferson City thence to St Louis."[8]

While Sterling Price wrote of his success of the raid through Missouri, it is generally considered to have been an unsuccessful foray northward. This was the last major offensive action by the Confederate Trans-Mississippi Department.

Additional communications from Thomas Hawley ceased or are lost to history because only one remaining letter exists for the remainder of the year, but it held a description of the Battle of Nashville. After the pursuit of Price was concluded the 11th Missouri Infantry traveled to Nashville departing Missouri on November 24, arriving on December 1.

The events which led up to the Battle of Nashville began with Sherman's success in capturing Atlanta. The Confederate Army defending Atlanta was commanded by General John Bell Hood. The Battle of Jonesboro, Georgia, fought on September 1, resulted in the Union Army cutting the last rail supply line into Atlanta. Realizing it was fruitless to defend the city any further, Hood abandoned Atlanta to the Union Army. While Sherman was continuing his "march to the sea," Hood's Army of Tennessee moved to northwest Georgia and then to Florence, Alabama. On November 21, Hood began the Tennessee Campaign which included battles at Spring Hill, Franklin and finally Nashville. Hood's objective was to cut the supply line to Sherman and also to attempt to cut off and destroy either Major General George Thomas' force (19,000 men) in Nashville or Major General John Schofield's force (20,000 men) dispatched from eastern Tennessee. Hood's army totaled greater than 30,000 men.

During his advance on the Union forces in Tennessee, Hood fought a small battle at Spring Hill, Tennessee, and then threw his army at the Union forces at Franklin, Tennessee. The Battle of Franklin was a bloody battle and a decisive Union victory in which Hood lost 6,500 men compared to 2,500 Union losses. In addition, Hood lost 15 generals and 53 regimental commanders. Despite the loss and being outnumbered, Hood marched on Nashville where he threatened the city and planned to defensively defeat the Union Army. It was this situation which resulted in the 11th Missouri Infantry being called to Nashville.

The Battle of Nashville was fought on December 15 and 16, 1864, and the 11th Missouri Infantry was instrumental in the Union victory. The regiment attacked the left flank of Hood's army on December 15 assisting in forcing the withdrawal of Hood's line. On December 16, Hood concentrated his line along an excellent defensive position, but had too few men to withstand the Union attack in the afternoon. Again, the 11th Missouri Infantry was part of the attack which broke the Confederate line around Shy's Hill and a route ensued. The flag staff of the 11th Missouri Infantry bearing the regimental colors was shattered into three pieces so great was the Confederate fire during the attack, but the attack was successful. The cost was high for the 11th Missouri Infantry with about 90 casualties of the 325 men who participated in the attack. Three soldiers of the 11th Missouri were awarded the Medal of Honor for their efforts in the attack.

Unfortunately, Thomas Hawley had many friends wounded in the battle and he mentioned two of these in his letter written on December 20 — Captain William Notestine and Lieutenant Colonel Eli Bowyer. These were names repeatedly mentioned in Hawley's letters throughout the war. As regimental surgeon, Thomas Hawley provided immediate medical care on the battlefield and then moved the wounded to the divisional hospital in the rear. William Notestine was shot in the leg, shattering his femur on December 15. His leg was amputated after he reached the hospital. Lieutenant Colonel Eli Bowyer was shot in the arm by a Confederate sharpshooter while positioning the regiment prior to the attack on Shy's Hill on December 16. Thomas Hawley did not detail his activities but he mentioned he was busy for four days dealing with the numerous wounds which occurred.

Hd. Qts. 11th Mo. Inf. V. V.
Near Spring Hill 10 miles
below Franklin, Tenn. Dec 20th 64
Dear Father and Mother,

I know your anxiety to hear from me, especially after a severe battle as we have just had at Nashville. So I hasten to write but you may think 4 days after is not much haste. But I could not write before. We had all we could do day and night after the fight. Next day after had to pick up in haste and follow Corpl. Hood after he was badly thrashed. I suppose you have heard that our special friends in this gallant regt. were wounded enduring the severe fight. Capt. Wm. Notestine in the left thigh above the knee. I examined the wound on the battlefield as best I could, fixed it up in rough splints from rails. Wrapping well with bandages, put him in the ambulance just before dark, have not seen him since. He bears it like a true hero, as he is. I shed tears of deep sympathy for these dear brother soldiers. I did and do love them as brothers. The orderlies just from Nashville last night, saw both at the Officers' Hospital, well cared for. I deeply feel the cruel pain of parting with these dear fellows. Just as they are wounded I asked the privilege of going to see them but the Divs. Surg. would not permit. Capt N. was wounded on the 15th while in command of skirmishers gallantly charging the Rebs. Our boys did not go to suit him. He rushed in front of all calling them to follow up the steep hill. They had just captured a fort with some guns and prisoners, had fought the Rebs back over two miles.

The col. was wounded about 10 o'clock on the 16th, was riding in front of the regt. coolly giving commands while the Reb sharpshooters kept up a constant hot fire just across a long cornfield. The col. was urging a charge at the time a minnie ball struck him 4 inches below the elbow on the outside of the left arm and I cut it out 2½ inches below the elbow on the inside, lodged just under the skin. Poor man, he was so brave, did not want to leave the battlefield after I brought him off in the ambulance. He wanted to go back and make the charge but I knew it would not do, was suffering [so] much and almost fainting sometimes after the ball was extracted. He rested some and had taken some stimulants, arm bandaged up, sent him 2½ miles near town to the divis. hospital in charge of our Divs. Surgeon and several officers of the Division Surgeon. All the wounded were sent there. I could not leave the field just then as wounded kept coming in all the time. After a lull I jumped on my horse and galloped to the hospital. Dr. Murta was just operating by enlarging the wound and removing fragments of bone of which there was about 20 he has there. The col. stood the operation under the influence of chloroform was humming the Red, White and Blue part of the time. About an inch and half of ulna was removed leaving the bone in a pretty good condition to heal but it will take some time. I left him feeling cheerful, walked to the ambulance that took him to town. [He] ate some tea & crackers, said he wanted to come back to the field but must submit to Dr. Murta and I, just the men he wants to attend him. I fear but have strong hopes he will soon be able to go home. Capt N. is cheerful and doing well but both in the same room with our officers. The hospital is a large, strong building in a good situation. Capt. N limb is off just half way of the thigh. I wrote to col. to send for his wife, thinks it would help cheer him up. He did not want to go to the hospital but there was no other place. I am writing in haste for I think we will start soon, just stopped here last night. No further orders. Rained all day. Yesterday, cold and wet today. Your, Pa and Myra's letter of the 1st came today, the first since I saw Ma's. I shall come if possible this spring. Health good but fingers cold. Pardon the scribble. I think you had better see Mrs. B. and tell her if you think best [she] know the truth. She knows how I love the Col. and will do all I can but for the present I am too far off. Cheer her up and give her my kind regards. I may write to her if I can soon. Give my love to all and especially to the dear family circle which I am one. Thanks for the dear, good letter. I'll answer Myra soon and come if I can soon. Oh, so much love from your affct. son,

Thomas

Thomas Hawley finished the year working diligently trying to save the lives of the men he had come to know and respect. The Battle of Nashville was a day of glory for the 11th Missouri Veteran Infantry, but it was one of great loss and pain. At the conclusion of 1864, many events had occurred in the past twelve months. Thomas Hawley, although only the assistant surgeon of the regiment, was in charge of the medical department of the 11th Missouri

Infantry and had held this position throughout the year. He had medically pulled the regiment together after the Vicksburg campaign and made it as healthy as possible. In 1864, he lost many friends when approximately 100 non-veterans left at the expiration of their term of enlistment in August. The final six months of the year tested the resolve and fighting ability of the regiment as they campaigned without stop from July to the end of 1864. The regiment had been involved in the Battle of Tupelo, the expedition to Oxford Mississippi, including the skirmishes at Abbeyville and Hurricane Creek, the expedition to DuValls Bluff, the pursuit of Price in Missouri, and finally the Battle of Nashville. Along the way many friends were lost, including, Zeba French due to resignation, and William Notestine and Eli Bowyer due to wounds. Thomas Hawley had yet to be granted his promotion and despite his pledge to leave the regiment if he was not appointed regimental surgeon, still he remained. By his own words, he knew the regiment had no medical professional and he refused to leave them. The year was ending and Hawley looked to the future, he looked to his familial obligations and he looked to his obligations to the soldiers of the 11th Missouri Infantry. He remained, hoping the interminable war would soon be over. He felt only one more battle and finally, the peace he desired would be the reward. The reward was yet to come.

FIVE

1865

Spanish Fort, Occupation of Alabama and Postwar Life

In January 1865, the Civil War was entering the final chapter and the Union armies slowly subdued the Southern resistance. The 11th Missouri Infantry, as part of A. J. Smith's XVI Corps, pursued Hood's defeated army south from Nashville until December 28 and then went into winter quarters at Clifton, Tennessee, and Eastport, Mississippi, until February 7, 1865. The war was not over for the Thomas Hawley and the men of his regiment as they had one final conflict ahead of them. The regiment received an infusion of soldiers from the Seventh Missouri Infantry prior to the Battle of Nashville only to lose about 90 men in the conflict; however, the regiment began receiving conscripts. Over a six month period the 11th Missouri Infantry received about 500 draftees or substitutes which filled the ranks.

The effects of the Battle of Nashville carried into the new year. Tragically, Thomas Hawley's friend, Captain William Notestine, died in February of exhaustion resulting from the amputation of his leg. Hawley's best friend in the regiment, Eli Bowyer, remained away from the regiment until May recuperating from his wounds.

In January 1865, the Confederate government was facing a difficult year — General Robert E. Lee was besieged by Grant at Richmond, General Joe Johnston was trying to defend the Carolinas from the relentless William T. Sherman, and Hood's defeated army was attempting to avoid the wrath of George Thomas after the defeat at Nashville. Hood's Confederate Army had been soundly defeated and began its retreat from Nashville beginning on December 16, 1864, and the Union Army followed closely the cold, wet, hungry and tired Rebel army until it crossed the Tennessee River on December 27. At that point General John Bell Hood resigned command of his army.

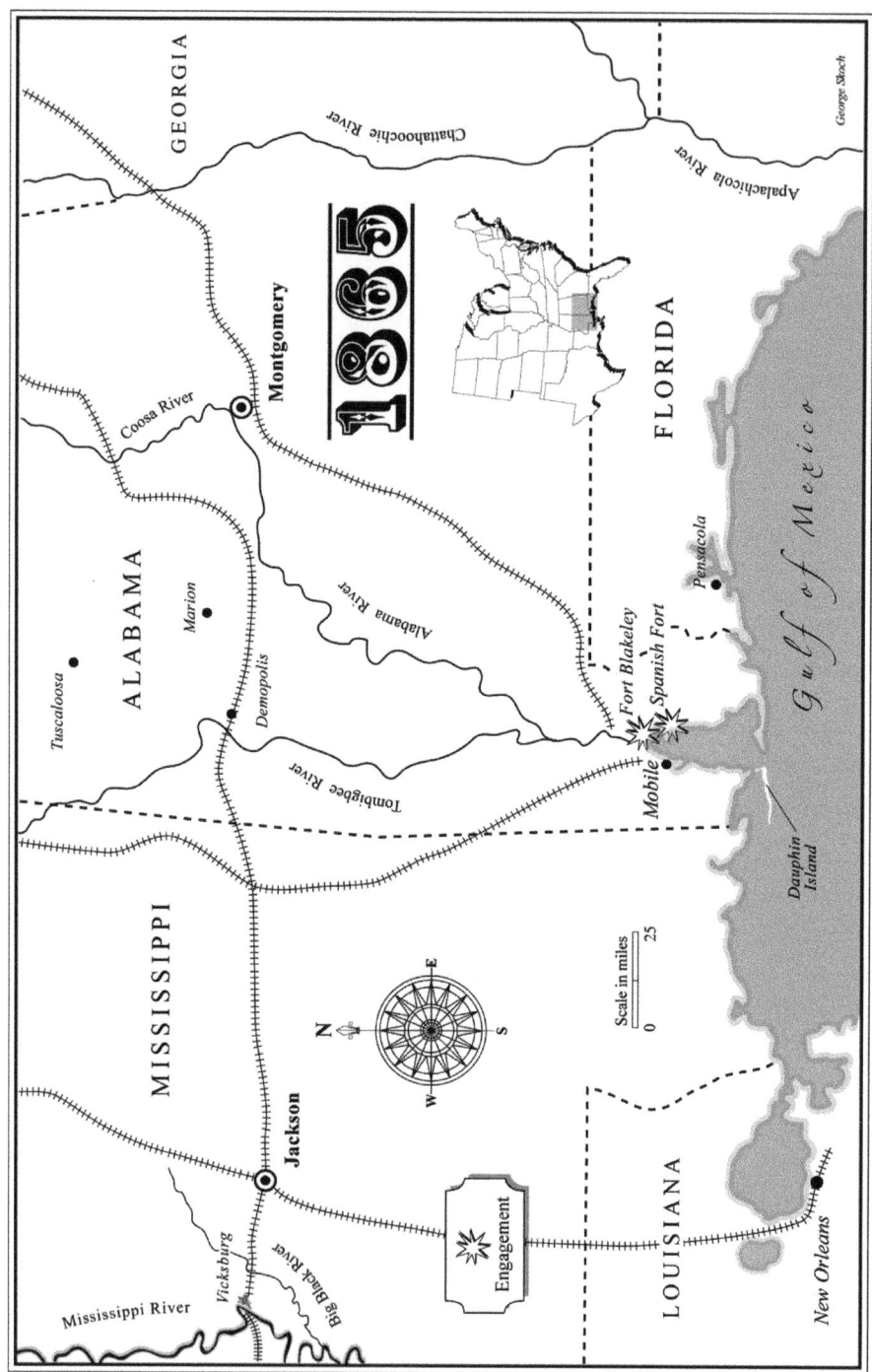

Five. 1865

The Confederate Army had lost the ability to replace losses in men and matériel and the seemingly unstoppable Union Army moved steadily against any concentration of Confederate troops. One of the larger Confederate concentrations of troops was located at Mobile, Alabama, under the command of Major General Dabney Maury. Mobile was one of the last Confederate ports still in Southern hands and the forces at Mobile contained one of the last organized Confederate military forces which were not actively engaged. About 5,000 of Hood's troops were transferred to Maury's command, and at that stage in the war, any concentration of Confederate forces quickly drew the attention of the Union commanders.

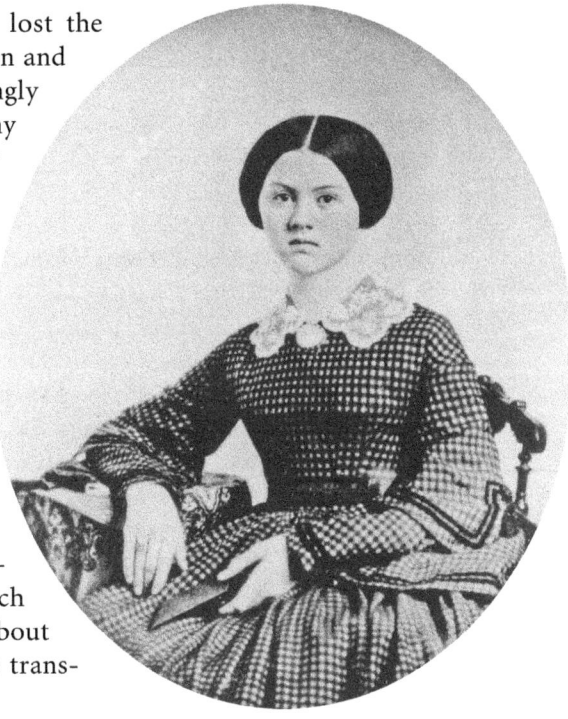

Caroline Joy Hawley (courtesy Joan Garvin).

On February 3, Thomas Hawley wrote a letter to his sister Myra regarding her impending marriage, but Thomas revealed his intention of marrying Miss Carrie Joy if he could gain the necessary approvals from the army for a leave of absence.

Camp 11th Mo Inf. Vet. Vol.
Eastport, Miss. Feb 3, 1865

Darling Sister

With the cordial approval of the officers and their good wishes, I forwarded this morning an application for leave of absence and openly avowed, as it was necessary to give a good and sufficient cause why leave should be granted, that I wished to fulfill an engagement made sometime ago and as it will take several days to pass the judgment of Genl. Smith and Maj. Genl. Thomas and return. I earnestly desire to get there in good time to attend your nuptial festive scene and if all is right, your plan may yet be carried out to the letter. I could not be mus-

tered out as I and Col. B and other officers thought, with the fair prospect of a speedy peace.

I asked Carrie what she thought of still carrying our plan even if I could not remain with her for a very long time. She consented, bless her dear heart. So if all is well when I come to see you made happy, you may be with me in the happiest hours of my life.

Some think and say it is foolish to be married during the war or while one is in the army. I once thought so. Let each one qualified to judge, if this places themselves in my position, whether is it easier to part with one loved dearer than life only known as bethrothed or as wife when if the latter you can freely sympathize and if afflicted openly visit without calling forth the scandal of the hard hearted world. I cannot consider our vows any more binding than they are at present. Why not let the world know of them by the short legal process. Besides we in the army can often send for our wives. They can come to us when we cannot go to them when in Memphis or some city. But dear Sister, I need not argue my, or rather our, cause with you. In your circumstances the case is clear. Perhaps Pa and Ma may not think so just now. I am satisfied they will not seriously object at least. Carrie is a warm advocate and says her parents consent to abide by our good judgment. Kind ain't they, never having seen me? She desired to know what Pa and Ma thought of this change in affairs. [I] Confessed I had not written soon enough but had confidence they would decide in our favor as they thought I was a tolerable good boy. So you see it is all left in the hands of our generals and if they decide all right, we will be happy. If I cannot get permission to leave, hope to bear the disappointment as a good soldier and trust to providence in that all is for the best. I need not assure you it would be the hardest trial I have had for a long time. The major just stepped in, said he had taken my papers to Col. Hubbard commanding 2nd Brigade, brevetted Brig. Genl. for meritorious conduct at the Battle of Nashville. He said he thought I would get it for the novelty of it. The major will now take it to Genl. McArthur, Cmdg. 1st Division. The gallant Major Green, Ma knows him, is you see warmly elicited in my cause. Let us hope and pray for the best.

Many of these brave friends of ours often inquire for the gallantly good Col. Bowyer. I know you will show him all the friendship possible. He is beloved by officers and men. God grant his speedy recovery. We mourn the hour that Capt. Notestine our former school mate is or was at the point of death. I loved him and shed tears when the noise of the battle was hushed and all was quiet, saw the remains of the wounded. I am pleased to hear Bro. A is doing so well. Well Sis, remember I come if possible, shall telegraph you from Cairo. Much love to all the dear ones at home. Hoping, praying again and again for your happiness. I am as ever your affectionate Bro.

Thomas

Five. 1865

There is a rumor that we will soon move, don't think so.

We may move in a few days down the river or east. This makes my cause rather uncertain. I'll telegraph from Cairo.

Doctor Thomas Hawley and the 11th Missouri Infantry began the Mobile Campaign on February 7, 1865, when the soldiers boarded river transports and were carried to Vicksburg, Mississippi, arriving on February 14. On February 19, the regiment was again transported by river transports to New Orleans and arrived on February 21. After a two-day sea voyage, the regiment finally arrived at Dauphin Island located in Mobile Bay on March 7. The exit from New Orleans was a relief to many in the regiment and was expressed by Sergeant Charles Treadway, "I have seen enough of New Orleans to do me. One has to be very careful whare he puts his foot or he will mire or get snake bit. Snakes and alligators are thick as rabbits in the barns."[1] So, on March 7 the 11th Missouri was close enough to see Mobile, a fortified city with three circles of earthen works that surrounded the land approaches to the city. Floating batteries and shore batteries protected the bay exposure. The city of Mobile was not the target of the Union advance, but rather the two formidable defensive forts located about seven miles from the city on the eastern side of the bay—Spanish Fort and Fort Blakeley.

Rainy weather and swampy conditions made the advance on Spanish Fort a difficult march. On March 27, the XVI Corps marched to initiate the siege of the two forts in conjunction with the XIII Corps. Once the two corps were in position, Union commander Major General Edward Canby pushed to encircle Spanish Fort but the advancing Union troops were surprised when soldiers of the Louisiana Brigade charged out of Spanish Fort and temporarily pushed regiments of the XIII Corps backward. By March 28 Spanish Fort was fully encircled and the siege had begun.

The mile and half long defenses at Spanish Fort were formidable, "... trees had been cleared and obstructions placed for the oncoming Federals. A tangled abates stretched about 15 feet deep along the whole front, and in front of the breastworks ran a ditch 8 feet wide and 5 feet deep. Rebel sharpshooters manned rifle pits scattered in the front of the six batteries or redoubts that crowned the crest of a red bluff running along the line."[2]

On March 27, the 11th Missouri attacked with their division, and the Confederate defenders threw the full might of their artillery against the Union soldiers. The Confederate artillery was devastating to the Union troops besieging Spanish Fort. The artillery included 6 heavy guns, 14 field cannons and 12 Coehorn mortars. The Southern defenders lost 5 killed and 44 men wounded on March 27, and in this unsuccessful attack, the Union XVI Corps lost 91 men killed and many others wounded.

The Union Army continued a siege for 13 days at Spanish Fort, and artillery duels and sharpshooting were common occurrences. The constant exchange of fire resulted in several casualties within the regiment including future chaplain, George Brown, and Captain William Erwin. The casualty list for the 11th Missouri is not definitive, but regiment reported 4 killed and another 17 wounded during siege.

In the April 9, 1865 letter, it was reported the fall of Spanish Fort occurred early in the morning of the day the letter was written. Thomas Hawley began this letter "Dear Darling Wife." Since the Battle of Nashville, Thomas Hawley was furloughed home and was married to Carrie Joy on February 21, 1865, and then returned to the regiment in Alabama. The wedding service was performed by Thomas' father, Nelson Hawley.

April 1865 was one of the most significant months in Unites States history as several major events occurred, including, the fall of Richmond, Lee's surrender at Appomattox, the Union victory in Mobile, the assassination of President Abraham Lincoln, and the Confederate surrender in the Carolinas. By the end of April, the Civil War was over for all practical purposes. Thomas Hawley's letter echoed the impending peace as he stated, "This peace, as looked for through 4 years of suffering and privation, becomes the priceless boon of our desires."

No. 13 Camp 11th Mo. Inf. V. V.
Near Blakely Fort
Sunday Night April 9, 1865
Dear Darling Wife,

Since I last wrote you two days ago some very important changes have taken place. Spanish Fort was captured last night at 1 o'clock with all its munitions of war. Ammunition, guns, commissary stores, etc., about 500 prisoners. About ten we crossed the small river near Sp. Fort and marched to this camp half a mile from Blakeley, leaving one brigade of the 13th AC [Army Corps] to garrison the fort. And just now it is officially reported that Blakeley is captured with 5000 prisoners and they say we can march directly into Mobile, but there are several rivers intervening, bad roads, etc. However, I think we will continue onward to Mobile tomorrow at dawn, and this, the next if not the last, strong hold of Rebelldom, must succumb to the power of these United States. Is not this a glorious inheritance we are trying to keep safe from harm? I feel the burning of a patriotic heart, occasionally and am almost wild with joy as the sweet hope brightens of a speedy peace. This peace, as looked for through 4 years of suffering and privation, becomes the priceless boon of our desires, and now to me and mine it means so much. Words fail to express half the emotions and hopes of a loving heart, a bright and blissful home with the dear wife of my bosom. Our hearts' spirits blending until they are unspeakably welded by the glue of fervent love. All the joys and endearments of home springing up around us. Happy each by always striving to render one another so, and those around us. These are some of the bright pictures canvassed to my mind's eye by the prospect of an early honorable peace.

    The chief character in all these daydreams is my dearly beloved wife, for whom my love goes on, increasing every day of this beautiful bright spring time. May your happiness, joys, and hopes be as fresh and joyous as the rosey spring of life. Most of the officers in good health. Maj. Green, Capt. Kendall and Capt. McMahan, just at my left elbow, writing to his betrothed now at Chicago. The last three days have been rather cool for comfort but today's was more pleasant. Our gunboats are still down [in] the bay.

    We enjoyed divine worship neath the solemn pine trees this quiet twilight eve. The minister, a private soldier, was quite eloquent, drew a large audience of orderly soldiers. The singing was spontaneous and heart-cheering. I felt happy from the love of God. We hear rumors of more good news, letters, Richmond, gunboats, etc., all mixed. Please give my brotherly love to your present host & hostess, kissing Gracie for me also and sent by letter as Dear Bell says, my love, whether I tell you or not, to our dear Parents, bros. and sisters, aunts, uncles & cozs. Dearest of these scribbled love missives come too often [to] send them to some other less unfortunate fair lady, or in reverse. Send just as many back as you dare spend time with. You know this heart, this arm, this all is thine. We are one flesh now and ever. I love the fairer part of the one, so fondly, so dearly, so truly and ever kiss thee many, many times ere we journey to the fairy land of dreams to dwell in amnesial bower.

Yours truly, Yours wholly, Your husband,

T. S. Hawley

There have been various dates offered as the end of the United States Civil War, but President Andrew Johnson pronounced the end of the war to be May 10, 1865. When Thomas Hawley wrote his letter on May 29, the war was over although the last armed conflict continued in some places until as late as June 1865. There were only a few more Thomas Hawley letters written after the Battle of Spanish Fort in April 1865.

By the end of the Civil War the state of Alabama had lost civil authority and for a time anarchy reigned. The Union Army was called to fill the void left by the absence of civil law. On June 7, 1865, the Military Division of the Tennessee was commanded by General George Thomas, who had commanded this territory since 1863, and Thomas had administrative authority over Alabama. In 1865 the Department of Alabama was placed under the command of General C. R. Woods headquartered at Mobile. In early summer 1865, cities

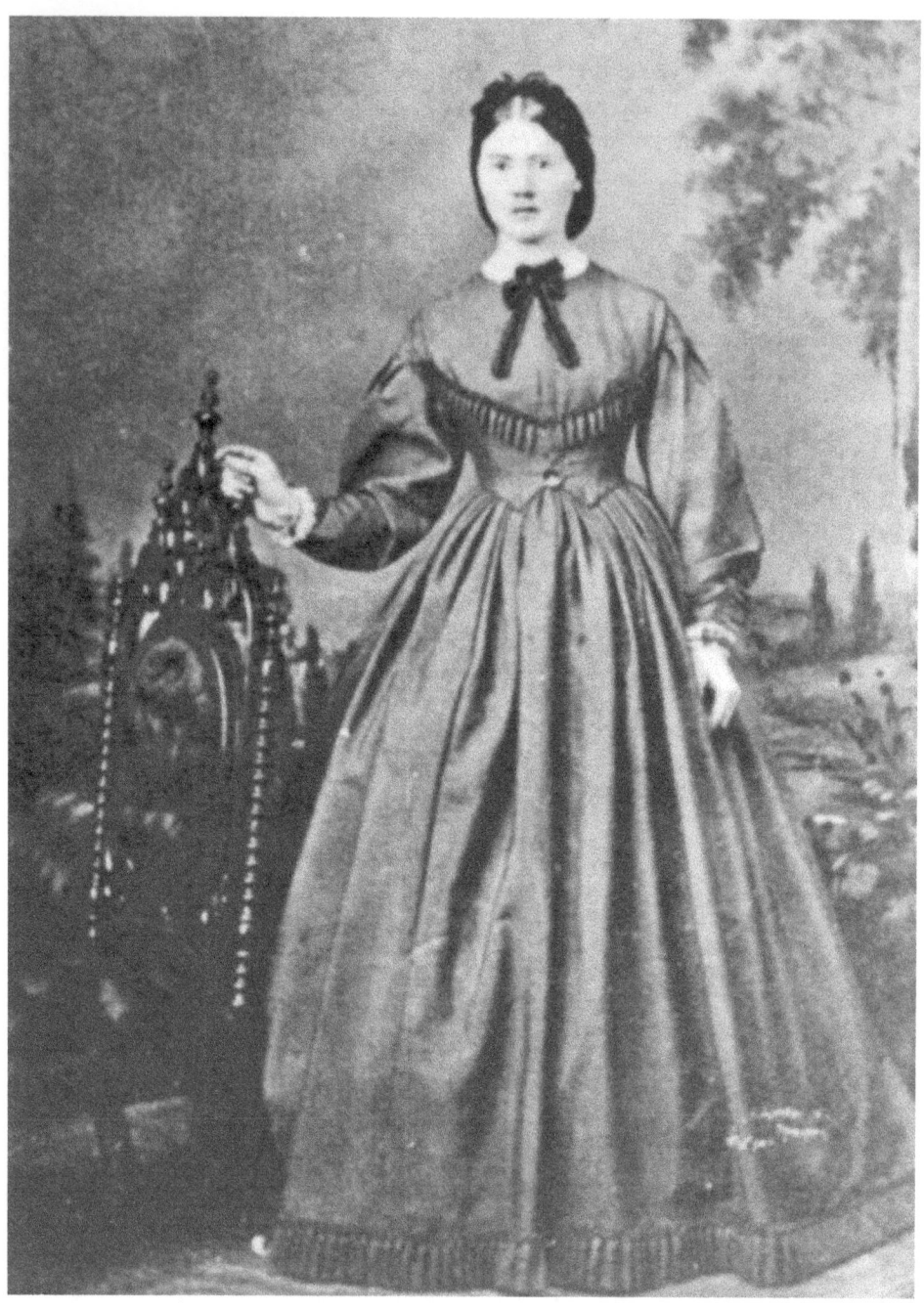

Caroline Joy Hawley, ca. 1860s (courtesy Kathryn Breuer).

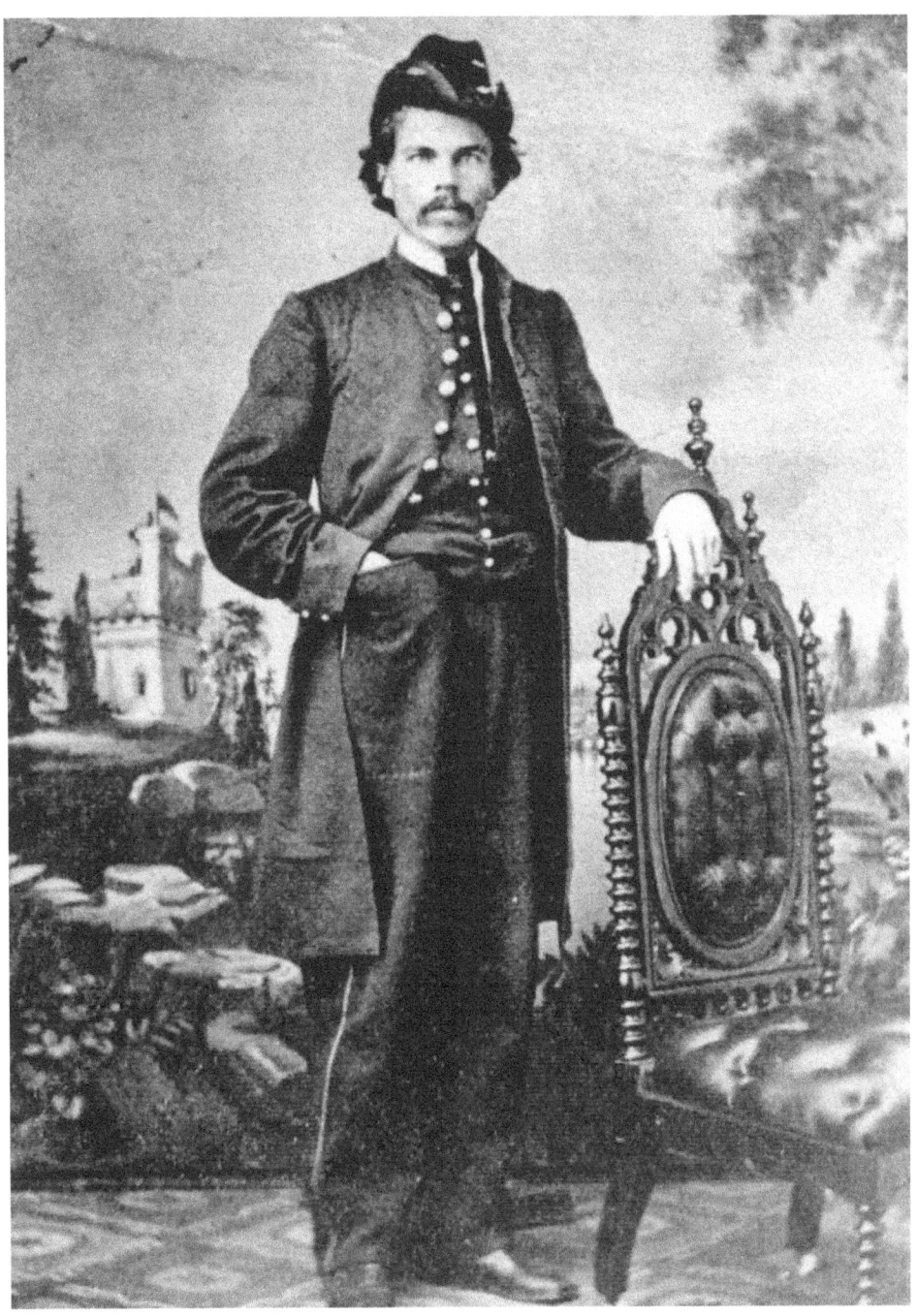

Dr. Thomas Hawley, ca. 1860s (courtesy Kathryn Breuer).

and the surrounding territory were formed into four military districts, Mobile, Montgomery, Talladega and Huntsville, reporting to General Woods. Under military control, the type of authority, either good or bad, was reflective of the character of the commander in charge of a specific geography. Fortunately, President Andrew Johnson appointed Lewis Parsons as the provisional governor of Alabama on June 21, 1865, which was an important first step in establishing civilian rule in the state.

The 11th Missouri Infantry's term of service was not over with the conclusion of the war. The conditions in Alabama, one of the most staunchly supportive states for the Confederacy, caused the United States government to station Union troops to maintain order until civil law was reestablished. The regiment and Thomas Hawley were stationed at a small town, Demopolis, located in south central Alabama. The interactions between the occupying Union Army, now United States soldiers, and the local citizens initially were pleasant. Even the interactions with the ex-Confederate soldiers were peaceful. Hawley remarked in his May 29th letter about the situation between ex-slaves and ex-masters and expressed a concern and the need for the population to care for their crops. He wrote he hoped to return to the north during the next three to four months. Finally, the local citizens spoke with him about the number of local residents who died in the recent war and he wrote about his wish the nation could reconcile and heal old wounds.

Hdquarters. 11th Mo. Inf. Vet. Vol.
Demopolis, Ala. May 29, 1865
Dear Mother,

Your dear, kind letter was welcomed by me 4 days ago. It left Olney on the 18th of April. So you see it was over one month on the long trip. Lt. Col. Green says the mail will start through via Vicksburg tomorrow. This will shorten the distance over one half, and I hope the time also. It seems so long to be without hearing from the loving ones at home. One can imagine many changes taking place in that time. I received a good letter from Sister Myra dated the 1st inst., was well satisfied and happy.

The weather here is fine and nature looks refreshing. Most of the citizens are agreeable and kind, changing for the better since our arrival. Their preconceived opinions of the Yankees was not very favorable to us, but the soldiers and officers by their kind, gentlemanly bearing are teaching them things never thought of before. As a general rule the Reb soldiers treat us courteously, and so far, we have not heard of one single instance of violence of their part. No rebel marauders or guerillas. Some of the Negroes are committing depredations on the plantations. Their idea of freedom is a life of ease and comfort without restraint or labor and most of them will not believe their former masters and run off the first opportunity to see and stay with the Yankees. They almost worship us. Some say "Hiss do Lord now we's free. We prayed for it a long, long time, now he's come, we knowed he would." If their masters have always treated them well, by persuasion and promises, they generally keep most of their hands and this is a matter of almost total importance. Just now the large corn crop must be tended or it is lost for this year, and it is their only hope of sustenance or source of income as but little cotton was planted this year.

I also hope Pa can finish the house before winter. Wish I could be there a time to assist him, but present orders indicate we will be kept here three or four months yet, until civil law is established and the old order of things ordained, minus slavery. I am well persuaded the best policy to present towards the masses of the southern people is kindness but firmness, and they will yet make good loyal citizens of the United States, better than many north. We must make a great allowance for the political and social teachings. Their supposed bound primarily allegiance due the state and only secondary to the Union. I do hope all the bitterness and hatred will forever be removed. I was told by a citizen last evening that we had no idea of the number of men kill[ed] in this part. Deserted houses and plantations are very common.

It was two months after the May letter when Thomas Hawley wrote specifically to his mother who was feeling lonely and depressed as the children were starting lives of their own and her husband continued his educational and religious efforts. Hawley wrote he had been fortunate to have the friendship of Eli Bowyer to help him through the difficult and emotional days of loneliness and absence from his family. On August 17, Thomas Hawley wrote from Marion, Alabama, in the south central part of the state. The frequency of receiving letters was slow and the last letter from his wife, Carrie, was about three weeks late.

Lieutenant Colonel Modesta Green took a portion of the regiment for garrison duty at Tuscaloosa while the remainder of the 11th Missouri performed similar duties in Marion. It was clear the soldiers were tired and ready to go home. Thomas Hawley wrote the number of desertions was high and, in fact, about 197 men deserted from the regiment, most during the occupation in Alabama and over 70 percent of the desertions were draftees and substitutes. Sensing the situation within the regiment in Alabama was reaching a critical stage, Colonel Eli Bowyer petitioned the Secretary of War to allow the regiment to be mustered out of service. This was not to occur soon and by all indications, the soldiers and officers of the regiment were not informed when they could be expected to be mustered out of service. Thomas Hawley concluded in his letter by stating he wanted his wife to come to Marion. He also stated he shared his mess with the new regimental chaplain, Rev. George Brown.

There is an addendum in this letter which noted several officers were going to send for their wives, including Colonel Eli Bowyer, Lieutenant Colonel Modesta Green, and Captain Constantine McMahan. Hawley also announced his promotion to the rank of major finally arrived and he was officially the regimental surgeon.

Hospital 11th Mo. Inf. V. V.
Marion, Ala. Aug 17th 65
Dear Mother,

I have just finished rereading your loving letter of the 1st inst. written while Pa and Sister F[annie] were in Mt. Carmel. Think I can feel some of your loneliness and sympathize with you. When all the family have left you, and Pa so much of the time in the district. It is also very true you do not look for comfort or society outside of your own family, but under the circumstances would it not be a help to have one or two true confidential friends in whom you can always place an explicit confidence? Such are hard to find and much to be valued. I have always found it necessary to my happiness and as you know, in whom I place my reliance, that is the col. Besides we each have a friend who sticketh closer than a brother. I too feel that it has been a long time since my visit home. Indeed my last one was hardly a visit home because the time there was so short but it was a very happy one for me. I do assure you, we will live in full hopes of a happy reunion at an early period, then for a long, full, joyful visit.

I feel quite sure we will see you before the holidays and we must have a good long visit together. I heard from Sister M. not long ago, all well at that time, also from Carrie up to the 28 July, quite well and able to write good loving letters, without which I would be lost. The letter from Bro. A[mos] has not made its appearance yet. I was indeed surprised to hear they were all safe in St. Louis again, after so long a time. Hope they are doing well. I will write H. by return mail. I have always been much attached to the family and always kept up a regular correspondence with Harry, although the letters often delayed and some now lost. The other members of the family I have not heard directly from for a long time.

The 6th Ills. Cavl. is being stationed in this portion of Ala. Col. Linch [Lynch] is going to Demopolis, I heard, and some are coming here. The 9th Ills. Calv. are going to Tuscaloosa Ala. 50 miles northeast of this, where the companies H, I & B of our regt. have been stationed since we left Demopolis, Al., Lt. Col. Green Cmdg. We do not yet know whether this means to relieve us or only as a support to our forces. The soldiers are growing dissatisfied and exceedingly anxious to get home. I almost fear sometimes they will rebel and go any how. Several, who are although good soldiers, have deserted. The last three months have been the hardest they ever served, according to their estimate, that is some of them. Others try to be contented and more cheerful.

The col. has petitioned the sectr. of war to have the regt. mustered out of the service just so soon as the interest of the service will permit it. The officers have joined him in this petition stating the facts in the case. I hope it may do some good. We are indeed scarce of news, only once in a great while see a northern paper. These you so kindly send me, I appreciate. The medical journals have come quite regular recently and afford some relief. We have had a long dry spell. Today, the whole town was filled with a cloud of dust penetrating into every nook and corner. I am two squares off the main road but the fine dust found its way here. So far the sick are doing quite well. I have 12 in hospital and 20 in quarters who are able to walk half a mile every day for medicines. So you see, these at least are not dangerous. The col. and adjt. are in usual health. Adjt. has offered his resignation. It may or may not be approved. Col. Green thinks of going home if he can this month on leave of absence if we remain here in act[ion]. I want my dear wife to pay us a visit. I think it would be pleasant, as the place is so healthy, people sociable and that season of the year just the right time to come south. But as I said before, I much rather we could all go home before that time and be made fine American citizens.

And now dear Ma as I have no news of importance and must write to Carrie yet tonight and it's after 9 o'c, permit me to shorten this epistle after I repeat again my words of cheer and comfort to the best of mothers. At present they are the best I have but a long chat, face-to-face, with a stolen kiss occasionally would be far preferable. Be of comfort, all things work together for our good and we will one day be there, happy for our suffering here below. Just now I am messing with the Chaplain, Mr. Brown, and two of the boys in here, a pleasant time. Yet I often think no one can prepare a meal like my Ma. Then comes the strong wish to be there and try one, and gaze longingly up [at] the dear circle of smiling faces. Please give my best love to E. Bell and ask her to answer my letter with many kisses. Love and lots of etc. to Sister Fannie with the French & music. Best brotherly love to Bro. Amos with good wishes for his success. True filial love to Father and earnest prayers for his success and health, but please remember the flesh is weak. Ma, I send you in son's warmest purest, truest love,

Yours affectionately,

T. S. Hawley

If we stay here some months yet and communications are open, some of us officers think indeed will send for our wives and at present all indications are favorable to this visit just now and we think they would enjoy the trip and we will soon be within a few days communication of Illinois besides we expect to furnish an escort. Col. Bowyer will send for his wife and daughter. Lt. Col. Green *for his wife. Adjt. Finch, also Capt. Mc. will go for his and I shall be happy to see Carrie here if all the good friends think best and I think they will. I need not assure you, home would be far more desirable to me and I guess the others but as the land is at peace, railroads open and all things pleasant and favorable, a visit of a few weeks or months would be most pleasant. This is a quiet, healthy little town in a fine country but I will tell you more of this trip when it is sure, which cannot be for some weeks. Capt. Kendall will muster out in June as he is then three years, and officer. The col. thinks my commission will come some of these days. I will then muster as major as it will not keep me any longer than my present work. But it may not come as my time is so near out. I have just finished rereading your good letter of the 18th ultimo. Many thanks for this good letter. I have tried to write as usual but often could not send them, and I guess some have been lost. I have tried to answer all inquiries. If I have not always, ask fully. It does my heart good to hear all the dear friends speak so endearingly of my darling wife and especially my loving mother. I hope we can ever be a source of happiness and comfort to our dear parents. Carrie often speaks in the most affectionate terms of her new mother & father. I have no help yet and a number of men sick, thirty or more, none bad. I use a small house as hospital. All your friends are well. I send much love and kisses for papers. You was always the best of mothers to me. My love to you is ever growing stronger, nearer and dearer. Much best love to Pa, Ma, bro. & sisters.*

Your very affectionate son,

Thos. S. Hawley

On August 25, Thomas Hawley wrote his weekly letter from Marion, Alabama, and he reported the weather was hot and dry. The dust permeated everything. The attitude of the soldiers was poor and they were becoming more insubordinate as the summer progressed. Thievery was rampant in the countryside as civil law was being restored. Hawley wrote he did not trust the Alabamans with the full control of the law, but on a positive note several of the wives of the officers were scheduled to arrive at the post.

Thomas Hawley's letter of August 25 may be one of his most prophetic letters as he predicted someday someone might want to capture his experiences of the war and he wrote a message to the readers. If he wrote 200 letters as he mentioned, about half of the letters have been preserved which is an amazing accomplishment. The message he wrote in this letter to future generations was a tribute to his character. He was devoted to his duty and he was very human as he was swept through the war years in some of the darkest days in American history.

Hospital 11th Mo. Inf. V. V.
Marion, Ala. Aug 25th 1865

Dear Father & Mother,

This is to be the usual weekly letter about the fifth volume and number over 200. I suppose if all these ever collected, written during my five years of absence, rather think I would hardly follow all of them. Some breathing cheerfulness, hope and warm with love. Others full of strong desire and firm determination. Many almost with repetitions of former letters, some dull and are barely readable. Yet they have all been under peculiar circumstances. We are all creatures of circumstances. So of course these notes, by the way, must partake somewhat of the surroundings.

If I have ever said anything wrong or calculated to wound any one's feelings, I chance pardon. If I have been amiss in duty, it was not through want of desire to do it, but because the body was weak or weary. I have always tried to comply with my promises and perform my duties near as possible. Often weak, weary and sick at heart. These 4 years of terrible war have been trying ones to me. Yet thank the Lord, his grace has always been sufficient for me. His shield has ever been over me in the hours of danger. How much I am indebted to the prayers of the righteous ones at home I can never tell, but I shall always try to be thankful for them and strive to visit them so far as able.

My health is quite good for this climate this time of year. The weather is quite cool this morning, promising rain, which rain is needed very much. Everything is parched and dried up. The dust is fine as flour flowing into everybody's eyes, ears, nose & mouth, penetrating into the most secluded nooks & cranny of these abodes. The soldiers are inclined to be insubordinate and discontented, want to go home and leave these rebels to themselves. Indeed I think it would make but little difference as social life is in discord and every man fears his next neighbor. Law and order has given place to chance and anarchy. Thieves mature their plans at day time and carry them into effect at night. I never saw or heard of such a state of things. Almost all kinds of valuable property is unsafe. Stock and cotton especially is changing hands rapidly at this time.

And I suppose we must stay to keep the thieves in abeyance until civil law reigns again all over the distracted land. Perhaps all winter, it looks so at present. I fear we cannot trust the Reb task masters in full power of the law, just yet. They do not manifest the spirit of repentance and loyalty enough to entitle them to any favor. The officers & men in usual health. Mrs. Col. Green will be here tomorrow. Mrs. Lt. McNeal from Springfield, Ohio, came Monday. I hope somebody else will come from Ohio soon. Col. Green has applied for leave of absence and Mrs. Green surprises him in this wilderness of rascals. I have not heard from Carrie for about one month. If we stay I want her to come or start about the middle of Sept. It is almost hoping against hope to think of coming home before Dec. Nevertheless I hope we will. Much best love to all the dear ones at home. Fannie, Eva Bell, I send kisses for a letter. Please all write soon and remember me to all kind and inquiring friends.

Your affct. son & bro.,

Thomas

By October 1865 the remaining time in Alabama for the 11th Missouri Veteran Infantry was short, but no one of the regiment was aware of this. Some of the officer's wives had arrived, but Carrie Hawley had not yet arrived. The regiment had moved back to Demopolis and in the opinion of Thomas Hawley, this location was not as favorable as Marion, Alabama. He made the acquaintance of a Doctor Bailey, originally of Palmyra, Missouri, who had served in the Confederate Army and was impressed with him as an individual. As the civil authority in Alabama was forming it was decided the state should have a militia, but this concerned Hawley. The thought of armed Southerners so soon after the last war was disturbing and he felt the newly freed slaves would again be at risk of losing what had been so dearly won during the war. He also pointed out the new unscrupulous, scourge to the Southerners, the carpetbaggers, who the held power in the newly forming government.

Thomas Hawley recorded the soldiers of the regiment were still discontented. The supplies, food, clothing and discipline were lacking. He concluded his letter with hopes the regiment would soon be mustered out of service.

Demopolis, Alabama
October 8th 1865

Dear Parents,

I have been rather postponing writing to you because I thought Carrie would be here by the 5th inst. George Adams saw Capt. Mc[Mahan] last Monday and informed us when he arrived Friday that Mc. would start Wednesday. So we look for them positively Monday or Tuesday. If they do not come tomorrow, I will go to Meridian and meet them. I have not heard from home or Carrie for a long time. I cannot account for it as the mails arrive much earlier now than formerly by the Ohio & Mobile Railroad.

Thanks for [the] opportune arrival of the medical journal and the Cincin[nati] papers.

I commenced a letter some days ago and after all only wrote a hasty note which I was ashamed to send. Col B[owyer] is not looking for his daughter, does not want her to come now, since we left Marion, as the school advantages are all lost and this a much more unpleasant place to live in and the society and accom-

modations much poorer. The aristocracy are rampant rebels, and will not care for the poorer and suffering classes. Finch and I had quite a time to get boarding. I have a nice place, very pleasant family, and am at home with pleasant fix ups.

Dr. Bailey from Palmyra, Mo. has been the medical purveyor in the Confederate Army. I esteem him as quite a gentleman and estimable Dr. in the profession. His wife is a fine, kind hearted lady. They do not put on much style nor take boarders to make money. The civil authorities are organizing the state militia by consent of the President and authority of the provisional governor. I fear there may be a clash between them and the regular U. S. soldiers and that, if in their power, they will oppress the "poor Niggers." Yes, they will shoot and grind down the darkies that try and are succeeding. The grand, grand quality of this place found a true bill against one enterprising darkie because he had kept a restaurant of small, though neat dimensions, a few days after the municipal law had been established, although not published. As he could not give bail for $200 was sent to the county jail 18 miles away from his defenseless wife and children. All this while thousands of poor white-trash steal and commit all forms of crimes without being brought to justice. One, a dubbed Brig. Genl., Dustan, once commander of a few worthless militia at Memphis, Tenn., an ex-cotton agent, says he made over $50,000 at this place in less than three months. Boasts he has curtailed expenses in the last few weeks, as he now only spends $2,500 in one week and [you] must know this money comes from what rightfully belongs to Uncle Sam. Yet this rascal goes unhung, rides his fine horses and goes in the best society. Horses, mules, cotton and other property is being stolen almost every night near us. The weather has been very dry for some weeks about Demopolis. The dust is fine and penetrates in every nook and corner.

The rainy season sets in soon, then the roads are next to impassable. Mud, mud for [tear in letter]. I could not be compelled to live in this county for any consideration, i. e., just in or around Demopolis.

I think they can dispense with our services as soldiers in this state in three months at the farthest. All military organizations are confused, most confounded, all the officers and soldiers think Uncle Sam is not fulfilling his part of the contract with us and they are not disposed to do duty or suffer from poor clothing, lack of pay or poor rations without complaining & murmurings.

If this state militia are permitted to keep up their organization and do well, they may eventually take our place and we [will] be permitted to go home. Oh Bright Hope, to see the dear ones and enjoy all the blessed privileges of civil life to be again a "Free American Citizen" If we must stay some time longer with Carrie, my darling wife here, I will be very happy as under our circumstances here, could it be otherwise. I am all anxiety—and desire to see and be with her, the choice of my heart, of my friends, bosom companion for life, through its adversities and prosperities, the sharer of my joys and sorrows, my life, my beloved wife. My heart is overflowing with thankfulness and gratitude. My health is good as usual. So of the others. Please give my love to all, Fannie, Evie Bell, Bro. Amos, Sister Myra, Bro. Will, Coz Dode. Compliments to Mr. & Mrs. Geo. Gunn and other friends. I hope you enjoyed conference and remain as best suits you. I am as ever your loving and affct. son,

Thos. S. Hawley

The last letter written by Thomas Hawley in a Union uniform was written on December 22, 1865, and although he was unsure of the reason for moving from Demopolis to Memphis, he and the rest of the 11th Missouri Veteran Infantry were scheduled to be mustered out of service on January 16, 1866. This concluded four and half years of service. Hawley wrote, "Our hearts leap with joy at the idea of going home." Although his wife was with him, he was finally going home to start a life as a simple United States citizen. Thomas Hawley was only 28 years old, but he had lived a lifetime in the past four years. He had done his duty and matured. He had medical experiences which he might never have had in a career as a civilian doctor and he had helped preserve the Union. No one could have asked for more.

Demopolis, Ala.
Dec. 22, 1865

Dear Parents, Bro. and Sisters,

At last we have marching orders to report to Maj. Genl. Jno. E. Smith at Memphis, Tenn. Nothing said about mustering out, but we hope for the best. By the time this reaches you, you may know something about it. We hear there is a prospect of some trouble with England and some timid ones fear this is the cause of our order in haste to Memphis. The order came by telegraph from Genl. Woods at Mobile. Col. Eli Bowyer is at Montgomery attending a court martial as witness for some of our officers, but is expected back soon, as he was telegraphed today. Dear Wife and I will bring up our command in a few days, will go by rail to Meridian & Corinth. The order implied more haste than was consistent with just a muster out, as we could of course take our time for it. Most all the sick are able to go, indeed, but two confined to their beds at this time. Co. A, Capt. McMahan cmdg., will remain behind until relieved by other troops. Some say Negro troops and we are glad of it. For these citizens deserve to be ordered around by darkies, who they so much despise and indeed have despised us and treated us most shamefully by reports, most false & slanderous, to the gov[ernor] and he to the cmdg. general who was foolish enough to believe it.

I need not tell you our hearts leap with abounding joy at the idea of going home, if we were only sure it was so. Demopolis is not large enough to hold us

all. All the boys go around with smiling faces. The prospect is brightening to all you see, but all the time will come up the fear this is not as it should be. They may perhaps keep us still longer in the service. We will trust all is working for the best, look on the bright side of the picture.

Oh! how we would like to clasp each of the dear home friends in our arms, sit down among and be one of you for an infinite time when none dare to molest or make us afraid of military orders, court martials, etc. To be or not to be again a free American citizen by our own orders, march to our own time and music, halt at will, camp at pleasure, etc. One thing makes us glad, this we are sure of being relieved of this place—mud, mud and secesh cornbread, without one ray of unionism, are not congenial to good tempers and healthy digestion. We hope to leave them behind without many tears, shaking the mud from our feet as a testimony of their many sins, moral and national. Darling wife will write a few lines. We cannot possibly quite spend [the] holiday with you. May come soon after, hoping for the best. We congenially send a world of hopeful, endearing love to all. Will write soon as we arrive in Memphis, before, if time. Each in good health and in fine spirits. Yours affectionately,

Thos. S. Hawley

On January 16, 1866, after four and half years of service to his country, Thomas Hawley was mustered out of service in Memphis, Tennessee. Along with the remainder of the 11th Missouri Infantry he returned to civilian life. At the end of the Civil War, Thomas Hawley was rewarded for his service in the Union Army by settling in St. Louis with his wife Carrie, just as he had predicted in his letters written during the war. Thomas and Carrie Hawley lived a happy and contented life in St. Louis and the couple had six children: Martha (May) May, Elizabeth (Lizzie) Phelps, Nelson Joy, Thomas Goodale, Wilder Hayes, and Carrie Belle.

Of Thomas' siblings, Amos Augustus Hawley died on April 4, 1867 at the age of 27 years. He was an unhealthy man and no cause of death was recorded. A letter from Carrie

Dr. Thomas Hawley, Grand Army of the Republic photograph, ca. 1900 (Missouri History Museum, St. Louis, Missouri).

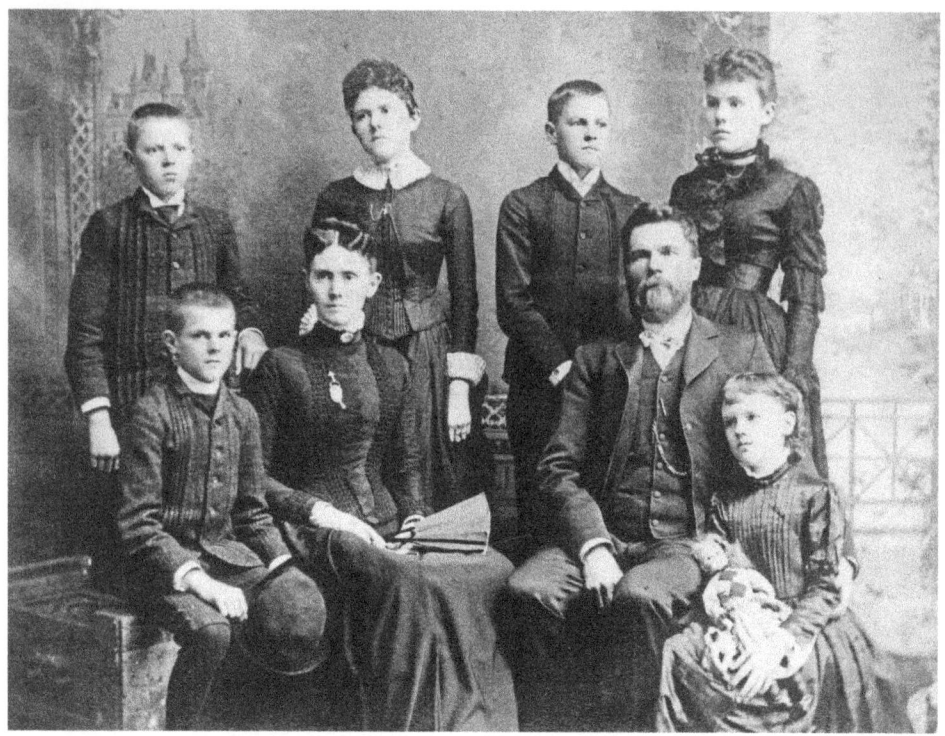

Thomas Hawley and family (courtesy Kathryn Breuer).

Hawley stated Amos died suddenly, presumably of the aliments which plagued him during the time of Thomas' correspondence. He was buried at Haven Hill Cemetery in Olney, Illinois.

Maria (Myra) Denning Hawley (1842–1914) lived until 1914. Maria and William Reed were married in 1865 and the couple moved to Middletown, Ohio. William Reed was a successful businessman in various trades. Reed operated a general merchandise business for 25 years. In 1890, the couple moved to Chicago where Reed operated a livery business. Maria and William Reed had five children — Nelson, William, Rella, Eugene and Frank. While Marie had a successful marriage, she experienced much unhappiness in regard to her children. Maria's son, Nelson died in infancy, Rella was born in 1868 but died while attending the Louisville Female Seminary in Louisville, Kentucky in 1887. Frank also died at young age in 1893 at the age of 19 and Eugene, a successful businessman, died in January 1909 at the age of 28 in Chicago. Maria outlived four of her children and only one child, William, remained alive at the time of her death. Maria died on December 28, 1914 and her husband William died in 1925.[3]

Helen Frances (1848–1874) married Harvey Johnson and she died at the young age of 26 on July 4, 1874. Helen died within days of giving birth to her first child. The child also did not survive more than a few months. Helen (Fanny) was buried at Haven Hill Cemetery in Olney, Illinois.[4]

Eva Belle (1856–?) married Frank Turner in Chicago, Illinois, and the couple had three children — Frank, Hawley and Maud. Frank Turner was an attorney, businessman, successful real estate agent and the couple lived in Chicago in 1900. Unfortunately, Maud died at the age of 9 in St. Louis of the enlargement of the heart. In 1910 the family lived in Pasadena Ward in Los Angeles.

Thomas's father, the Rev. Nelson Hawley, lived until December 24, 1876, and his mother lived with Thomas in St. Louis after the death of Nelson. Elizabeth Phelps Swearingen Hawley died on December 3, 1886, of a cerebral hemorrhage in St. Louis and was buried in Olney, Illinois.

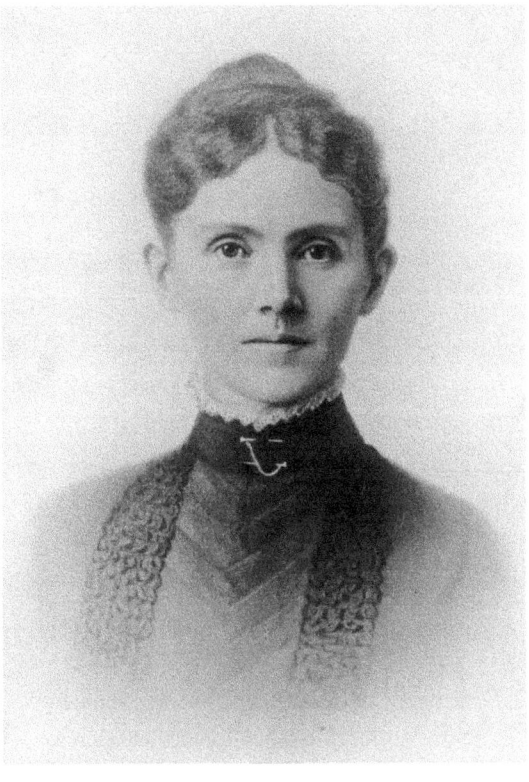

Caroline "Carrie" Joy Hawley (courtesy Kathryn Breuer).

The love of Thomas Hawley's life Caroline Joy Hawley died on January 11, 1890 in St. Louis of pneumonia and Thomas never remarried.

Thomas remained part of the Republican Party and was active in the 11th Congressional District Republican Committee. He was member of the Ransom Post of the Grand Army of the Republic and served as a medical review professional for pensioners. He established his practice at 247 Carr Street in St. Louis. He also served on the Board of Pension Examiners in St. Louis where he guided physicians as they dealt with requests from Civil War soldiers for government pensions. Thomas Hawley lived a quiet and productive life as a physician and was recognized as one the "notable men of St. Louis."

Being a religious person Thomas Hawley was asked about entering the

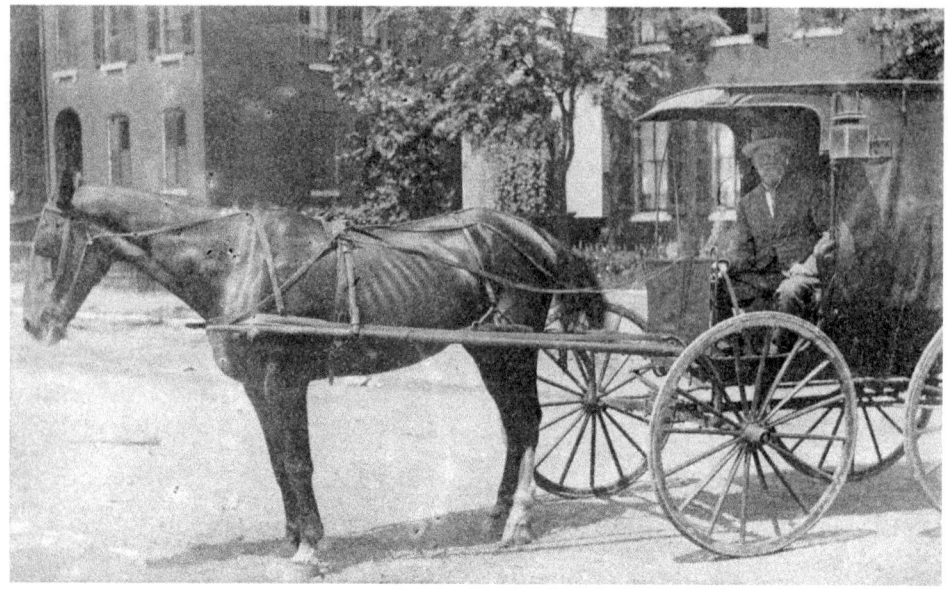

Thomas Hawley and horse and carriage (courtesy Joan Garvin).

ministry, he answered, "I wanted to do good in the world, so chose the medical profession rather than the ministry, as I felt I could then help people both physically and spiritually."[5] Thomas also stated his ambition was his six children should have a good education. Although he desired to leave each of his children $5,000, he was unable to do so.

Thomas Hawley so loved flowers he was never without them and he boasted a beautiful garden at his home after the war. He also liked woodworking and working around the house. The Hawley family lived in a home on Easton Avenue in St. Louis. Thomas devoted his Friday evenings to "romp with his boys and girls," and played blind man's bluff, I-spy, pussy-in-the-corner in his fourteen-room home. As the children grew older, the home was a scene of more theatrical activities for the children, including, songs, speeches, and home theatricals. The Hawley home was also a menagerie of animals, including, dogs, cats, goats, chickens, horses, canaries and a mockingbird at various times.

Thomas Hawley died at his residence at 3065 Easton Avenue in St. Louis on July 24, 1918, at the age of 81. He died of cerebral apoplexy and was buried at Bellefontaine Cemetery in St. Louis.[6]

Fortunately, Thomas liked to sit for photographs and as a result several images of him and his family exist today. More importantly, Thomas Hawley compulsively liked to write letters which have remained his legacy by offering

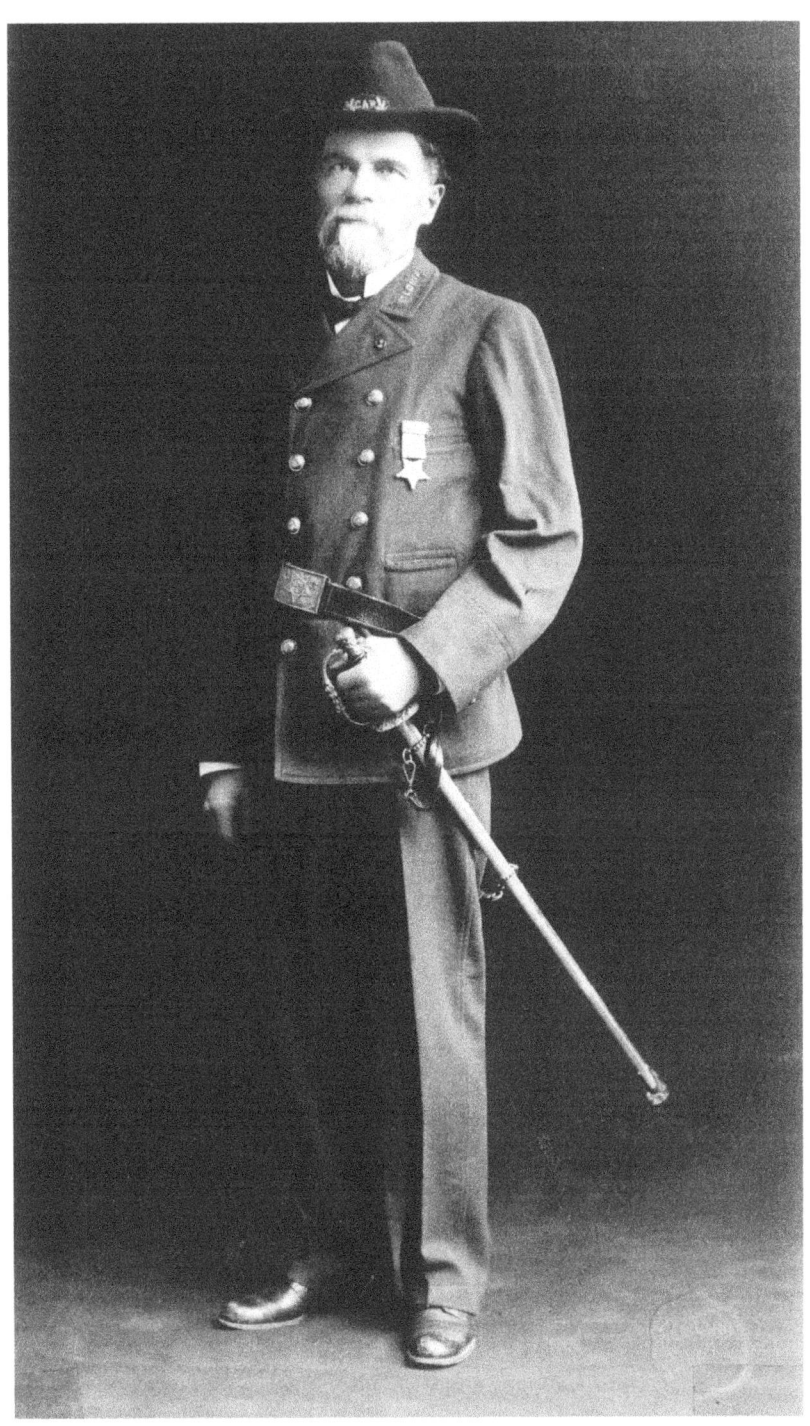

Thomas Hawley in uniform (courtesy Joan Garvin).

insight into a painful period in United States history. The Thomas Hawley letters offer a rare insight into the life of a medical professional in the western theatre of the Civil War. Hawley stated he felt he was a man of circumstances and in many ways was not in control of his life. Thomas Hawley knew his conscience required him to fight for his country in its hour of need and he gave four and half years of his young life to fulfill his life's calling. Because he was so faithful in his writing he was able to share his life with those who followed.

Chapter Notes

Preface Notes

1. Thomas Hawley, letter, August 25, 1865, Thomas Hawley Papers, 1856–1867, A0666, Missouri Historical Society, St. Louis, Missouri.

Introduction

1. William Parrish, *History of Missouri, 1860–1875*, Vol. III (Columbia: University of Missouri Press, 1997), p. 4.
2. Wiley Britton, *The Civil War on the Border* (New York and London: G.P. Putnam's Sons, 1899), p.1.
3. Parrish, p. 12
4. Thomas Hawley, family records, Hawley Papers, 1794–1953 (bulk 1857–1953), David M. Rubenstein Rare Book and Manuscript Library, Duke University. Durham, North Carolina.
5. Thomas Hawley, letter, August 25, 1865. Thomas Hawley Papers, 1856–1867. A0666. Missouri Historical Society, St. Louis, Missouri.

Chapter One

1. Stewart Sifakis, *Who Was Who in the Civil War* (New York, Oxford: Facts on File, 1988), p. 78.
2. Jefferson Davis, *The Rise and Fall of the Confederacy* (New York: D. Appleton, 1881), p. 417.
3. William Parrish, *History of Missouri, 1860–1875,* Vol. III (Columbia: University of Missouri Press, 1997), p. 22.
4. Nancy Williams, ed., *Arkansas Biography: A Collection of Notable Lives* (Fayetteville: University of Arkansas Press, 2000), pp. 41–42.
5. Clara Kennan, "Dr. Thomas Smith: Forgotten Man of Arkansas Education." *Arkansas Historical Quarterly.* Vol. 20, No. 4. (1961). pp. 309–310.
6. Eleventh Missouri Infantry, Descriptive Rolls, National Archives, Washington, D.C. 1861.
7. "Eli Bowyer," *Olney Times*, March 10, 1886.
8. Tom Kirkwood, *A History of Lawrence County Physicians and a Review of Medicine as Practiced 100 Years Ago* (Evansville, Ind.: Lawrence County Historical Society Unigraphic, 1975), pp. 19–20.
9. George Cullum, *Biographical Register of the Officers and Graduates of U. S. Military Academy, Vol. II* (Cambridge, Mass.: Houghton, Mifflin, 1891), pp. 85–86.

10. James E. McGhee, "'A Damned Tight Place': General Jeff Thompson Confronts the Federals at Fredericktown, Missouri," *Missouri Historical Review* (April 2009) pp. 150–154.

11. Eleventh Missouri Infantry, Descriptive Rolls, National Archives, Washington, D.C., 1861.

Chapter Two

1. William S. Stewart, papers, 1861–1864, (C2991), letter, January 12, 1862, Western Historical Manuscript Collection, Columbia, University of Missouri / State Historical Society of Missouri.

2. Thomas Smith, April 4, 1862, Compiled service records of volunteer Union soldiers who served in organizations from the state of Missouri, National Archives, Washington, D.C., 1962.

3. Compiled service records of volunteer Union soldiers who served in organizations from the state of Missouri, National Archives, Washington, D.C., 1962.

4. Melanchthon Fish, Civil War Pension Record, National Archives, Washington, D.C.

5. Eleventh Missouri Infantry, Morning Reports, National Archives, Washington, D.C., May, 1862.

6. Thomas Hawley, letter- August 1, 1862. Compiled service records of volunteer Union soldiers who served in organizations from the state of Missouri, National Archives, Washington, D.C., 1962.

7. Russ A. Pritchard, Jr., *Raiders of the Civil War: Untold Stories of Actions Behind the Lines* (Guilford, Conn.: Lyons Press, 2005), pp. 66–69.

8. Robert Murphy, *The War of the Rebellion: A Compilation of the Official Records of the Union and Confederate Armies, Series I, Vol. 24* (Washington, D.C.: U.S. Government Printing Office, 1880–1901), p. 509.

9. Anne Razey Gowdy, *A Sherwood Bonner Sampler, 1869–1884* (Knoxville: University of Tennessee Press, 2000), pp. xiii–xiv.

10. Frank Moore, *Rebellion Record: A Diary of American Events*, Vol. 6. "Richmond Dispatch Account" (New York: G. P. Putnam, 1863), pp. 280–2.

Chapter Three

1. Samuel Baldridge, resignation letter, November 12, 1862, Compiled service records of volunteer Union soldiers who served in organizations from the state of Missouri, National Archives, Washington, D.C., 1962.

2. Stephen Morse, "Historical Perspectives of Modern Bioterrorism," in *Microorganisms and Bioterrorism*, Burt Anderson, Herman Friedman, and Mauro Bendinelli, eds. (New York: Springer, 2006), p. 16.

3. Joseph Brooks, letter, April 1, 1862, compiled service records of volunteer Union soldiers who served in organizations from the state of Missouri, National Archives, Washington, D.C., 1962.

4. Baldridge, letter, November 12, 1862. Compiled service records of volunteer Union soldiers who served in organizations from the state of Missouri, National Archives, Washington, D.C. 1962.

5. Andrew Brown, "Sol Street, Confederate. Partisan Leader," *Journal of Mississippi History*, Vol. 21, No. 3 (July 1959), pp. 155–173.

6. William Oathcart, *The Doctrines, Ordinances, Usages, Confessions of Faith, Sufferings, Labors, and Successes, And Of the General History of the Baptist Denomination in All Lands* (Philadelphia: Louis Everts, 1881), p. 913.

7. William Notestine, letter, June 12, 1863, Civil War Pension File, National Archives, Washington, D.C.
8. Duncan McCall, *Three Years in the Service: Record of the Doings of the Eleventh Reg. Missouri*. (Springfield, Mo.: Johnson & Bradford, 1864), p. 26.
9. Joseph Johnston, *The War of the Rebellion: A Compilation of the Official Records of the Union and Confederate Armies*, Series I, Vol. 36 *(Washington, D.C.: U.S. Government Printing Office, 1880–1901), p.* 215.
10. "Another Disaster on the Mississippi; Explosion of the Ammunition Steamer City of Madison," *New York Times*, August 26, 1863.
11. T.E. Vineyard, *Battles of the Civil War*, (Chicago: Hammond, 1914), p. 110.
12. Thomas Hawley, Hospital Casualty List: Vicksburg. Thomas Hawley Papers, 1856–1867, A0666, Missouri Historical Society Archives. St. Louis, Missouri.
13. Edward Nelson, ed., *Quinquennial Catalogue of the Ohio Wesleyan University, 1842–1886* (Delaware, Oh.: Ohio Wesleyan Publishing, 1886), p. 101.

Chapter Four

1. Eleventh Missouri Correspondence Book, Special Field Order No. 14, March 6, 1864, National Archives, Washington, D.C.
2. Galusha Anderson, *The Story of a Border City During the Civil War* (Boston: Little, Brown, 1908), pp. 309–314.
3. William Sherman, *The War of the Rebellion: A Compilation of the Official Records of the Union and Confederate Armies*, Series I ,Vol. 76 (Washington, D.C.: U.S. Government Printing Office, 1880–1901), pp. 16–17.
4. Michael Ballard, *The Battle of Tupelo, Mississippi: July 14 and 15, 1864* (Tupelo: Northeast Mississippi Historical and Genealogical Society, 2009), p. 5.
5. Charles Treadway, *The Letters of Charles Wesley Treadway: Foot Prints: Past and Present,* Vol. 9 (Olney, Ill.: Richland County Genealogical and Historical Society, 1986), pp. 140–141.
6. Ballard, p. 10.
7. Compiled Service Records, Field and Staff record, Compiled service records of volunteer Union soldiers who served in organizations from the state of Missouri, National Archives, Washington, D.C., 1962.
8. Treadway, pp. 145–146.

Chapter Five

1. Charles Treadway, *The Letters of Charles Wesley Treadway: Foot Prints: Past and Present*. Vol. 9. (Olney, Ill.: Richland County Genealogical and Historical Society, 1986), p. 148.
2. Sean Michael O'Brien, *Mobile, 1865: Last Stand of the Confederacy* (Westport, Conn.: Praeger, 2001), p. 45.
3. *Manufacturing and Wholesale Industries of Chicago* (Chicago: Thomas B. Poole, 1918), p. 327.
4. H.H. Sweringen, *Family Register of Gerret Van Sweringen and Descendants* (Muncie, Ind.: privately printed, 1906), p. 10.
5. Elizabeth Hawley Locher, *Memoirs of My Beloved Father, Dr. Thomas Hawley*, unpublished, Hawley Family Archives.
6. Thomas Hawley, Death Certificate 791–25089, July 25, 1919, Missouri State Board of Health, Bureau of Vital Statistics.

Bibliography

Anderson, Galusha. *The Story of a Border City during the Civil War.* Boston: Little, Brown, 1908.
"Another Disaster on the Mississippi: Explosion of the Ammunition Steamer City of Madison." *New York Times.* August 26, 1863.
Baldridge, Samuel. Resignation letter. November 12, 1862. Compiled service records of volunteer Union soldiers who served in organizations from the state of Missouri. National Archives. Washington, D.C., 1962.
Ballard, Michael. *The Battle of Tupelo, Mississippi: July 14 and 15, 1864.* Tupelo: Northeast Mississippi Historical and Genealogical Society, 2009.
Britton, Wiley. *The Civil War on the Border.* New York and London: G. P. Putnam's Sons, 1899.
Brown, Andrew. "Sol Street, Confederate. Partisan Leader." *Journal of Mississippi History,* Volume 21, Number 3 (July 1959).
Brooks, Joseph. Letter, April 1, 1862. Compiled service records of volunteer Union soldiers who served in organizations from the state of Missouri. National Archives, Washington, D.C. 1962.
Compiled service records of volunteer Union soldiers who served in organizations from the state of Missouri. National Archives. Washington, D.C., 1962.
Cullum, George. *Biographical Register of the Officers and Graduates of U.S. Military Academy. Vol. II.* Cambridge, Mass.: Houghton, Mifflin and Company, 1891.
Davis, Jefferson. *The Rise and Fall of the Confederacy.* New York: D. Appleton, 1881.
Eleventh Missouri Correspondence Book. Special Field Order No. 14. March 6, 1864. National Archives, Washington, D.C.
Eleventh Missouri Infantry. Descriptive Rolls. National Archives, Washington, D.C., 1861.
Eleventh Missouri Infantry. Morning Reports. National Archives, Washington, D.C., May, 1862.
"Eli Bowyer." *Olney Times.* March 10, 1886.
Fish, Melanchthon. Civil War Pension Record. National Archives, Washington, D.C.
Gowdy, Anne Razey. *A Sherwood Bonner Sampler, 1869–1884,* Knoxville: University of Tennessee Press, 2000.
Hawley, Thomas. Death Certificate 791-25089. July 25, 1919. Missouri State Board of Health, Bureau of Vital Statistics.
Hawley, Thomas. Family Records. Hawley Papers, 1794–1953 (bulk 1857–1953).

David M. Rubenstein Rare Book and Manuscript Library, Duke University. Durham, North Carolina.

Hawley, Thomas. Hospital Casualty List: Vicksburg. Thomas Hawley Papers, 1856–1867. A0666. Missouri Historical Society Archives. St. Louis, Missouri.

Hawley, Thomas. Letter, August 1, 1862. Compiled service records of volunteer Union soldiers who served in organizations from the state of Missouri. National Archives, Washington, D.C. 1962.

Hawley, Thomas. Thomas Hawley Papers, 1856–1867. A0666. Missouri Historical Society Archives, St. Louis, Missouri.

Johnston, Joseph. *The War of the Rebellion: A Compilation of the Official Records of the Union and Confederate Armies.* Vol . 36. Washington, D.C.: U. S. Government Printing Office, 1880–1901.

Kennan, Clara. "Dr. Thomas Smith: Forgotten Man of Arkansas Education." *Arkansas Historical Quarterly,* Vol. 20, No. 4 (1961).

Kirkwood, Tom. *A History of Lawrence County Physicians and a Review of Medicine as Practiced 100 Years Ago.* Evansville, Ind.: Lawrence County Historical Society, Unigraphic, 1975)

Locher, Elizabeth Hawley. *Memoirs of My Beloved Father, Dr. Thomas Hawley.* Unpublished. Hawley Family Archives. Undated.

Manufacturing and Wholesale Industries of Chicago. Chicago: Thomas B. Poole, 1918.

McCall, Duncan. *Three Years in the Service: Record of the Doings of the Eleventh Reg. Missouri.* Springfield, Mo: Johnson and Bradford, 1864.

McGhee, James E. "'A Damned Tight Place': General Jeff Thompson Confronts the Federals at Fredericktown, Missouri." *Missouri Historical Review* (April 2009).

Moore, Frank. *Rebellion Record: A Diary of American Events.* Volume 6. "Richmond Dispatch Account." New York: G. P. Putnam, 1863.

Morse, Stephen, "Historical Perspectives of Modern Bioterrorism," Burt Anderson, Herman Friedman, and Mauro Bendinelli, eds. in *Microorganisms and Bioterrorism.* New York: Springer, 2006.

Murphy, Robert. *The War of the Rebellion: A Compilation of the Official Records of the Union and Confederate Armies,* Vol. 24. Washington, D.C.: U.S. Government Printing Office, 1880–1901.

Nelson, Edward, ed. *Quinquennial Catalogue of the Ohio Wesleyan University, 1842–1886.* Delaware, Oh.: Ohio Wesleyan, 1886.

Notestine, William. Letter, June 12, 1863. Civil War Pension File. National Archives, Washington, D.C.

Oathcart, William. *The Doctrines, Ordinances, Usages, Confessions of Faith, Sufferings, Labors, and Successes, And of the General History of the Baptist Denomination in All Lands.* Philadelphia: Louis Everts, 1881.

O'Brien, Sean Michael. *Mobile, 1865: Last Stand of the Confederacy.* Westport, Conn: Praeger, 2001.

Parrish, William. *History of Missouri 1860–1875,* Vol. III. Columbia: University of Missouri Press, 1997.

Pritchard, Russ A., Jr. *Raiders of the Civil War: Untold Stories of Actions behind the Lines.* Guilford, Conn.: Lyons, 2005.

Sifakis, Stewart. *Who Was Who in the Civil War.* New York, Oxford: Facts on File, 1988.

Sherman, William. *The War of the Rebellion: A Compilation of the Official Records of the Union and Confederate Armies,* Vol. 76. Washington, D.C.: U.S. Government Printing Office, 1880–1901.

Smith, Thomas. April 4, 1862. Compiled service records of volunteer Union soldiers who served in organizations from the state of Missouri. National Archives, Washington, D.C., 1962.

Stewart, William S. Papers, 1861–1864 (C2991). January 12, 1862. Western Historical Manuscript Collection, Columbia. University of Missouri/State Historical Society of Missouri.

Sweringen, H. H. *Family Register of Gerret Van Sweringen and Descendants.* Muncie, Ind.: Privately printed, 1906.

Treadway, Charles. *The Letters of Charles Wesley Treadway: Foot Prints: Past and Present,* Vol. 9. Olney, Ill.: Richland County Genealogical and Historical Society, 1986.

Vineyard, T. E. *Battles of the Civil War.* Chicago: Hammond, 1914.

Williams, Nancy, ed. *Arkansas Biography: A Collection of Notable Lives.* Fayetteville: University of Arkansas Press, 2000.

Index

Numbers in **_bold italics_** indicate pages with photographs.

Abbeyville, skirmish at 2, 202, 205, 220
Adams, Capt. George 236
Alabama Infantry, 37th 128
amputation surgery 31
Anderson, William 209, 212

Baker, H.C. 36–37, 50, 96, 103, 112, 114
Baldridge, the Rev. Samuel 78, 80–81, 83, 89, 91
Banks, Gen. Nathaniel 172, 187
Barney, Cal 103–104, 109
Barnum, Col. William 153–154, 162, 173–174, 176, 182–183, 187, 196, 199–200, 202–**_203_**, 214–215
Bayles, David 21–22, 26, 29, 34–38; rumor of arrest 29
Belleville 11, 13, 51, 62, 104, 178, 204
Belmont, Battle of 42
Bentley, Clark 27–28
Big Black River Bridge, Battle of 118–120
Black, Charles 17
Black, Col. 69, 131, 157–158, 196
Blair, Frank 6, 122
Blew, Lt. Jacob 103, 105, 200
board of examiners (medical) 62
Bond, Dr. 14
Bonner, Sherwood 72
Boonville, Battle of 23
Bouton, Col. Edward 188
Bowyer, Dr. Eli 32–34, **_33_**, 36–37, 40–41, 47, 51, 54, 57, 59–62, 69–70, 87–88, 90, 95, 97, 128–129, 131, 134–135, 139, 141, 145–147, 149–151, 153–154, 156–157, 175, 177, 179–180, 190, 200, 202, 205, 207–208, 211, 215, 218, 220–221, 224, 231–233, 238
Brice's Crossroads, Battle of 186, 188–189, 191, 193; firsthand accounts 189

Brooks, Chap. Joseph 18–20, 26, 34, 37, 48, 89–90
Brown, Benjamin Gratz 14–15
Brown, the Rev. George 226, 231, 233
Burnes, Dr. 31–33
bushwhackers 27

camp hash 68
Camp Jackson Massacre 13
Canby, Gen. Edward 225
Cape Girardeau: Union garrison 34–36, 38, 40, 42–43, 45, 47, 49, 51–52, 54, 56–57, 212–214, 216
Carter, Capt. Charles 69–70, 87
Carthage, Battle of 23
Central Christian Advocate 18, 89
Champion Hill, Battle of 118–121, 124, 133, 139, 163
Charley, ex-slave 44–46
Chickamauga, Battle of 152, 158
City of Madison explosion 150–151
Conrad, Samuel 33, 136, 140, 141, 148–149
Copperheads 86, 97, 141, 146–147, 165, 208
Corinth, Battle of 63, 71, 128, 175
Corinth, Siege of 58, 65, 74, 105
Cowperthwait, John 47–48, 193, 195

Davis, Gen. Jefferson C. 62
Dollahan, Capt. Thomas 37
Donald (Donnell), Samuel 33, 136, 148–149
Doughtery, James 11, 13

Edwards, Dr. 94, 96, 99, 109
Elliott, Cyrenus 36
Elliott, Dr. 16, 19, 56, 77, 141
Emancipation Proclamation 69, 74
erysipelas 98–99

251

Filley, Oliver 6
Fish, Melancthon 57, 62, 129–130, 133–135, 137, 141, 143, 145, 176–177, 180–182, 189, 191, 200, 207
Forrest, Gen. Nathan Bedford 101, 159, 181–182, 186, 188–189, 191–195, 197–198, 201, 205–207
Fort Blakeley 225–226
Fort Donelson, Battle of 52, 57
Fort Henry, Battle of 52, 54, 57
Franklin, Battle of 217
Fredericktown, Battle of 42
freemasonry 101–102, 157, 169
French, Zeba 42, 44, 46–48, 56, 103–104, 107, 109, 129–130, 132, 135, 137–138, 149, 152, 154, 157, 166, 168, 176–177, 179–185, 187, 109, 129, 130, 132, 135, 137–138, 149, 152, 154, 157, 166, 168, 176–177, 179–185, 187, 190–191, 194–196, 200, 203, 220
Friese, Dr. Robert 77, 104, 116, 180
Fuller, Dr. A.B. 24–25, 27, 30–33

Gaddy, George 155–156
Glaze, Col. H. 104, 130, 132, 143
Grand Gulf, Battle of 114, 119–120
Grant, Gen. Ulysses 37, 42, 52, 64–66, 71–72, 86–87, 95, 99–100, 110, 112, 114, 118–124, 128, 131, 137–138, 142–143, 145–146, 152–153, 158, 175–176, 179–180, 182, 206, 210, 221
Gray, Dr. John 103, 162
Gray, Lewis 33, 162, 164
Green, Maj. Modesta 137–138, 140, 224, 227, 230–233, 235
Gregg, Gen. John 118
Griffin, Bow 23
guerrillas 101, 118, 153, 213

Halleck, Gen. Henry 43, 45, 47, 51, 54
Hamilton, Dr. James 11, 13–14, 16
Harney, Gen. William S. 17–18
Harney-Price Truce 17–18
Hassen, Dr. John 20
Hawley, Amos 7, *15*, 16–17, 35, 37, 44, 51, 55, 67, 71, 80, 83, 85–86, 88, 96–98, 104, 124, 140–142, 146, 148, 152, 155, 157, 164–165, 169, 172, 182, 185, 201, 204, 207, 233, 238, 239, 240
Hawley, Caroline "Carrie" Joy *155*, 165, 182, 184, ***223***–224, 226, 231–237, 239, ***240, 241***
Hawley, Elizabeth "Ma" "Mother" 7, 17, 20, 25, 36, 41, 44, 48, 51, 54, 59, 68–69, 71, 74, 77–78, 83, 85–88, 90–93, 96, 102–103, 105–108, 113–115, 127, 134, 136, 140, 142–143, 145–146, 149, 152, 157, 162, 165, 172, 179, 185–186, 188, 200–201, 205, 207, 218–219, 224, 230–235, 239, 241; Death of sister 82–83
Hawley, Eva "Evie" 7, 10, 17, 49, 51, 56, 59, 65, 71, 80, 83, 85–88, 91, 96, 100, 124, 140, 142, 146–148, 152, 162, 179, 185–186, 212, 236, 238, 241
Hawley, Helen Frances "Fanny" 7, 10, 17, 19, 35, 44, 50–51, 59, 60, 66, 69, 71, 83, 85–88, 96, 99, 100, 106–107, 124, 131, 134, 136, 140, 142, 145–146, 148, 152, 156–157, 162, 165–166, 169, 178, 180–187, 196–197, 207, 212, 233, 236, 238, 241
Hawley, Maria "Myra" 7, 10, 17, 19, 27, 30, 35–36, 39, 50–51, 55, 58, 60, 71, 83, 86–88, 91, 96, 100, 103, 106, 124, 128, 131, 134–135, 140, 142, 145–146, 152, 155–156, 162, 165, 172, 185, 187, 195–197, 201, 207, 212, 219, 223, 230, 238, 240
Hawley, Nelson "Pa" 7, 15, 17, 20, 35, 37–39, 41, 48, 51, 54–55, 59–60, 65, 67, 71, 77, 83–91, **89**, 95–97, 102, 104, 106, 109, 126, 133–135, 140, 142, 146–147, 152, 157, 162, 164, 169, 179, 181, 185, 207, 211, 216, 219, 224, 226–227, 231–232, 234, 241
Hawley, Theodocia 7
Hendee, Clark 25–28
Hicks, Col. Stephen 15, 26, 141
Hoffman, Dr. F.H. 136, 139, 143, 150–151
Hoffmiester, Dr. Augustus 156
Hollister, Capt. Charles 49, 59
Holly Springs, Raid on 71–75; burning of hospital 74
Holt, John 48–49
Home Guards 7, 30–31; skirmish at Rolla 30
Hood, John Bell 217–218, 221, 223
Hospital No. 3 LaGrange 77–95
Hoyt, William 23
Hubbard, Lucius 202, 224
Hurricane Creek, skirmish at 2, 204–205, 220

Illinois: 2nd Cavalry 73; 5th Cavalry 143; 6th Cavalry 86, 102, 161, 232; 7th Cavalry 108, 163; 7th Infantry 11, 14; 9th Cavalry 232; 13th Illinois Infantry 19, 24, 27–28, 30–31, 50; 22nd Illinois Infantry 11, 14; 26th Illinois Infantry 94, 153; 29th Illinois Infantry 73; 30th Illinois Infantry 139; 40th Illinois Infantry 15, 94–95, 114, 153; 45th Illinois Infantry 85; 48th Illinois Infantry 97; 49th Illinois Infantry 97, 170, 187; 61st Illinois Infantry 210; 62th Illinois Infantry 73 ; 63rd Illinois

Infantry 94; 72nd Illinois Infantry 63, 66; 111th Illinois Infantry 2, 7, 62, 66–67, 69, 71, 74, 81, 87, 88, 93, 95–97, 99, 125, 128–129, 131, 133–135, 143, 157, 164; 130th Illinois Infantry 104
Indianola 118, 120
Ing, Stanford 27
Iowa: 2nd Artillery 175–176; 6th Infantry 96, 153; 8th Infantry 156
Island Number 10 57, 74
Iuka, Battle of 63, 71, 128, 148, 175

Jackson, Claiborne Fox 6, 7, 17, 18
Jackson, Battle of 118, 137–138
Jann, Jasper 133, 135
Johns, Ellis 37
Johnson, Daniel 208–209, 212
Johnson, Harvey 241
Johnston, Gen. Joseph 122–123, 129, 137, 194, 221
Jonesboro, Battle of 208, 217

Kaley, Henry 33, 147–149
Kansas-Nebraska Act 5
Kendall, Capt. 212, 227, 234
King, Edward 209, *211*–212

Lee, Gen. Robert E. 221
Lee, Gen. Stephen Dill 160, 194, 197
Lexington, Battle of 38, 40
Lincoln, Abraham 6, 7, 65, 70, 210, 226
Little Dixie 6
Livingston, Maj. Benjamin 35–36, 195
Lookout Mountain, Battle of 158
Lymans, William 84–85
Lyon, Nathaniel 7, 13, 18, 23, 34

malaria 34, 137, 139
Mann, Samuel 37, 140, 141, 148–149
Maria Denning 62–63, 83–84
Marmaduke, John S. 23, 208
Martin, Col. James S. 62, 103, 131
Maury, Gen. Dabney 223
Mayberry, Maj. 66, 68
McCall, Duncan 132
McClernand, Gen. John 65–66, 68, 112, 114, 118, 122
McClure, Capt. 130, 145
McKay, Martha 20
McMahan, Capt. Constantine 227, 232, 238
McNeely, William 19
measles 38, 45–47, 52, 56, 95,
Meily, George 121, 133
Mills, Dr. Madison 119, 121, 125
Minnesota: 5th Infantry 154

Minor, the Rev. Simon 108
Missionary Ridge, Battle of 158
Mississippi Infantry, 36th 122, 128
Mississippi Valley Sanitary Fair 181
Missouri Compromise of 1820 6
Missouri Compromise of 1850 6
Missouri: 3rd Infantry (CSA) 122; 7th Infantry (US) 173–174, 187, 200, 221; 8th Infantry (US) 11; 11th Missouri Infantry (US) 2, 7, 10, 20, 32, 34, 36, 42, 43–44, 47, 49, 50–52, 54, 56–64, 66–67, 69–71, 74, 78–80, 83–84, 87–91, 95, 97, 99, 103–5, 108, 114, 122, 128–130, 132–134, 137–138, 140–143, 145–146, 148–149, 151, 153–156, 158–160, 162–163, 165–166, 168, 171–176, 178–179, 181–183, 186–188, 191, 193, 197–202, 205, 207–208, 210, 212–213, 216–221, 223, 225–226, 230–232, 235–236, 238–239; 33rd Missouri Infantry (US) 89, 172, 182, 186
Missouri Military Act 17
Missouri Rifle Battalion, First 2, 7, 16, 18, 20, 22, 24, 30–32
Mitchell, Brother 14
Morgan, Gen. John Hunt 140–141
Morrison, Brother A.B. 77, 81, 83–84, 87, 95, 103, 105, 138
Mott, P.E. 84–85
Mower, Gen. Joseph 62, 128, 133, 140, 154, 175, 177, 187, 191–192, 198–199, 207–208, 214
Murphy, Col. Robert 71

Nashville, Battle of 2, 10, 217–221, 224, 226
Notestine, Finley 59–60, 136
Notestine, Jim 33, 147
Notestine, William 129, 179–180, 189, 195, 204–205, 211, 218, 220–221, 224

Ohio: 27th Infantry 128; 53rd Infantry 114; 70th Infantry 114
Okolona, Battle of 193
Olnick, Dr. 94
Oxford Expedition 2, 10, 200–207, 220

Palmsteer, James 37, 40, 130, 132–133, 138
Panabaker, Lt. Col. William 36, 54, 56, 133
Pemberton, Gen. John 64, 118, 121–123, 131
Phelps County courthouse 20, *29*
Phillips, Dr. James 63, 67–69, 133–134
Pillow, Gen. Gideon 42
pleurisy treatment 98–99
Plummer, Dr. 31
Plummer, Col. Joseph 38–43, 46, 50, 52, 55, 57

254 Index

Porter, Adm. David Dixon 100, 113–114
Prentiss, Gen. Benjamin 37
Price, Sterling 2, 17–18, 20, 23, 38, 40, 71, 209, 213, 216–217, 220; 1864 raid 213–217
Priunns Family 11

Rainey, Dr. John 67–69, 95
Raymond, Battle of 118–120
Red River Campaign 172, 175, 178–180, 186, 189
Reed, William 240
Reynolds, Thomas 6
Ridgely, Elmore 33, 137
Risley, Father 23
Rolla Union garrison 2, 10, 18–32
Roman, Dr. H. 11, 13–14
Rosecrans, Gen. William 112, 152, 158
Ross, Annie 75, 77–78, 84, 86, 88, 130
Ross, Dr. B.W. 75

Sam Young 116
Sappington, Mark 27–28, 48–49, 95, 97, 147, 184–185, 190, 195
Saxton, Rufus 22, 26
Schofield, Gen. John 217
Sheppard, Charles 181–182, 209, 212
Sherman, William 64, 72, 118, 122, 128–129, 137, 146, 152–153, 160, 175–176, 181–182, 185, 188, 193–194, 207–208, 210, 217, 221
Shiloh, Battle of 58, 65, 107
Sixteenth (XVI) Corps 197, 201, 209, 221, 225
smallpox 56, 84, 86, 103
Smith, Gen. A.J. 181–182, 187, 189, 191, 193–194, 197–199, 201–202, 205–207, 209, 212–213, 221, 223
Smith, Dr. Thomas 16–21, 23–25, 27, 30, 34–42, 47, 51, 54, 56–57, 89–90, 129
Southern Illinois Conference 40
Spanish Fort, Siege of 2, 10, 225–227
Spring Hill, Battle of 217–218
Stewart, William 52
Stockade Redan 122–123, 128–129, 155, 162

Stooky, Widow 13
Street, Sol 101–102
Sturgis, Gen. Samuel 50, 186, 188, 193, 195, 197–198
Stuz, Rudoph 43, 149
Swearingen, Lincoln "Link" 35, 69, 141, 143–145, 149, 151–152, 156–158

Thomas, Gen. George 193, 217, 221
Thompson, Gen. M. Jeff 42, 47, 103, 105
Throp, Peiper 17
Treadway, Sergeant Charles 197, 216, 225
Tupelo Campaign 2, 10, 193–199, 220
Turner, Frank 241
typhoid fever 34, 38–41, 45–47, 52, 59, 137

United States: 1st Infantry 175; 4th Reserves 14
United States Sanitary Commission 110, 130, 181
Updegraff, Col. 41
USCT, 55th Regiment 188
USCT, 59th Regiment 188

Van Dorn, Gen. Earl 2, 71–75, 78, 164, 203
Vicksburg Campaign: attacks at Stockade 122–123, 128–129, 155, 162; Hawley's account 119–121, 124–126, 127–129, 130–133; mine explosion 131; surrender 132; Yazoo River Expedition 98–100

Washburn, Gen. 163, 176, 180, 182–183, 203
Weber, Col. A.J. 91, 132–133, 154; death 132–133
West, Bennie 13, 17
West, William 17
Wilson, James 48, 199, 200
Wilson, John "Dock" 156
Wilson's Creek, Battle of 34, 38–39
Wirtz, Dr. Horace 74, 78, 80
Wisconsin: 8th Infantry 71
Woods, Gen. C.R. 227, 230, 238
Wymans, Col. 19

www.ingramcontent.com/pod-product-compliance
Ingram Content Group UK Ltd.
Pitfield, Milton Keynes, MK11 3LW, UK
UKHW041934140426
5217IPUK00014B/476